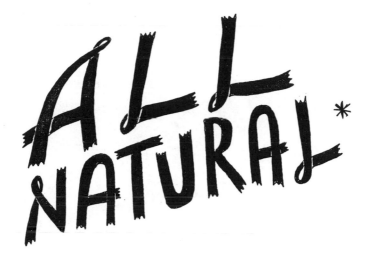

ALL NATURAL*

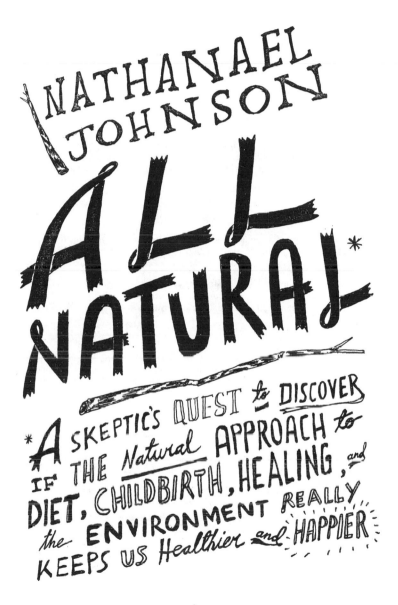

NATHANAEL JOHNSON

ALL NATURAL*

*A SKEPTIC'S QUEST to DISCOVER IF THE Natural APPROACH to DIET, CHILDBIRTH, HEALING, and the ENVIRONMENT REALLY KEEPS US Healthier and HAPPIER

RODALE.

© 2013 by Nathanael Johnson

All rights reserved. No part of this publication may be reproduced or transmitted in any form or by any means, electronic or mechanical, including photocopying, recording, or any other information storage and retrieval system, without the written permission of the publisher.

Rodale books may be purchased for business or promotional use or for special sales. For information, please write to:
Special Markets Department, Rodale, Inc., 733 Third Avenue, New York, NY 10017

Printed in the United States of America
Rodale Inc. makes every effort to use acid-free ⊗, recycled paper ♺.

Portions of this book were previously published in *Assembly*, *Eldr*, and *Harper's* magazines, and in the collection *Sierra Songs and Descants*. *E. coli* DNA images used by permission of the California Department of Public Health.

Book design by Amy King

Library of Congress Cataloging-in-Publication Data

Johnson, Nathanael.
    All natural: a skeptic's quest to discover if the natural approach to diet, childbirth, healing, and the environment really keeps us healthier and happier/Nathanael Johnson.
        p.   cm.
    Includes bibliographical references and index.
    ISBN 978—1—60529—074—4   hardcover
    1. Organic living.   2. Environmental health.   3. Human ecology.   I. Title.
GF77.J64   2012
640—dc23   2012029538

Distributed to the trade by Macmillan
2   4   6   8   10   9   7   5   3   1   hardcover

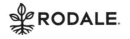

We inspire and enable people to improve their lives and the world around them.
rodalebooks.com

To Mom and Dad. We turned out all right despite/because of all this.

Contents

INTRODUCTION

My inspiration for this book began when I was 7, as I sat huddled with my little brother on the covered porch of our house in the pines outside Nevada City, California, our backs against the door, watching the rain fall. It was cold that day, the kind of cold—just on the verge of freezing—that somehow cuts more deeply than it would if the temperature dropped another five degrees and wet turned to snow.

That was 1986, and we were out there because my parents had just bought a computer, an IBM 286. The screen was two-toned black and amber, and the machine produced a grinding noise when it was processing information, as if it were gnawing on the floppy disks we fed it. Nonetheless, my brother, Tim, and I were fascinated to the point of obsession. It was like a starship had materialized in our house—the magnetism of futuristic coolness was just as irresistible, which was precisely what my parents were worried about.

For most of our young lives, they'd managed to shield us from technology. They were determined to raise us in an Edenic natural setting, so we moved to a town in the hills of Northern California surrounded by communes and spiritual retreats, where many people lived off the electrical grid and foraged for food in the forest. As babies, we'd crawled around naked because Dad had determined that all diapers, even the organic cotton kind, were an abhorrent corruption of nature's plan. We were fed a diet of organic brown rice and garden vegetables. We visited naturopaths and chiropractors. There were no televisions in our house, and we were not supposed to watch TV when we visited friends because, as my mother explained with an unsatisfying lack of specificity, it would rot our brains. But my parents, for all their idealism, also had a pragmatic streak. They knew that they couldn't hold back the rising tide of technology forever. When the computer first entered the house it was strictly off-limits. But then, under heavy lobbying, and with the understanding that a computer-dominated culture was inevitable, they agreed to a compromise: For every three hours we spent outside we were allowed to play Space Quest for half an hour. Which is why my brother, and I were outside in the wet, wrapped together in an old blanket.

I don't remember all of what was going through my head that day, besides thinking, *I'm cold,* and frequently fighting the urge to check the time. I know I wondered whether the frigid outdoors was really healthier than a warm seat in front of a computer. I fantasized about that image for a few moments. Then I asked my brother how far we'd gotten. Tim fished the clock out of his pocket. "Almost eight minutes," he said.

Perhaps my parents' precautions outweighed the risk, but to them the 286 was inseparable from the open pit mines, fiery smelters, and factory lines that had called it into being. It represented the piecemeal conversion of the world—from a colorful place that fostered life into a gray place that fostered mechanical efficiency. And my parents worried that the computer could cause a similar conversion in our brains. By the same rationale, all technologies—that is, all attempts to control, improve, or otherwise meddle with nature—were suspect. Factory farming, food processing, pharmaceuticals, and hospital births were, in their eyes, all products of the same industrial force and, therefore, were liable to do more harm than good in the long run.

According to family ideology, good health resulted from forming connections with the surrounding world rather than controlling it, from finding harmony with nature. But when I encountered nature as a kid, instead of granting me health, it generally wanted to eat me: It wanted to lay eggs in my cereal, to fly clumsily into my ear, to skitter across my pillow and disappear into the blankets. It's easy to point to aspects of nature that are annoying or dangerous, but that's not enough—it turns out—to win you unlimited Space Quest privileges. My parents had no trouble acknowledging that some parts of nature were bad and some kinds of technology were good, while maintaining their preference for the former and suspicion of the latter. And even I had to admit that there was something weird about the desperation that came over me when my time at the computer was up. Even I had to admit that there was something about the natural world that made me feel good.

My family went backpacking in Yosemite every summer—a kind of pilgrimage, to be completed regardless of difficulty. The year I was born, I rode atop Dad's backpack, and two summers after that my little brother joined me in this palanquin. From then on, Tim and I paid back this service, taking a larger burden each trip. Strangers on the trail used to gape at us—this pair of heavy-laden toddlers, bandannas around our necks, red felt hats on our heads, trudging resolutely into the backcountry. I loved those trips. For some reason the mosquito bites and sunburns, the exertion and the grime, all seemed insignificant. Each day I felt my pack grow a little lighter, my stride a little surer. Each evening my brother and I teetered out into the shocking coldness of a new lake to dog-paddle in little gasping ellipses. Each night the family sat together, sipping tea, and watched the alpenglow fade from a new set of peaks.

The same year that Tim and I had sat in the sleet to earn our computer time, we hiked over Koip Peak Pass. We'd camped just before the trail grew steep, where a glacier dripped into a shallow pool. As the sun rose I made out a jagged line rising improbably up an escarpment of rusty scree. I'd never seen a trail that simply hurled itself up a cliff face in that way, but when we began the ascent I found we were following the same line I'd traced from below. At the end of one switchback, which

seemed to traverse out over nothing, I paused. To one side I could lean
into the mountain, my hand splayed across the talus tiles; to the other
was sky and wisps of cloud. Below, there was a rock outcropping, then
air for 5,000 feet, and then the flat pan of Nevada desert stretching out
until it met the sky again. I thrilled, just for a second, at something like
the sensation of flight, then felt the greasy skid of vertigo and pulled my
head away. My family was on the trail below: Dad following Tim closely,
and Mom—with her two-ton fear of heights—behind, placing each foot
with the fanatical concentration of a firewalker.

When we reached the top of the pass, a lake shimmered on the other
side a few thousand feet below, and beyond: peak after peak to the limit
of sight. We huddled in the lee of a rock pile, chewing dried pineapple and
laughing over nothing but the wild sense that we had just done the impossible. I felt tough—suntanned, windburned, and strong. It was pretty
much the opposite of the way I felt when my half hour on the computer
was ticking down (furtive, compulsive, weak). Up there it seemed self-
evident that a healthy environment—untainted by technology—made
healthy people.

<hr />

Back down at sea level, twenty-plus years later, it's not self-evident at all.
In this age of global warming, killer germs, and obesity, it's easy to feel
as if we've somehow slipped out of synch with the global ecosystem. But
it's just as easy to dismiss that feeling by pointing out all the good that
our industry has brought. We've got more stuff. We live longer. Everything gets better and easier.

I suspect most of us are actually stuck somewhere in the middle: We
recognize the good that technology has conferred, but also have a gnawing sense that something is missing or awry. This sense is persistent, but
frustratingly vague. Call it "ecological anxiety." You know you've got it if
you are occasionally concerned that hormone-mimicking chemicals are

leeching from takeout containers into your food, but have found that plastic is too useful and too ubiquitous to avoid; if you're left cold by encounters with the medical system, but aren't really sure you believe in that alternative practitioner your friend recommended; if you sporadically pay more for food marked "GMO free" or "All Natural," but only if it's not too much more; if you use eco-friendly laundry detergents, but still dry your clothes with an energy-guzzling machine rather than a line, and travel on airplanes and basically just *live* in the oil-hungry civilization you were born into, because: What are you supposed to do? Go all Ted Kaczynski and move to a shack in the woods?

This book is a sort of imaginary shack in the woods, not for building mail bombs—just the opposite: It's a comfortable refuge from the people driven to such extremes, quiet enough that you can pull at the thread of ecological anxiety until it reveals the deep place where it's tangled. Come on in, have a seat by the potbellied stove. The water's almost ready. It's a polarized, all-or-nothing world out there. The interesting nuances in the middle ground tend to be neglected. Which is too bad, because many of us are agnostic, and curious.

At least I am. I'm utterly seduced by the distant descendants of that golden-screened computer, and by the ability of progress to bring nature under control. I can't do without technology: I'm not willing to give up antibiotics, or movies, or ice cubes, or germ theory, or space exploration. But I'm also dismayed by the way faith in technological progress tends to trade away beauty, and wonder, and joy, and all of those slippery, unquantifiable things that—in the end—make life worth living.

—•—

This question about the relative merits of nature and technology has been under debate for about as long as there have been people to debate it. The first recorded disagreement in the Bible is over whether humans should try to improve their lot, or leave Eden alone. British philosopher

Stephen Toulmin, who recorded the history of this argument in his book *Cosmopolis,* has shown that if you look back across occidental history you can see the pendulum of popular opinion swinging from one extreme to the other. Toulmin picks up his inquiry in the 17th century, with Europe's descent into the Thirty Years' War. This bloodbath seemed to prove that people with opposing ideas (in that case Catholics and Protestants) couldn't live together peacefully, and that the only way forward was to determine who was *right*—for the technology of rational philosophy to trump human nature. And so French philosopher René Descartes devised a proposal to achieve incontrovertible facts. Descartes's solution was to turn away from the biological messiness of nature and focus on a system of rationality, built on the firm foundation of the one thing he knew with absolute certainty: "I think, therefore I am." Cartesian rationalism insisted that truth comes not from observation of the outside world but from turning inward and building abstractions upon *cogito ergo sum.* So, in the 17th century, as the pendulum swung one way, Descartes lay in his sickbed (alone), chopping logic up into more and more exquisite forms—working to escape nature's chaos by forging certainty from thin air.

In the late 18th and 19th centuries, the weight slowed, then swung back: Rather than looking for truth in abstract logic, people looked for it in the stars, in the daffodils, and in the unmarked spaces on the map. They searched for meaning by playing with electricity, inhaling unknown gasses, and drifting (sometimes plummeting) in hot air balloons. They made nature their textbook. Paintings of this time put visual pleasure before precision, and music favored grand gestures over symmetry. Replacing Descartes was William Blake, naked in the garden (with company), beset by visions, and declaiming poetry to the roses. As this period was drawing to a close in the early 1900s, Einstein showed that the straight lines of Newton's simple geometric universe were in fact curved and complex; Heisenberg's Uncertainty Principle established there were questions without answers, that mystery was at the very core of nature;

and Freud kicked down the brickwork Descartes had laid between emotion and rationality.

As the 20th century progressed, the pendulum careened back toward its Cartesian apex. Two world wars renewed the desire for irrefutable certainty, and certainty—it seemed—could be found in industry. Ford's assembly lines helped win the wars, then made the victors rich. The artists who rode the Zeitgeist to glory in this period were those who turned their work into a species of geometric proof. Piet Mondrian's squares, Arnold Schoenberg's mathematical music ("How the music sounds," Schoenberg said, "is not the point"), and the concrete massifs of architectural brutalism were exalted.

My parents grew up in the 1950s, during this age of technological rapture: They'd watched as the first TVs gathered up vibrations (not from a pipe, or a wire, but out of the air!) and turned it into a moving picture in a box. They were told that there would be no end to such wonders. The atom would supply electricity too cheap to meter, and laboratories would supply better living through chemistry. They would colonize Mars. They would beat death. They would have jetpacks.

Then it all soured. The atomic promise became the cold war. Better living through chemistry became a "Silent Spring." There were no jetpacks. The pendulum swung back in the other direction and, at the age of 29, my father rode it from the East Coast to the West. He arrived in Berkeley—in a baby-blue VW bus, with hair down to his shoulders—where my mother was already a lawyer's wife concerned with cocktail dresses and dieting. I was a result of history's momentum, produced in the heady rush toward romantic primitivism.

———

Although any attempt to reduce half a millennia to a few paragraphs is bound to oversimplify it, there is some rough truth to the generalization that people tend to oscillate between two fundamentally different ways of understanding the world: the technological perspective, which sees a mechanical universe of separate parts; and the all-natural perspective, which sees a living universe in which nothing can ever be fully separated from the influence of the larger, ever-changing whole. The technological perspective favors small facts that can be known with certainty. Its method for understanding nature is often a sort of autopsy, conducted under the klieg lights of reductive science. It's generally defeated by a lizard-tail trick: Researchers are left holding a tiny wriggling piece of data, while the larger whole slips off into the darkness. The natural perspective intuitively gets the big picture, but tends to fudge the details: Romantics travel out into the wilderness to experience nature as a whole, then return to rhapsodize poetically while expurgating encounters with leeches and dysentery.

The technological perspective is more precise, but when followed with blinkered fixity, it leads to strange destinations. As I began my research I found myself stumbling over paradoxes: Americans are the most rational dieters in the world—we often pay more attention to nutritional data on labels than to the way food makes us feel—and yet, the more we diet, the fatter we become. As medical technology has improved in labor and delivery units over the past decade, the risk that a woman will die in childbirth has increased. Our successes protecting ourselves from germs have made us more susceptible to disease. More Americans now die from too much medical care than from too little. One in ten Americans is medicated for depression, and yet the more antidepressants we take, the sadder we become, and severe, disabling depression has reached record highs.

Paradoxes are interesting because they indicate a glitch in the system, a portal through which one may escape conventional thinking. The term *paradox* comes from the Greek: *para*, beyond, and *doxa*, belief. Rather than implying something that cannot possibly be true, it suggests something is amiss in the orthodoxy: *ortho*, straight, or right, and *doxa*, belief. Paradoxes are the wrinkles where the cloth of belief does not fit the shape of things as they truly are.

The breakdown in communication between the people who favor nature and those who favor technology is at the foundation of these paradoxes. It's this fundamental disagreement that allows Americans to get fatter and sadder each year even as we increase spending on healthcare. And, I believe, it explains our paralysis in the face of environmental decline.

———•———

Perhaps it's hyperbole to say that my inspiration for this book arrived when I was 7, but it's not an exaggeration to say that I've been hashing over this debate all my life, whether by arguing with my parents or with myself. By 7 I was already swinging between a faith in technology and faith in that soaring feeling I experienced in Yosemite's high country. I rolled my eyes at my parents' kookier notions and became known as the family skeptic, but I was never able to shake that romantic sympathy with natural beauty or its dark side: the gnawing ecological anxiety that our technological domination of nature was hurting me.

As a teenager I started reading whatever I could get my hands on about natural diets, natural health, and surviving in the wild. I was looking for some way to harness that feeling I'd had in high, uncivilized places. I searched for the insight that would transform me into a better, stronger mortal; insight that would tell me what foods to eat, what herbal tinctures to drink, or—to get right down to it—how a gangly young man with his nose in a book and his head filled with dreams of wilderness could get a girl to like him. But the advice I read wasn't very good (I probably would've been better off eating, rather than reading, one particular diet book, which made me first a convert, and then a stranger, to my own bathroom). I found that a lot of what had been written about this constellation of concerns was extreme—either dismissing the natural perspective without a hearing, or credulously embracing it—once again—without evidence.

There were, however, a few writers bringing evidence to the question of natural health. Evolutionary biologists, starting with Stephen Jay Gould, showed me that humans might indeed be especially suited to the environment that shaped us. Every book or scrap of science I picked up led me to two more, and feeding my curiosity in this way only made it grow. My fascination continued throughout college and into the years when I began working as a journalist. As a reporter, I've found the same big questions lurking behind my little stories about food, health, and the environment. Again and again, we knock our heads against the same paradoxes, the same assumptions, the same philosophical blind spots.

In the last 20 years I've become something of an amateur expert, an observer of the space where food, medicine, and environment meet. It's a space fragmented by disciplines, and understanding how we've messed it up requires a broad perspective, one wide enough to see the themes common to industrial forestry, end-of-life medical care, and the obesity epidemic. In each of these fields, there are real experts who know them far better than I do, and so I come to this project humbly. The book you're holding isn't a polemic; my purpose in trying to unravel the confusion surrounding technology and nature is not to convince, but to wonder. Wonder, I think, describes the place shared by the rigorous science of the technological perspective and the creative free thinking of the natural perspective. And that's the place where I've attempted to lay the foundation for this book.

CHAPTER ONE

A HEALTHY START

BIRTH

Hanging on the wall beside my desk is a photograph from my first morning on earth, and as I've endeavored to organize my thoughts on natural childbirth—and on the wisdom of trusting nature in general—my eyes have strayed to this image so often that it has taken on iconic significance. The family is captured in black and white, lounging on homemade corduroy pillows, which lean against the dark grain of a redwood wall. A mobile hangs half out of frame—balls of yarn dangle from a coat hanger. The two preteens in the picture are unfamiliar to me: They are my half brother and half sister, but I remember them only as adults because their father, from my mother's first marriage, took them into his custody a few years after this picture was made. I'm the baby in the center, contorted into a posture of spastic newborn disorientation. My brother smiles down at me; my sister looks into the camera from under a Cal Bears visor; Dad, thickly bearded, long-haired and leonine, lies with an arm around me; Mom lounges in back, radiant and beautiful, which is a bit staggering since she'd recently delivered me to that bedroom. What sets it apart from most newborn photos, however, is not what's in the picture, but what's missing: There

are no IV towers, no ID bracelets, no hospital-issue blankets, or bassi-
nets of industrial plastic to interrupt the natural-fiber aesthetic. In this
family—the picture says—we don't fear nature, instead we embrace it,
moving in harmony with its cycles. It was taken on October 9, 1978.

I only got around to asking my parents about the photo a few
months before my wedding. That's probably because I'd never thought
much about birth or babies until Beth, my fiancée, made having children a precondition to her acceptance of my marriage proposal. Father-
hood, which had been a theoretical possibility, assumed an onrushing
inevitability and, suddenly, it seemed important that I develop a position on progeny politics, starting with birth. Beth had no bias against
hospital births. We came from opposite sides of the cultural divide:
While my father had made his living as a psychotherapist—exercising
extrapolations from Jung on dreams and ephemera—her father had
worked as an orthopedic surgeon, exercising concrete mechanics on
bone and muscle. A few months after I was born at home, she was born
via scheduled Caesarean section. If I was going to insist on homebirth
and breastfeeding and all the other natural practices my parents had
embraced, it seemed only fair that I discuss this with Beth while she still
had the option of finding a less doctrinaire partner in parenting. And,
if I was going to articulate my position on these issues, it no longer
seemed acceptable to base it on the hazy warmth I got from a picture. I
started my remedial education by calling my parents and asking them
to share their recollections.

My mother, Gail, had given birth to my brother and sister in a Berkeley hospital. Brent was her first, born in 1966, and it had taken nine
hours and forceps to convince him to exit. She'd been left alone during
most of her labor and perhaps it was the resulting memory of neglect, or
perhaps the way the forceps had cut and welted Brent's head, or perhaps
the general feeling of helplessness associated with being a patient in any
hospital—whatever the reason, the experience felt unnecessarily traumatic. My sister, Erin, was born at the same hospital in 1970, and though

that birth was uncomplicated, it had left Mom with that same vague sense of wrongness.

By the time I came along, things had changed. The agent of that change was a six-foot-two poet with blue eyes, a swimmer's body, a declamatory basso voice that rumbled up from his belly, and wavy brown hair that cascaded down between his shoulder-blades. He had a name like some fictional frontiersman: Belden Johnson. Dad swept into Mom's life like a flood, overflowing her banks and casually demolishing the contours that had contained her. She exchanged her tightly restrained role as immaculate hostess and lawyer's wife for the liberty and chaos of the counterculture. The photographs from this time show a luminous woman, smiling, with straight hair to her waist over simple tunic dresses.

After my parents began living together, they would periodically rent a cabin in the California wine country where they'd hole up for days on end with a grocery bag of food and occasionally a few tabs of LSD. My conception was very likely buoyed on that psychedelic tide. They both remember feeling, that night, in that cabin in Sonoma County, the utter certainty that they had just made a baby. Though it's unlikely that the chemicals would have altered the dance of the gametes in any biological sense, this event does seem metaphorically significant: My parents, who would become so committed to safeguarding their children from the corrupting influence of modern technology, had unwittingly undermined themselves, baptizing my first moments of mitosis in Timothy Leary's bioluminescent broth. They thought they were raising an earth child, but my ecosystem was already polluted with synthetics.

My parents, like all parents I suppose, later tried to put from their minds the possibility that they might have ruined their child. When I pressed Dad on this point he managed to recall only vague trepidation.

"But, Dad," I said, "if you were, you know, um, *tripping*, weren't you worried that you were going to get a really messed-up baby?"

"That certainly did cross my mind," he said, hesitantly, before settling on a flip response: "and obviously it was true."

Somehow, the knowledge of this contamination was less disturbing than the shadowy dangers of environmental pollution and industrial toxicology of California in the 1980s, over which my parents had little control. Teasing aside, from the moment of conception Dad did everything he could to shelter my newly formed embryo from all insults—chemical, psychological, or physical. I would be his first child, and he threw himself headlong into parenthood.

Realistically, however, there wasn't much he could do before birth and absent any practical outlet for his creative paternal instinct, he became ferociously and dubiously helpful. He read poetry and sections of the *Iliad* to Mom's abdomen. He built a deck off the bedroom so that when I emerged, I could lie in the sun. He played music for me and made up snatches of a lullaby in French (*Mon petit bébé, tu es très joli*), which he'd sing over and over. The pinnacle of Dad's efforts, however, was the "beasty-yeasty": a concoction of brewer's yeast, yogurt, and granola, blended until smooth. The idea was to prevent morning sickness—brewer's yeast contains vitamin B, which seems to ease some women's symptoms—but the beasty-yeasty was where Mom drew the line.

"You couldn't exactly drink it," she said. "You kind of had to gag it down." No matter how unpleasant the retching, Mom would explain to Dad, the expulsion of vomit was preferable to drinking it in this ersatz form.

Behind all this action were hours of study. Many people were becoming alarmed enough by the state of childbirth around that time to write books about it, and Dad read everything he could get his hands on. *Birth Without Violence,* by Frederick Leboyer, had just come out, suggesting that, rather than enduring the bright lights and cold metal of a delivery room, babies should be placed into warm water to mimic the environment of the womb. And Suzanne Arms's *Immaculate Deception* made the convincing case that many of the technical birthing interventions were not employed out of necessity, but because a historically male medical culture presumed that women's bodies were inherently dysfunctional.

None of this was foreign to my father, who'd been born without medical assistance. His parents—a Washington bureaucrat (father) and professor of English (mother)—were in many respects conventional citizens of the buttoned-down 1950s, but they had occasionally indulged their own attraction to nature's way: in birthing babies, in growing their own food, and in milking their own goats. There was another even more powerful factor working to convince Dad of the superiority of home-birth. He explained matter-of-factly to Beth and me over breakfast one morning that while in therapy he'd relived his own birth—he'd actually felt sensations and emotions that he interpreted as neonatal memory. "I know," he said, looking at me with a little rumble of bass merriment. "I can tell, that's got your skeptical mind going."

Some of the details he'd recalled from his birth were specific enough for him to check. Most convincingly, he remembered experiencing the panicked feeling that his shoulders had become stuck in the birth canal, a detail that his mother supposedly later confirmed. "She was shocked," he said. "She asked me how I could possibly know that had happened." Dad lifted his hands heavenward at this revelation, as if to say, "How else can you explain it?" For him, the experience of reliving his birth had been so profound that he became a therapist, leading others on the same journey into memory. The tenets of this practice, called primal therapy, hold that the psychic scars of birth and babyhood often form the foundation of self-destructive habits in adults, and that healing this residual infant pain is the way to dissolve the emotional stumbling blocks people end up tripping over throughout their lives. The experience of leaving the womb, Dad was convinced, was formative. Babies born via Caesarean section, he said, often become adults who drift along without taking initiative, letting others determine their direction in life.

I'd always avoided thinking too deeply about Dad's belief in the power of neonatal psychology because the whole business made me a little queasy. It just didn't square with my experience of the way the world worked. My friends who were born via Caesarean were not detectably different than those who had passed through the birth canal. And the idea that a person's emotional architecture is defined by his experiences on day one was, for me, uncomfortably similar to the notion that personalities are determined by the stars under which they are born. Most of all, it bothered me that I had only my father's non-verifiable experience as evidence.

In the decade before I was born, however, my father's theory must not have seemed as far-fetched as it does today. Back then—when young men were being drafted to firebomb villages in Vietnam; and all the writers seemed to be drinking themselves to death in the suffocating normalcy of the suburbs, or dropping out and joining communes; and every inspirational leader was being assassinated; and the police were firing tear gas at the rioters a few blocks away in Berkeley—the idea that the psychic trauma of medicalized birth had created a generation of damaged people seemed plausible to a lot of well-respected psychologists and sociologists. Mom was also immersed in the literature of counter-cultural birth. She read the stories of doctors performing Caesareans in order to make their tee time. She saw a film, shot to prepare Navy wives for birth, full of searing images: women strapped into stirrups, drugged, and casually cut open fore and aft to hasten birth. She was convinced that she (and I) would be safer at home. "It seemed like a hospital birth was insane and inhumane," she said. "There was no question in our minds."

My parents would not be dissuaded. They had found a doctor who was just as radical as they were: Lewis Mehl, who had published one of the first peer-reviewed studies on modern-day homebirth in the United States. When my due date came and went, Mehl explained that the risk of stillbirth increased for babies who stewed for too long, but my parents, confident in their choice, simply smiled and said that I would emerge when I was ready.

I was ready three weeks later. It was early October, when the heat spills over the coastal mountains into the San Francisco Bay. In autumn it's as if someone has opened the oven door to California's Central Valley, and plumes of summer-forged air flood down the delta to cut back the fog. Flowers burst into bloom again in this weather, and Mom must have noticed them as she walked down Benvenue Avenue. It was a quiet neighborhood, where trees shaded tall houses. She had recognized the pattern of contractions, and had asked a friend to come over and look after Erin and Brent. When she returned, she found that they had baked a heart-shaped birthday cake. Mom called the midwife, then went upstairs. There were a few hours of intense labor, and some pain: Years earlier she'd hurt her back horsing around with the kids, and the contractions triggered spinal spasms. The night fell and brought slips of cool ocean air through the windows. Someone lit candles. When progress seemed to slow, Dad went looking for upbeat music. He put a Chieftains record on the turntable, and I emerged to an Irish hornpipe. My brother cut the umbilical cord. My sister wiped the sweat from Mom's forehead. As a neo Nate, I was massive: They weighed me on a fish scale, and it was clear that I exceeded 11 pounds, though it was hard to judge by exactly how much because the load was close to the instrument's limit. (Nine pounds is a lot of baby, 11 pounds is an orca.) Mom held me and I began to nurse.

What came next spoiled, or at least complicated, the moral of the story. The scene had become quietly celebratory as the newly enlarged family crowded into the room. The sun rose. A family friend took the photograph that now hangs on my wall. But the midwife was nervous. It's normal for some blood to come with the afterbirth, but the flow was not tapering off. Dr. Mehl, who arrived shortly after the birth, said that it looked a lot like a postpartum hemorrhage. My parents didn't know it, but postpartum hemorrhage was the leading cause of maternal death (and it still is, due to the lack of skilled birth attendants in the developing world).

Mehl saw that he quickly had to decide whether to take Mom to the hospital or act on his own. He took a coin from his pocket and flicked it into the air. Heads. He cleaned one arm, then reached up into my mother's uterus to scrape away the bit of placenta that had not delivered and was preventing the blood vessels from closing. The pain was severe, worse than any part of the birth. Mom closed her eyes and relaxed, willing herself out of her body to a place where she could observe the sensations from a detached remove. She was so successful, so serenely still, that everyone watching panicked.

"Oh my God, she passed out," someone shouted. "Stay with us, Gail," the midwife urged.

Mom was thinking, *Shut up, I'm fine!* When she told me the story, she laughed ruefully and said, "It's just pain."

Birth Today

Some 30 years later it was a bit destabilizing to learn that there had been an element of danger in my otherwise idyllic birth—especially since it was around this same time that my wife and I learned that our first tentative foray toward parenthood had been successful. My birth research, which had been a pleasantly abstract exercise, gained the consequential heft of reality.

All things being equal, a candlelit homebirth sounded far more tranquil (not to mention affordable) than a gadget-packed delivery room. But, after hearing the full story of my own birth, I began to wonder if my aversion to the sterile ambience of fluorescent tubes and whooshing heart monitors was based less on questions of medical safety than on a dislike of hospital decor. And, however strong my opinions were, they would not count for much if Beth disagreed. It was her body after all— and she had been raised with a very different set of assumptions about hospitals. While I'd rebelled by questioning the tenets of my parent's natural ideals, she'd rebelled by moving to liberal San Francisco and voting a straight Democratic ticket. The equal and opposite force of our de-nesting ejector systems had propelled Beth and me to stake our claim on the same turf.

It looked as if the political terrain we were homesteading would not shelter a homebirth. A quick glance at historical maternal mortality rates had been all I needed to convince me of the value of obstetric intervention. The graph showing U.S. maternal mortality over the last hundred years plunges from Himalayan heights down to a gentle plain. In the early decades of the 1900s, between 600 and 900 women died from pregnancy-related complications for every 100,000 births. By 1997 that maternal mortality rate had fallen almost 99 percent to 7.7 deaths per 100,000 births. The most obvious change in the intervening years was that birth became more technological. Some have argued that this industrial revolution in the delivery room has saved more lives than almost any other medical innovation.

The rise of Caesarean surgery was a significant part of this change. In 2011 about one in every three pregnant women wound up having a Caesarean, making it the most common surgery in America. There is no hard data to indicate how many of these surgeries are performed due to actual emergencies, but doctors have estimated the number might be around 5 percent. The percentage of women requesting Caesareans is probably even lower: Despite scores of stories in the media about the rise in elective operations, surveys that actually asked the opinions of mothers, rather than their doctors, found very few who preferred surgical birth. The vast majority of Caesareans are nonemergencies done for medical reasons that often fall into a scientific gray area—some clinicians will insist on planning the surgery before the due date if a woman has had a previous C-section (though this is controversial), or if the baby is breeched (supported by randomized clinical trials), or if the baby seems too big (again, controversial). Many Caesareans are neither planned nor emergencies, but are done because the doctor and patient decide during labor that the operation seems safer than the uncertainty of a questionable fetal heart rhythm, or a cervix that remains closed hour after hour.

Birth presents a basic problem: There's a baby inside, which needs to get out. A C-section is not usually the *best* solution to this problem, since it leaves mothers immobilized during the most challenging weeks of infancy and can have longer-term side effects, but it is the most *reliable* solution. The surgery is a literal shortcut, easy to teach and easy to perform, and it produces standard results. The same goes for the other technologies that have streamed into maternity hospitals. They've all worked to replace the unpredictable complexity of the body with uniform mechanical simplicity. It seems obvious from the rarity of death in modern childbirth that this industrial logic was improving health.

This might have been enough to convince me if I had been engaged in a disinterested inquiry: Historical statistics show that technology has made us safer—case closed. But when it came to my own family, this kind of broad-brush actuarial reasoning left me unsatisfied. This would be our first major family health decision and could very well determine our path going forward. I suppose I wasn't ready to completely toss out my parents' way of life. There was a part of me that, despite the persuasiveness of the raw numbers, could not be swayed from the sense that there was something wrong—fine, I'll say it, something unnatural—about one in three women delivering their babies surgically. Another part of me scoffed at this prejudice. Why cling to primitive ways? Suppose we lived in a future in which babies were delivered by *Star Trek* beam-me-up technology, which has been shown to actually *improve* the health of both the baby and the mother. Wouldn't I opt for the baby to appear effortlessly in a column of sparks and a splatter of amniotic fluid? I would, though not without a begrudging sadness to be giving up birth as a fundamental fact of life, as something that connects us to our ancestors and to our more distant animal relatives. Once I'd established that I'd accept that loss in exchange for easier births, however, all that was left for me to do was determine if we had already reached the glorious future. Had medical technology trumped our evolutionary biology?

There is, in fact, a vigorous debate over medical intervention in birth, and not just between the fringe and the medical establishment, but within the establishment. No one is suggesting that we revert to the practices of the 1900s, but many clinicians and scientists are warning that the medicalization of birth has gone too far. When I took a closer look at the data, I found one seemingly impossible statistic after another. Progress in reducing the infant mortality rate had advanced through the 20th century, but had stalled in the 21st century. This plateau, "has generated concern among researchers and policy makers," according to a 2008 brief from the National Center for Health Statistics. "The U.S. infant mortality rate is higher than those in most other developed countries," wrote the statisticians, "and the gap between the U.S. infant mortality rate and the rates for the countries with the lowest infant mortality [Japan, Sweden, Spain, and others] appears to be widening." In addition, the numbers of preterm and low birth-weight infants had actually risen (a part of this increase was due to a higher number of twins and multiples, perhaps from the rise of fertility treatments, but the increase remained when researchers only looked at singleton births).

When it came to the health of mothers, the trends were even more troubling. A paper published in the *Journal of Obstetrics and Gynecology* noted a marked increase in severe injuries to women during birth: kidney failure, pulmonary embolisms, respiratory failure that required patients to be put on a breathing machine, and more. This increase had occurred between 1998 and 2005, including a 92 percent rise in the percentage of women who needed blood transfusions. Mothers hadn't become less healthy in that period. The study had adjusted for the effects of hypertension, diabetes, age, and multiple births, but weeding out these problems hadn't made much of a difference. What did make a difference was controlling for the mode of delivery: "For many of these complications," the authors wrote, "these increases were associated with the increasing rate of cesarean delivery." Most disturbing of all, national vital statistics showed that the maternal mortality rate was climbing.

This, in particular, seemed too bizarre to be true, and most researchers initially chalked it up to "statistical noise"—the result, they said, of several states adding a checkbox to death certificates to note if a woman had been pregnant a year prior to her demise. But then the state of California made an inquiry that adjusted for these changes and revealed that there was still a consistent upward trend in maternal deaths. "After several decades of declining rates of maternal mortality in California, rates began to rise in 1999 and proceeded to double in the next seven years," the researchers reported. Part of this rise was due to the fact that mothers had become older, sicker, poorer, and more obese—but not all of it.

The total number of women dying was still minuscule compared to the turn of the century: Maternal mortality had gone from 6 deaths per 100,000 births in 1999, to 14 per 100,000 births in 2006. But more troubling than the total number of deaths was the implication that the best efforts of obstetrical medicine to improve health had perhaps done just the opposite. When the California researchers, speaking at a conference, got to the slide showing a graph of this increase, there were gasps from the audience of obstetricians.

These numbers hit home when I did the math and found that it had been safer to give birth in 1978 (when I was born), than it would be for Beth to deliver in 2011, if the upward trend continued. The popularization of supposedly safe and reliable techniques like the Caesarean were meant to improve outcomes. In just the last decade, the Caesarean rate had increased from 22 percent to 32 percent, which amounted to half a million additional surgeries each year—an extraordinary investment of money and medical resources. And yet, when I asked experts what that investment had bought us, they said that there had been no corresponding improvement in the health of mothers or babies. The conventional wisdom has held that, while C-sections may hurt mothers, they reduce the number of babies who might develop cerebral palsy or die due to lack of oxygen. But cerebral palsy rates, like infant mortality rates, have been flat.

"If you look at the statistics, we don't see much improvement in the last ten years," said Debra Bingham, the executive director of the California Maternal Quality Care Collaborative, a partner in the state's ongoing inquiry on maternal deaths. "What we do see is more women dying, and more women suffering birth-related injuries than we have in decades."

I met with Bingham in her office on the Stanford University campus. She had worked for years as a nurse, and then as an administrator of a labor and delivery unit in New York City, before earning her doctorate in public health. Her short, neatly coiffed white hair framed an unlined face that radiated grandmotherly warmth. When I asked why our efforts weren't improving health, she cleared her throat delicately. Administrators and clinicians were allowing their faith in progress to guide them toward presumptively beneficial technology, Bingham said. What they were not doing—for the most part—was allowing the numbers to change their minds when the evidence suggested the technology didn't help. For example, she said, "Clinicians adopted electronic fetal monitoring with the hope that it would improve outcomes. Even after it became known that continuous fetal monitoring does not improve outcomes clinicians continue to use the technology."

Bingham herself had been an early advocate of fetal heart monitors. The rationale for these machines made sense: Watch babies closely enough and you should catch a certain number whose hearts are slowing because they are desperately low on oxygen. She became an expert interpreter of fetal heart rhythms and spent much of her career teaching these skills to nurses. But when the actual data from randomized controlled trials came out, the comparisons among thousands of births showed that the babies who had received continuous heart monitoring were no more likely to survive (nor have less risk for cerebral palsy) than those who had not. The birth industry in the United States basically ignored this evidence, continuing to buy machines for hospitals and routinely using them in every labor (while other countries heeded the science). Years later, after looking at the evidence anew, Bingham began to suspect that in most cases these machines had done more harm than good: They tethered women down (a problem because the inability to move freely can make labor more uncomfortable), they provided fodder for frivolous lawsuits, and they prompted unwarranted surgeries with frequent false alarms of fetal distress.

Despite the lack of evidence to support them, some traditions in obstetrics perpetuate obstinately, Bingham said. She first began to question these traditions in 1981 after she herself gave birth in the hospital where she worked as a maternity nurse. Another nurse had taken her son away to the nursery shortly after he was born, as was routine. Bingham had done the same thing hundreds of times herself, but this time it felt unmistakably wrong. For months she'd been waiting eagerly to see and hold her newborn baby and, lying there without him, she felt a suffocating loneliness. She still gets emotional thinking about it. She waited anxiously, wondering if her son was crying, trying to hold the contours of his face in her memory until, after two hours, she'd had enough. She walked into the nursery and, despite the entreaties of her coworkers, refused to go back to her room until they agreed that she could take her son with her.

Bingham knew there was no scientifically valid reason to separate healthy mothers from healthy babies. There was overwhelming evidence, in fact, that babies who stay with their mothers do better (they cry less, stay warmer, and have lower levels of stress hormones). But, when she returned to work, she continued enforcing the hospital policy and telling mothers that the babies would be better off in the nursery. Years later, when Bingham reached a position of authority, she helped revise policies at several hospitals to keep mothers and babies together, but she was still troubled by the fact that she'd essentially lied to mothers to convince them to submit to a practice that she knew made no sense. Institutional inertia is powerful, she said. As of 2005, half the babies born in the

United States were being taken away from their mothers before they were an hour old.

"My best explanation is that everyone involved, from me to the mothers, fathers, and loved ones, have been indoctrinated to be submissive in the face of authoritative hospital policies and practices," Bingham said.

It seemed obstetrics had gotten stuck, awkwardly astride the fence between craft and industry. It had resolved to give up the artisanal excellence of the craftsperson in exchange for the logic of mass production, but its leaders had never stopped thinking like craftspeople, allowing their hunches, their traditions, to trump data. In a 1978 ranking of medical specialties according to their use of solid scientific evidence, obstetrics came in dead last. In her 2007 book, *Pushed,* journalist Jennifer Block compared the obstetric practices supported by evidence to the practices actually used and showed that a yawning chasm still separated the two. And, in 2011, the American Congress of Obstetrics and Gynecology published a paper showing that only 25 percent of its own clinical guidelines for obstetrics were "based on good and consistent scientific evidence." The rest of the recommendations were based on evidence that was limited or inconsistent, or on opinion. The industrial logic, it seemed, had a momentum of its own. I wondered if this momentum was ultimately responsible for at least part of the rising maternal mortality rate.

Bingham suggested that, if I really wanted to explore the full complexity of this issue, I needed to look at the problem in context. Specifically, she thought it might be helpful if I listened to the stories of women who had almost been killed by childbirth, who could tell me with some authority what had happened and why. For every death there are dozens of near misses, and hundreds of women who are left with severe, life-altering injuries, she said. "This increase in deaths is just the tip of the iceberg."

NEW DANGERS

Michelle Niska has a friendly face marked by Scandinavian ancestry: straight blond hair, a high forehead, and a plumpness high on her cheekbones that squeezes her eyes to slits when she smiles, which is often. Her disposition is steeply inclined toward sunny guilelessness, which suits her role as an elementary school teacher (she teaches English to immigrant children) and as a Minnesotan.

I found Michelle in the pages of the *Anoka County Union*. The story was written with spare, newspaper bluntness, a style that derives its power through presenting both the incredible and the mundane in the same matter-of-fact tone. Michelle's story was so extreme that I began to wonder if the facts were simply wrong. When Beth, who was working as a nurse, came home that evening, I asked her how unusual it was for someone to lose 115 units of blood.

"Fifteen?" she said, "Um, well, that's more than most people have in their bodies."

"No, one hundred and fifteen."

"Don't be ridiculous," she said briskly.

Michelle had had a normal pregnancy, her second. Her first child had been delivered by Caesarean three years earlier, and the doctors recommended scheduling a C-section for this birth as well, which she did. This once-a-Caesarean-always-a-Caesarean rule is debatable, but it makes sense if you see the surgery as a nearly risk-free procedure. When Michelle's contractions started (a week early) she checked into the hospital and the nurses rolled her straight to the operating room. Her obstetrician, Jeff Raines, was out riding with his cycling club, so it was his partner, Cephas Agbeh, who performed the operation and presented the eight-pound baby girl to Michelle. It was only when Agbeh reached into the incision to remove the placenta that he realized something was wrong. The placenta is a one-pound purple tangle of branching and rebranching vessels. It carries a prodigious volume of blood—a tenth of all the blood from each heartbeat flows to the organ. Usually, hormones cause its vessels to contract after birth, and the placenta separates cleanly away from the uterus. But this time, when Agbeh pulled, he felt resistance—a bad sign.

"It hits you very quickly," Raines said. "It's one of those things where the bottom just drops out of your stomach."

Agbeh gave a few terse commands. Everyone started moving very quickly. The anesthesiologist held a mask up to Michelle's face.

"We're going to have to put you under," he said.

There was a curtain over Michelle's chest, screening her from the sight of her own viscera, but she knew something was wrong.

"That's not good, is it?" Michelle asked.

The anesthesiologist searched for the right words, then settled on terse honesty: "No." He pressed the mask over her mouth and nose.

Raines was still cycling when his pager buzzed. He called back and explained that he was at least an hour away, "Do you still want me to come in?" he asked. When the affirmative answer came without hesitation, he knew the situation was dire. He rode hard to his car, pulled on a pair of jeans, and went straight to the hospital. The sweat from the ride had barely dried when he jogged into the operating room.

Michelle was bleeding profusely. Her placenta had grown through the wall of her uterus, Raines said, snaking blood vessels into her abdomen, and these conduits acted as open spillways. Cups of blood gushed out with every heartbeat. The doctors were applying pressure with gauze to slow the flow, then removing the pads to close off the arteries. But as soon as they relaxed the pressure, Michelle's blood pressure would fall to a whisper and the wound would flood before they could do much cutting or clamping.

"It's kind of like walking up a sand dune," Raines said. "Each step you take you slide back almost as far. The blood is pouring up and the suction device—you can hear, it's not sucking air—she's bleeding as fast as it's sucking."

More doctors were summoned to the operating room. A pair of trauma surgeons cracked open Michelle's chest. One of them reached down, wrapped his hand around her main blood vessel, the aorta, where it curved down from the heart, and—in an effort to staunch the flow to her lower body—closed his fist tight.

Raines went to find Michelle's family. Diane and Jim Niska, her parents, had been in the middle of a lake, fishing, when Michelle called them to say she'd gone into labor. They were still on the road when they got another call and learned that a little girl had been born and Michelle was still in the operating room because there was some bleeding. By the time Raines spoke to them they'd been in the hospital for hours and knew something was terribly wrong.

"She's hemorrhaging," Raines told them. "It doesn't look good."

After four hours in the operating room, Michelle was still bleeding heavily. The doctor squeezing her aorta closed had felt his hand slowly go numb with pain. There were seven surgeons working on her. They had removed her uterus completely and were cauterizing other points of internal bleeding, stemming the flow.

"We had gone from a fire hose to a garden hose," Raines said.

The doctors were recycling blood—suctioning it out and pumping it back into Michelle—but it wasn't enough. They were using up bags so quickly that it soon became clear that they would exhaust the hospital's entire blood bank. Someone called the Red Cross, and police cruisers began shuttling blood from other hospitals. Nurses formed something like a bucket brigade to move the blood to the operating room. All told, they would use 110 units (the newspaper story I'd read had come out before the tally was completed)—more than all the blood circulating in the bodies of 11 large adults.

At 11:00 p.m. the physicians decided they needed to try something new. Michelle's parents saw the gurney pass through the hall but, so thickly clustered were the doctors and nurses, they could not catch a glimpse of their daughter. Michelle was taken to the interventional radiology room, where another doctor fed a probe up through the blood vessels in her leg to her abdomen. There, it released a gel to stop up the leaks in her circulatory system. This artificial clotting worked. The bleeding slowed to a trickle.

Raines went to find Michelle's parents. When Diane saw him, she stopped breathing. Raines simply nodded and smiled. "I've never been so happy to see a nod in my life," Diane said. At 2:00 a.m. Raines collapsed in a bed at the hospital and tried to sleep. He was awakened by his cell phone at 7:00 a.m. Michelle was bleeding again.

———————

When I began to talk to obstetricians, some of them stopped here. What we needed, they said, were more hospitals like the ones that Michelle was in, more blood banks, more expertise in interventional radiology, more surgeons. This was logical, but after Bingham's admonition to be aware of the tendency to seek improvement through technology despite—rather than because of—the evidence, I was wary. It was only after I'd talked to the Niskas long enough to learn Michelle's full medical history that I saw the problem with a knee-jerk impulse for more technology: Such recommendations are blinkered by a limited perspective—a tight focus on the catastrophe itself. To understand what had happened to Michelle Niska you have expand the scope of focus to encompass her previous pregnancy.

At the first indications of labor for her first child, three years before, she'd rushed to the hospital, where the nurses admitted her, got her set up in a bed, and then pretty much left her alone. Someone would come in every 15 minutes or so to take measurements and check the fetal heart monitor. They added Pitocin, a synthetic version of the hormone oxytocin, to her intravenous drip, which increased the force of her contractions. The doctor ratcheted up the dosage slowly. Even though Michelle had an epidural, the contractions were still intensely uncomfortable. And this discomfort only increased as the hours ticked by. With the catheter and the epidural, an IV in her arm, and the fetal heart monitor around her belly, Michelle was immobilized. Holding any position for hours is hard, she said. "Even when you sleep, I realized, you roll around. And when you are in pain and you can't move, you just lay there and think about how much it hurts." A survey of mothers found that 77 percent of those who were able to change position during labor said that movement was at least somewhat helpful in relieving pain (by comparison, 75 percent said the same of narcotics). Michelle had labored for 21 hours when the doctor asked if she'd thought about a C-section. She had been thinking about it for the last 10 hours or so. "If you don't do it, I'll cut him out myself," she quipped.

The Caesarean has always held a certain conceptual attraction for me. I've often experienced an uncomfortable twinge when I see a massively pregnant woman. This feeling doesn't spring from sympathetic pain, but from something like a simpleton's thunderstruck disbelief: The notion of that entire bulging mass passing through pelvis and the vagina so utterly violated my sense of anatomy that I could not entirely believe it occurred. Birth seemed no less improbable than levitation. No wonder we have fables about storks and fairies delivering children. To the cultural theorist, Camille Paglia, the mystery of the female anatomy is a threat, a reminder that we are all ultimately prostrate before nature.

"Woman's body is a labyrinth in which man is lost," Paglia wrote in *Sexual Personae*. "It is a walled garden, the medieval *hortus conclusus,* in which nature works its daemonic sorcery. Woman is the primeval fabricator, the real First Mover. She turns a gob of refuse into a spreading web of sentient being, floating on a snaky umbilical by which she leashes every man."

By this leash, nature draws us inexorably back to the earth: Birth rubs the primeval in our faces. It forces us to acknowledge the great mystery inherent in life-giving, the same mystery that inevitably overwhelms science and reason in the life-taking. The Caesarean incision is a stroke against the unknown. It makes what is invisible and circuitous, visible and linear. It replaces mystery with mechanics.

The use of the Caesarean goes back to mythic prehistory: Apollo (appropriately, the god of clarity and logic) used the technique to deliver his son, Asclepius, the god of healing. But it was historically the option of last resort, performed only when the mother could not be saved, because the operation nearly always killed her. Caesareans became safer after surgeons began to use antisepsis and anesthesia in the 19th century, so much so that some surgical authorities advocated for initiating the operation earlier, while the mother still had a chance of making it. But they still weren't very good: Late in the 19th century, Robert Harris, one of those surgical authorities advocating earlier Caesareans, found it instructive to compare the prognosis of pregnant women who had been cut by New York surgeons to those who had been gored by bulls. Women were six times more likely to die after a Caesarean; "a far better showing for the cow-horn than the knife," Harris wrote. As the years passed and surgical techniques improved (the discovery of penicillin provided a big boost), the survival rate increased dramatically. By 1970, Caesareans accounted for 5 percent of all births in the United States and had improved so much that doctors began using the surgery preemptively for breeched babies, for twins, and as time passed for women with chronic disease, and for women whose babies just seemed big. By the 2000s the likelihood that a healthy young woman would die during a Caesarean had fallen to less than 0.028 percent, making it one of the safest major surgeries performed. The operation had become so sure, so normal, that in 2006 a group of experts suggested that it might be an appropriate method for delivering the vast majority of babies.

The Caesarean has a simple Apollonian clarity in the operating room, but the risks and benefits grow complex in the months and years afterward. The surgery itself is an injury—women take between two and 12 weeks to recover, and the Caesarean wound becomes infected in 3 to 9 percent of cases. Then there are the adhesions, the internal scarring that develops in more than half of all abdominal surgeries. In rare situations these surgical scars can cause chronic pain, scramble organs, obstruct the bowels, cut off fallopian tubes, or—in subsequent pregnancies—increase the risk of stillbirth and of fetuses growing outside the womb. During Michelle's second pregnancy it was the Caesarean scar that provided egress for the placenta to snake out into her abdomen. This condition is called *placenta accreta*—or in Michelle's more serious case, *placenta percreta*. It used to be the kind of thing a doctor might see just once in his career, according to obstetrician Elliott Main, the principal investigator for California's maternal mortality inquiry. Main told me, "It's gone from being something that is extraordinarily rare to being something that is seen monthly at every large center." In the 1950s the incidence of accreta was one out of 30,000 births; now it's one per 533 deliveries. The risk of accreta increases with each subsequent Caesarean, Main said, adding that this epidemic of pathological placentas was caused by the rise in C-sections. On that point, there is scientific consensus.

We met at the California Pacific Medical Center, where Main is head of obstetrics. He rushed into his office, looking haggard, as if he were still keeping a medical intern's schedule, and he collapsed into a chair. His smile is warmly, sympathetic perhaps honed to help anxious families relax. Main wore a short beard—reddish brown, peppered with gray. He answered my questions with complete sentences that could have been lifted from the pages of a peer-reviewed journal, while staring intently at the floor, as if the carpet contained a medical teleprompter.

Accreta and related conditions (there's also placenta previa, where the placenta forms over the cervix, effectively blocking the exit) account for part of the rise in maternal deaths, he said, but how much is still unclear. When he'd started crunching the numbers, he'd first guessed that a suite of "usual suspects" might explain the increase in maternal mortality: obesity, heart disease, race, poverty, older mothers, fertility treatments—along with better accounting of deaths. But those factors had only made up for part of the increase. "That means," he said, "that we have to start looking at what else has changed in the last 10 years of obstetric practice." It's hard to ignore the fact that Caesareans increased

50 percent—representing an intensification of medical treatment during childbirth—in the same decade that maternal mortality had spiked.

Again, the numbers here are small: The review that Main had helped lead in California identified 98 mothers whose deaths in 2002 and 2003 were directly related to their pregnancies. That's about 50 more than expected based on the lower maternal mortality rate a decade earlier. A third of that increase was probably due to improved accounting, and at least a quarter was surely due to obesity and the rest of the usual suspects, which left between zero and 20 deaths that might be related to technological overreach. In the end, the reviewers firmly identified 15 deaths that were caused by some aspect of Caesarean surgery. It was a small number, but a small number with an extraordinary implication: An increase in medical care was killing people.

———

Jeff Raines was not optimistic when he began his second operation on Michelle Niska. She'd gone through a lot of surgical trauma; she'd received over 13 gallons of blood, which had surely put a lot of stress on her body; she was in a coma, and her systolic blood pressure had fallen to 30 (terrifyingly low). Raines sent word to her parents, who came down to say goodbye for the last time. Yet, somehow, Michelle held on. Over the next 24 hours the doctors twice more performed surgery to stop internal bleeding.

Michelle's mother, Diane, came in again the next morning with two nieces who had joined the family in their vigil. She stared at her daughter, intubated, perforated with needles, and wired to monitors. Chances were she'd never wake up. Then, Michelle opened her eyes. "I just about peed my pants," one of the girls remembered. Michelle tried to speak, but the breathing machine stopped her. Diane handed her a pen and paper. With a shaky hand Michelle wrote: *Am I going to die?* "No," Diane said fiercely. Then she wrote: *Did I almost die?* "Yes."

Protecting Women to Death

The most careful international comparisons of maternal heath show that the number of childbirth-related deaths are falling dramatically around the world. The United States, where the death risk is rising, is the one perplexing dark spot in otherwise sunny reports. We have a maternal mortality rate four times higher than Australia's, twice as high as Canada's and England's, and on par with Belarus'—the dictatorship where medical technology has not been significantly updated since the Soviet era, and where the fallout from Chernobyl has challenged the capacity of the health system. And yet, the United States was probably the country best equipped to handle the emergency of Michelle's second birth. After a six-month recovery (during which doctors monitored her fastidiously) she moved to New Mexico, where she is now thriving and raising two adorable children.

There are some problems the U.S. healthcare system handles very well: If you are going have a major medical emergency requiring high technology and the deft coordination of well-trained medical professionals who will not hesitate to make extraordinary interventions, you'd do well to schedule the crisis at a time when you happen to be in the United States. In a very real sense, the prevalence of surgical birth had saved Niska's life. It had also been the thing that put her in danger in the first place.

This paradoxical pattern repeats across the field. First, proponents of technological delivery justify the need for intensive care by pointing to injuries (e.g., the claim that vaginal birth damages the pelvic floor and causes incontinence). Then, the partisans of natural birth claim that the injuries themselves were caused by technological intervention (e.g., the claim that such damage is the result of drug interventions to speed up labor). The format for this debate was already set by the 1800s, when doctors were arguing that hospital birth was necessary to combat the high rate of fever after childbirth. In response, the Austrian professor of obstetrics Ignaz Semmelweiss proposed that doctors themselves were the vector of the disease. At the time it seemed utterly wrongheaded—dangerous even—to suggest that an agent of healing might be a spreader of disease (Oliver Wendell Holmes Sr. also proposed this hypothesis 3 years earlier in 1843 and was met with a similar scorn). Semmelweiss was mocked for taking this position, but it turned out that he was absolutely correct: Doctors rarely washed their hands in those days, even after examining cadavers and, despite their good intentions, they infected thousands of women.

In hindsight, it's clear that many of the attempts across history to assist women in labor have done more harm than good. When I looked up the causes of those sky-high maternal death rates from the beginning of the 20th century, it became apparent that the majority of the lives spared by obstetrical advances were not souls snatched back from nature's devouring maw, but women who had been saved from bad medicine. In a review of mother and infant health between 1900 and 1999, the U.S. Centers for Disease Control and Prevention concluded that early in the 20th century, "Poor obstetric education and delivery practices were mainly responsible for the high numbers of maternal deaths, most of which were preventable." Babies were delivered using "inappropriate and excessive surgical and obstetric interventions (e.g., induction of labor, use of forceps, episiotomy, and cesarean deliveries)."

Birth in Eden

All the evidence showing that human meddling can make birth more dangerous brought me back to my initial idea that birth was uncomplicated and safe until we mucked it up. There's a tendency, however, for this line of thinking to spiral into absurdity: If medicine falls under suspicion so must nutrition and culture and women, themselves. Modern women are too weak and fragile to give birth, the argument goes; they are too terrified by their physicality, "too posh to push." Perhaps it shouldn't be surprising that women are blamed for their difficult deliveries and for rising C-section rates, since that's essentially an updated version of the biblical position. The pain of childbirth, according to Genesis, is retribution for Eve's apple plucking.

The impulse to cast blame is understandable: It seems unlikely that nature, or God, would have designed women so that they or their babies cannot survive birth—after all, if a baby (or worse, the mother) dies, so do the genes. And so I set out to learn if birth was dangerous before medicine, religion, poor nutrition, or patriarchy began to muddy the waters. What was birth like in Eden?

Birth is a recent innovation in the grand scheme of things. For most of history, creatures reproduced by splitting off pieces of themselves—bacteria, sea anemones, and many plants operate this way. Variations on the theme produced spores, seeds, and eggs. But eggs are defenseless, and a number of species began sheltering them within their bodies until they hatched and could fend for themselves: There are fishes and reptiles that give live birth, along with most sharks, and Seychelles flies sometimes bear crawling larvae, but mammals became birthing specialists.

The next innovation, some 100 million years ago, was the placenta: a feeding system, oxygen supply, sewage treatment plant, and diplomat all wrapped up into one temporary organ. The placenta provided life support for babies, kept their waste from poisoning the mother, and prevented the maternal immune system from attacking this growth as it would any other foreign body. It allowed longer gestations so that some babies, like the giraffe, could run from predators moments after birth. But longer development in the womb also meant bigger babies, and this started to cause problems.

Evolution makes compromises. If increasing the size of babies raises the risk (a little) that some will die at birth, but also raises the survivors' chances (a lot) of going on to reproduce, then newborn babies will become bigger. Counterintuitive as it seems, the natural world is filled with examples of poorly designed birthing physiologies that cause death and injury. And of these examples, it was the spotted hyena that most thoroughly dashed my hopes of reclaiming Edenic natural birth.

The spotted hyena's birth canal heads almost to the complete rear of the animal before making a hairpin turn back toward the belly. When pups reach this point during birth their umbilical cord detaches—it is only long enough to provide oxygen to the pups for the first third of their natal journey—and the clock begins to tick down toward suffocation. The pups then pass through their mother's clitoris (!), which in hyenas comprises a seven-inch phallic tube. (This phallus is capable of erection and from some distance is nearly indistinguishable from a penis. Early biologists, including Aristotle, may be excused in thinking that the species was made up wholly of hermaphrodites.) The organ tears during the first birth, and maternal mortality among hyenas is as high as 10 percent. The fact that any animal must give birth this way seems the final proof that if nature had a designer, He—it seems unlikely, in this case, to have been a She—was vindictive or willfully negligent.

What recompense does nature provide for this horrible toll? Perhaps it has something to do with the relative value of testosterone: It makes the female hyenas masculine (the penis-like clitoris), but it also makes them fierce. The pups are born in pairs, and if both survive birth they immediately fight, often to the death. Under these circumstances, the aggression provided by high levels of testosterone would be indispensable. (Another hypothesis is that having a large phallus provides a social advantage in the hyena hierarchy; the scientists who proposed this were—what a surprise—male.)

Humans, of course, are not spotted hyenas. But, for me, the example of the hyena permanently exploded the argument that gentle birth was an evolutionary imperative. If natural birth requires tearing off the head of any phallus, count me out. Spotted hyenas, as a species, continue to thrive despite a maternal mortality 500 times the rate deemed unacceptably high for humans in America. The question is: How different are humans and hyenas? Each species appears to have made an evolutionary bargain, trading away the capacity for easy births for various other biological perks. Instead of testosterone, humans got larger brains and the ability to walk upright.

Authors making passing reference to the evolution of birth often explain that upright walking narrowed the pelvis. In fact, the exact opposite is true. The human birth canal is proportionally wider than that of a chimpanzee or any of the great apes, which have relatively effortless deliveries. Biological anthropologists who have studied the mechanics of two-legged striding think that walking stretched the hips wider from side to side, but in so doing, shortened the distance from front to back. The upright stature also required adjustment of the ver-tebrae, which went from being a horizontal beam—from which the body's architecture was suspended—to a vertical center post. This pushed the lumbar spine and sacrum forward, under the center of gravity, and further squished the birth canal into an oval, wider from side to side.

The notion that broad "childbearing hips" make for an easy birth is a myth because it's the front-to-back dimension of the hips that cre-ates the tightest squeeze. A woman's birthing conformation can be bet-ter judged by her height—a taller woman is likely to have more capacious pelvis. "I hate to say it, but it's sort of the classic Hollywood body," one experienced midwife ruefully admitted. Want to see what childbearing hips actually look like? Check out Heidi Klum.

Even in the best cases, birth is a tight squeeze for women, no matter how well hipped. Humans have the highest brain-to-bodyweight ratio of any mammal. The head of the average baby—4.4 inches by 3.7 inches—is close to the dimensions of the birth canal of the average woman—5 inches by 4.5 inches. Babies normally enter the pelvis side-ways (facing the hip), then rotate as they navigate their shoulders though the bones. The upshot of this tortuous journey is that birth is difficult for humans, more difficult than for most other animals, according to Wenda Trevathan, an anthropologist who has studied the evolution of birth. It would seem that evolution would have had to either sacrifice walking efficiency or sacrifice in utero development (and settle for smaller babies) but, instead, the species moved in a third dimension: Some 60,000 years ago early humans must have begun helping one another during birth.

"Mothers probably did not seek assistance solely because they predicted the risk that childbirth poses, however," Trevathan wrote with collaborator Karen Rosenberg. "Pain, fear and anxiety more likely drove their desire for companionship and security."

This insight has extraordinary implications. It suggests that women evolved to feel birth pains, that anxiety was not an impediment, but a vital tool. While monkeys seek solitude for birth, the adaptation of anxiety nudges Aristotle's social animal to seek help. Unlike the apes, we are literally built to require assistance. The terms of the hyena's evolutionary exchange had been as simple as a straight trade in baseball—lose survival in birth, gain survival in infancy—lose some pitching talent, gain some bats. But the exchange our ancestors made was more nuanced, because they had come up with the game-changing strategy of cooperation. By working together, the mothers of *Homo sapiens* were able to make redundant a number of traits—easy births among them—that previously had been vital for survival. It freed up room for evolutionary change. This innovation was radical   to extend the baseball analogy, it would be like devising a strategy that made pitchers unimportant, which would allow a team to trade its bullpen for power hitters. It's clear that social birth is one of the factors distinguishing our ancestors from their primate kin, which is to say that the practice of obstetrics is a fundamental part of what it means to be human.

The word *obstetrics* comes from Latin *obstetrix*, meaning a midwife, or "one who stays present." Trevathan noted, however, that there is not a high premium on remaining present in modern delivery rooms. If you

think of birth as a strictly mechanical process, prioritizing companionship seems perilously frivolous. But if evolution has truly programmed
emotion into the physiology of delivery, then managing feelings would
be the key to managing the physical process. Modern evidence bolsters
Trevathan's hypothesis. A 2011 review published by the Cochrane Col-
laboration, the foremost authority on evidence-based medicine, found
that women who had the support of another person throughout their
entire labor were 21 percent less likely to need Caesareans than women
laboring in places where companions were not permitted. It would make
sense from an evolutionary perspective that the cervix would remain
closed until the woman was able to assemble the people she trusted to
guide her safely through birth. "In other words," Trevathan wrote,
"women experience heightened emotion at birth, which leads them to
seek companionship, which in turn, leads to the ultimate outcome of
lowered mortality and greater reproductive success."

Curiously, while embracing some technologies that lack scientific
backing, modern obstetrics has resisted this older technology of simply
staying present, despite the strong evidence supporting it. The authors of
the Cochrane review wrote that "continuous support during labour has
become the exception rather than the norm. This may contribute to the
dehumanization of a woman's childbirth process. Modern obstetric care
frequently subjects women to institutional routines, which may have
adverse effects on the progress of labour." Trevathan's submission that a
woman's psychic state matters, that the creep of mechanical aid—to the
exclusion of the human touch—might be counterproductive, could
explain the paradox of increasing mortality in American births. But the
problem with studying the psyche is that it is invisible, impossible to
measure in any quantifiable way. To test this idea, I would have to find
some example of labor in which the birthing mother's emotions were
monitored as carefully as her vital stats. And that, I knew, would force
me to wade into dark waters, out into the realm of feelings and intuition,
far from the reassuring solidity of science.

PSYCHOLOGICAL LABOR

There aren't many birthing institutions in the United States that put emotional support first: Although administrators of every labor and delivery unit in the country would say they aspire to respect and honor their patients, respect is almost always trumped by the need to provide immediate access to the operating room, and by the economic imperative to provide beds and caregivers without going broke. As I asked around, I heard of a midwifery center in rural Tennessee that treated birth as almost a religious ceremony, as opposed to a medical treatment. This sort of thing would have been altogether too fruity for me, but Trevathan's theory and the center's exemplary (and blessedly non-mystical) statistics drove me onward. With some trepidation, I picked up the book *Spiritual Midwifery,* by the center's head midwife, Ina May Gaskin, and began to flip through accounts of births. These stories, told by mothers, often referenced the importance of feeling psychedelic, or being telepathic with a partner. Along with this mental contact, there was a lot of eyebrow-elevating physical connection as well: Pictures of men kissing their laboring wives and squeezing their breasts as they pushed. For one birth, the prescription for a stalled labor turned out to be an impromptu wedding—once husband and wife were bound with traditional vows, the woman relaxed and the baby shot out.

I began growing impatient as I flipped through the pages. It's not that I discounted this sort of thing—for all I knew telepathy was the key to facilitating birth. It's just that there was no purchase from which to assess its validity. It bothered me for the same reason I was bothered by my father's proclamations about birth therapy: Without some rational way to engage, I didn't know how to deal with it.

But in its second half, this book turned into something you might find in a medical student's backpack. The descriptions were unsparingly practical. And as I read onward I began to find some of those toeholds from which I could evaluate the far-out assertions in the first half: The stroking of skin, for example, and especially of nipples, causes women to produce oxytocin, whose synthetic analogue, Pitocin, is the most reliable obstetrical tool for prompting contractions. Was the Pitocin drip simply the crude mechanical override required by a culture unable to bring emotion—much less physical intimacy—into the delivery room?

The next morning, I happened to have an interview scheduled with Eugene Declercq, who studies birth at the Boston University School of Public Health, and I asked him if he'd heard of Ina May Gaskin. He had. "There's a tendency for people to blow her off because she's such a hippie," he said. "That's a huge mistake. She is able to read the science—and write it—as well or better than most academics in the field."

When I called her, I was glad to have Declercq's warning. Gaskin's husband Stephen answered the phone in a blissed-out drawl, called me "man," and squeezed in a reference to the military-industrial complex before handing me off. But the next voice to come on the line was different. It was a sharp, clipped voice that suggested a hard-bitten country pragmatism. By the end of our conversation I was convinced. I told her I'd like to visit her little pocket of Haight-Ashbury diaspora in Tennessee.

"Well, you'd be welcome," Ina May said.

I met Ina May and Stephen Gaskin in Nashville. They were both tall, lean, and gray, comporting themselves with the deliberate plainness that comes with a renunciation of superficiality. Both wore their hair in loose ponytails. Stephen's eyes were clouded with cataracts and mischief, while Ina May's were a clear and piercing blue. Her mien was terribly serious: "If you're not angry," she told me as we navigated the interstate out of the city, "you're not paying attention." When she smiled she did so with a ferocity that wrinkled her upper lip and revealed her canines in a sort of happy snarl. While Stephen was bent like a dry branch, Ina May stood ramrod straight. She wore batik-print pants gathered with a drawstring at the waist, and a sleeveless, blue, V-neck shirt.

I sat in the backseat of their coupe, and as we drove south through fields and woodlots, the couple told the story of how they'd first made their way along the same route to the place now called The Farm. They'd met in the 1960s in San Francisco, where Stephen had developed a following delivering freeform speeches on psychedelics and spirituality. (My father went to one meeting.) In 1970 Stephen left San Francisco on a lecture tour, and 300 of his friends came along, forming a convoy of school buses. Some of the women, including Ina May, were pregnant, and when they reached Northwestern University, near Chicago, one of them went into labor. Ina May assisted the delivery. That first birth, luckily, was easy. Stephen, who was lecturing, announced that a new consciousness was appearing in the universe at that very moment, and part of the audience rushed outside to watch through the windows of the bus.

When they reached Rhode Island, an obstetrician named Louis La Pere knocked on the door of Ina May's bus and asked if she would accept instruction. He'd heard that women were delivering babies on school buses and was hoping to prevent a tragedy before it happened. "He was just a wise man who'd read something in the newspaper about this woman with a master's degree in English delivering kids," she remembered.

La Pere spent the next few hours giving Ina May and two other women a crash course in delivery techniques, leaving them with an obstetrical textbook, a satchel full of medical equipment, and a sense of astonishment: Ina May and others had given birth previously in hospitals, and remembered their doctors without fondness. But this man was different—he instantly set the women at ease, comfortably joking and laying his hands on them with immediate intimacy.

"I've never seen someone touch Ina May that way," Stephen said. "Just petting her, and squeezing her."

"Touch was a big part of his practice," Ina May said. "He'd probably get sued for that today. I went to his clinic and it was clear he was much loved by the people in that community."

La Pere's bedside manner, and his technical instructions, provided a foundation for the women as they began building their own version of obstetrics. In the very next birth, the umbilical cord was wrapped around the baby's neck, and the mother hemorrhaged. Following La Pere's instructions, the women unwound the cord, suctioned the baby's airway, and gave the mother a shot of Pitocin from La Pere's satchel, which contracted her uterus and stopped the bleeding. The doctor had come just in time.

Ina May's own baby was the tenth to arrive on the buses, and the first to die. It was born two months premature and stopped breathing about 12 hours later. Ina May was grief-stricken, but didn't blame herself. The child had exhibited all the symptoms of hyaline membrane disease, she said. The lungs of babies with this disorder become so coated with mucus that they lose the ability to take in oxygen. At that time there was no treatment for it. The death didn't make Ina May question the wisdom of birthing on buses. Instead, she studied the obstetrical textbooks all the more avidly. It left her craving an infant to nurture, and she channeled that yearning into midwifery.

This reminiscing had carried us almost 70 miles south of Nashville, they talking over their shoulders, me craning forward to see, my legs folded sideways in the narrow backseat. We'd turned off the highway and were cruising between rolling green hills and the occasional farmhouse.

"When we first drove down this road, all the people came out on their decks to watch," Stephen said. "They were announcing our route on the radio: 'The hippies are moving down highway 20 now.' They were so relieved when we passed by."

"They thought we were the Manson family," said Ina May.

Eventually the two cultures learned to live in peace. The Tennesseans, especially those without medical insurance, employed the midwives. Many were Amish, who sometimes paid for their healthcare in furniture. About one-third of the babies the midwives delivered were the children of these rural poor, another third were children of The Farm, and the final portion were children of well-to-do women who had read Ina May's books and traveled from Atlanta or New York or places as far away as Hong Kong to give birth at the midwifery center.

We turned down the road leading to The Farm. Stately elms and bur oaks opened onto green-yellow fields of tall grass. The Gaskins lived at the end of a dirt road, in the house they'd built piecemeal around the tent they'd pitched in the 1970s—Stephen gleefully pointed to the original tent poles that had become part of the building. Above, at the ceiling line (and on almost every wall in the home) Stephen had built bookshelves into the walls. At the couches in the central kitchen-dining-living room were still more books in precarious stacks, strewn papers, and a silver laptop.

"Sorry about the mess," Ina May said. "I'm trying to finish a draft of this book."

She poked through the refrigerator and produced a pot of black-eyed peas, a cast-iron frying pan filled with cornbread, and some collard greens. We spiced the meal with nutritional yeast and liquid amino acids. It tasted unremittingly healthy. I felt right at home.

The Farm clinic, where the seven midwives practice, is a little yellow house shaded by tall oak trees and surrounded by a neatly mowed lawn. Ina May had arranged for another midwife to meet me there, and when I arrived a woman with gold wire-frame glasses and a pair of iron-gray pigtails resting on her broad chest was waiting. She beamed with pleasure and introduced herself as Pamela Hunt. Her manner was that of an especially kind school counselor.

On the inside, the clinic looked like a small-town doctor's office, though the usual utilitarian decorating scheme of cabinets, examining tables, and medical posters was muted by soft touches. There were embroidered pillows on the examining table, couches or rocking chairs in every room, and the light blue walls were decorated by framed photos of infants. In the largest room a four-foot square tie-dyed cloth—a kaleidoscopic image of concentric rainbows—dominated one wall. When women come for their prenatal visits, Pamela said, the midwives spend most of the time simply listening to them.

"We'll take their blood pressure, measure their fundal height, and all that, but most of the hour is spent sitting on these couches," she said. "We pay close attention to each individual and try to get to know her mindset—what makes her laugh, what makes her cry, specifically, how is her relationship with her husband?" In other words, the midwives pay more attention to a woman's relationships and emotional make-up than to her physical condition. In the course of labor, Pamela said, knowledge of the woman's fears and desires is generally more useful than her vital statistics.

Clustered around the clinic are tiny cabins, where women stay while waiting for contractions to start. Two of these buildings were occupied, but when I asked if Pamela would introduce me to one of these mothers-to-be, she looked shocked.

"That's a private space," she said, gesturing toward a cabin. Then she sighed and smiled the kind, long-suffering smile that teachers give to particularly slow students. "These women are going through a very intimate, vulnerable process. It's really not a good time to bring in strange masculine energy."

I felt my throat constrict. I'd flown to Tennessee to see for myself if these self-taught midwives had rediscovered something that the rest of civilization had forgotten. I couldn't very well make that assessment based on the impressions I got from this little tour. I'd known it would take a lucky alignment of stars to observe a birth, but I hadn't expected that the midwives would categorically reject the idea, or deny my access to their clients without so much as talking with them.

"But I'm not strange," I said, cocking my head in a way I hoped would look unthreatening and sympathetic, like a golden retriever.

"We just don't do that here," Pamela curtly replied, shaking her head. "Besides husbands, men usually don't attend births."

My gender would prove to be an unassailable barrier. Even classes for midwives in training were off-limits. The Farm's birthing operations, it turned out, were even more sealed off (at least to me and my masculine energy) than privacy-law-hamstrung hospitals. When I explained my predicament to Ina May, she offered a solution that would allow me to watch a birth from a distance. After digging into the back of several over-packed bookshelves, she produced a stack of VHS tapes. I could view these video recordings of deliveries without the danger that my mojo would intimidate anyone's cervix.

I stayed that night at The Farm's Eco-Hostel, a collection of buildings and campsites housing earnest young environmentalists who'd come to learn about organic gardening and green building techniques. Also visiting were a pair of young mothers, Diana and Brydget, who had brought a gaggle of tiny daughters from Nashville. I waited until the girls were safely asleep before I slipped one of Ina May's videos into the VHS player. A serene, Afroed mother named Janis appeared on the television, laboring to deliver a breech baby—the infant was sitting upright in the womb rather than diving out head first. Because of the danger associated with the head coming out last, breech babies are automatically scheduled for C-section in most hospitals. Yet, here was Janis, making an "Oh" of her lips to breathe, then smiling lazily at something one of the midwives must have said.

At that moment, one of the mothers, Diana, walked out into the living room. She choked on a horrified half laugh and asked, "What are you watching?"

I realized what she was seeing: Here was the tall bearded man who had seemed so nice at dinner, who had been so attentive to the little girls, so warmly solicitous of their opinions about the swimming hole, now sprawled out shirtless, sweating onto the grungy couch, while on the television a group of midwives in long dresses stroked Janis's bulging nakedness. "It's research," I stammered, pathetically tongue-tied. At that particular moment in the video, Ina May reached up from her position between Janis's legs to rub her nipples.

I was positively glowing with anxiety. Even if I had been alone I would have found it hard to watch the video with a purely clinical eye— there's no getting around the fact that birth is a culturally restricted event, and I felt as if I had been caught in tiptoeing trespass. But against all odds, Diana accepted my explanation and joined me on the couch. There commenced a period of awkward silence.

"Her cervix is dilated to seven centimeters," I finally said, like a sports fan updating the score. "It's a breech."

"Wow."

"Yeah."

Some long-hibernating defense system within my head, dormant since the ninth grade, woke with a start in the familiar glare of wincing sexual shame, and began trying to squirm out of the heat by offering up lame attempts at humor. We quipped back and forth, until we were joking convivially. By the time Janis had reached nine centimeters, Brydget had appeared, carrying a flask of vodka, which she passed around after settling in next to us. Alcohol wasn't allowed at the Eco-Hostel but over dinner the three of us had shared complaints about the Byzantine policies restricting activities on The Farm (as hippies age they seem to transform from defilers of the rules to scolding enforcers). The booze's illicitness made it all the more intoxicating, and the video kindled a thrilling sense of transgression.

In a way, it's odd that images of birth make people so nervous. We've all been there, after all. But in another way, this anxiety makes perfect sense. The portal between nonlife and life stands at the nexus of all our great taboos: Excrement and genitalia entwine with the possibility of death and with hints of sex. This last is especially disturbing, but birth is inherently sexual. The same female organs are engaged during birth and sex, of course. And the same chemicals surge into a woman's bloodstream, triggering a similar combination of agony and ecstasy, pain that can turn to pleasure and back again. Oxytocin—which floods into the bloodstream during orgasm, triggering feelings of love and contentment—is named from the Greek *oxus,* meaning swift, and *tokos,* meaning childbirth, a reference to its ability to accelerate labor by increasing the severity of contractions; *oxus* also translates as sharp, a coincidentally apt double meaning. Women have compared especially traumatic birth to rape, and others have experienced orgasms during delivery and while breastfeeding. It's no wonder we are reluctant to accept the sexual aspects of birth: Acknowledge that a kind of sexuality is at work during labor, and the intimation of incest is not far behind. Who knows what other terrors wait in the dark?

"I don't know how much more of this I can take," Brydget said after an hour.

I felt the same way. I cringed sympathetically as the women moaned and babies inched out on the screen.

"How are all these women so calm?" Diana marveled. "She's smiling! Oh, there's no way, look at her face, she's totally stoned." She turned to me. "You've got to do an exposé, and find out if they are feeding them some narcotic tree bark or something."

The beatific state of the laboring women was indeed striking. Whatever the midwives were doing to help them manage their psychic state, it was working. If there had been some psychoactive bark, then that would have made my job easier—physical interventions are more easily studied than the magic the midwives were working. I could understand, at least in part, why modern obstetrics gave short shrift to the psychology of birth. My eyes were tuned to physical action; I didn't know how to watch for feelings.

After Diana and Brydget went to bed, I stayed up assembling my impressions of these births. The first video had made the delivery of a breech baby look effortless. But, during the next recorded birth, something had gone wrong. The infant's shoulder had locked in the mother's pelvis behind the pubic bone, a shoulder dystocia. I'd leaned forward with interest. In New Jersey, an obstetrician had told me, juries consider shoulder dystocia so terrifying that, when sued, many hospitals have found it cheapest to simply sign the settlement checks without so much as contacting the lawyers. But there was no alarm in the video. The midwives asked the woman to turn over and crouch on all fours. Moments later, the baby slid free.

When I looked up the technique online I learned that it was called the Gaskin maneuver. The next day I asked Ina May if she was the eponymous Gaskin. She seemed a little embarrassed to admit that she was. She'd learned the trick from a Central American midwife who worked with Mayan women in the Guatemalan highlands.

"I didn't invent it," she said. "It really should be called the all-fours maneuver."

Birth attendants generally learn several other techniques for freeing shoulders: In the McRoberts maneuver, they push the woman's knees hard back to her chest while striking the area just above the pubic bone with a fist; in Wood's Screw maneuver, they snake a hand up into the woman and try to rotate the baby's shoulders; in the Zavanelli maneuver they push the baby back up and perform a Caesarean. All except the last are generally accompanied by what obstetric literature calls—with grim poetry—a "generous episiotomy," performed by inserting the open mouth of a scissor near the bottom of the vagina and cutting down toward the anus.

In each of these treatments the woman is passive. The secret of the all-fours maneuver is the unconsidered ability of the mother to take charge: When she turns over, gravity shifts the infant enough to allow first one shoulder, then the other to slide free.

This technique seemed preferable, at least worthy of trial. The one formal paper on the Gaskin maneuver showed that it took an average of two to three minutes and completely resolved the shoulder dystocia in

83 percent of cases—a better record than any of the other methods. There has been little further study of the technique, in part because it's hard for patients to turn once they are hooked up to an epidural (not to mention an IV, catheter, and fetal heart monitor). But Ina May thought the method hasn't spread due to an obstinate refusal by the medical establishment to cede any piece of authority to an outsider—to admit that Mayan elders know something the obstetricians should have been using all along. "Why couldn't you have the best of the modern world and not throw away what people used to know?" she asked.

The cultural amnesia extends even further when it comes to the psychology of birth, Ina May said. On her computer she pulled up a photograph of a sculpture: a human figure, smiling, and reaching under its knees to hold wide a gaping opening. Ina May found this figure carved in the roofline of Kilpeck Church in Herefordshire, England, built in the 12th century. These *Sheela-na-gigs,* as they are called, are scattered throughout the British Isles. Ina May thinks they are miniature visual obstetrical texts:

"I think this is a form of neurovisual programming; it would be tremendously helpful for women to see this," she said. "She's squatting, unladylike; her mouth and eyes are open. This is a woman who won't tear, because this is a woman who is smiling."

"Why is that?" I asked. "I don't see the connection."

"If your throat relaxes so will your cervix," Ina May said. "That's why holding your breath and pushing is so harmful."

No causal link between the throat and cervix has ever been documented, but it does make some sense that a woman who is calm enough to unclench her throat would be more able to allow loosening elsewhere. Obstetricians often learn that successful birth depends on the three Ps—the passage size, the passenger size (the baby), and the power available to push the latter through the former. But the metaphor is facile. It does nothing to illuminate the most opaque and, arguably, the most important part of birth: the fact that the passage changes in size. Pregnant women are literally shape-shifters—one birth hormone (named, awesomely, relaxin) softens the cartilage between the pubic bones, morphing the shape of the pelvis, while others ripen the cervix and stimulate contractions. And the release of these hormones may be slowed or intensified by emotions. At the very least, it seems safe to hypothesize that *Sheela-na-gigs* are a salute to the transformative power of the female body—a simple documentation of the fact that women can "get huge," as Ina May put it.

Ina May has found comparing reproduction to excretion is far more apt than comparing it to an overloaded tractor trailer charging toward a tunnel. To replace the three Ps, therefore, Ina May has proposed what she calls the sphincter law. Like the sphincters that control excretion, the cervix does not respond well to conscious commands, she said. Instead, like a sphincter, it responds to subtle cues that all is well in the world and that the moment is right (a locked door and a little running water perhaps). Sphincters contract when they are startled or frightened, Ina May said. Laughter helps them open.

I stopped her: "Laughter?"

"Yes," said Ina May; she paused. "But you really have to get to know the woman's sense of humor."

If the joke does hit the right notes, she said, it can provoke infectious giggling—teenage-sleepover laughter that grows until it overwhelms the conscious mind. I was intrigued. What is laughter, after all, but the release of tension? And what is a comedian if not the person you trust to see you safely through forbidding terrain, to trespass on taboos and then puncture anxiety with a well-turned punch line? In one sense, the midwife and comedian perform the same service, guiding their charges into forbidden territory while expertly dispelling fear.

"So, do you have any standbys?" I asked Ina May, fishing.

"Well, poop is usually funny," she mused. "And it's usually present. It's hard to relax down there without relaxing everything—I try to make it clear that it's no big deal, so the woman doesn't get embarrassed and tense up. Also, I've been working on my juggling act."

She waved me into the bedroom, fished around for a silken bag, and then, Ina May Gaskin, solemn matriarch of midwifery, high priestess of natural birth, and bitter critic of the medical establishment, began juggling plastic chunks of fake dog shit.

"These are hard, because they're uneven," she said, bending to pick up a fallen plastic turd. "I think they're the schnauzer model. Maybe I should go for something more like a fox terrier."

As wonderfully strange as they may seem, such techniques have served The Farm midwives well. After some 3,000 births, their Caesarean section rate stood at 3 percent (in these cases the midwives had driven the laboring woman to the hospital)—against the national average of 32 percent. Their infant mortality rate of 3.94 deaths per 1,000 births was also lower than the national average of 6.61, and their maternal mortality rate was zero. These statistics, however, were surely canted: The average woman who gave birth on The Farm was far less likely than the average American to be obese, and anyone with a serious condition like placenta previa would go to a hospital rather than The Farm. All the same, it seemed unlikely that these factors could increase the Caesarean rate tenfold.

There are other examples of midwives beating the national averages amid a much less healthy population. In the Navajo Nation, where obesity and diabetes are rampant, the local maternity services, which are midwife-centered, had a Caesarean rate of 13.5 percent as of 2007. And the midwives at the Family Health and Birth Center, who serve mostly low-income minority women in Washington, DC, had a Caesarean rate of 10 percent. Washington's infant mortality rate was 12.2 per 1,000—twice the national average, while the mortality rate at the Family Health and Birth Center stood at zero. There was also another example: the grandmother of all the American experiments in midwifery, a few hundred miles north, in Kentucky. As long as I was in the area, I figured I should visit.

BADASSED WOMEN ON HORSEBACK

As I drove northeast from Tennessee, the land on either side of the road grew steeper and greener, and by the time I reached Hyden, Kentucky, I felt I was at the bottom of a well with walls of beechwood and kudzu. This was true Appalachia, where dwellings clung to the rare plot of level ground—a doublewide up on a hillside ledge, a Dairy Queen in the bend of a river. The crook between hills provided enough resting place for the town of Hyden: a handful of brick buildings clustered around a crossroads. The house I was looking for was tucked a mile back into the forest, a manorial building of black logs and white chinking that stood above the Middle Fork of the Kentucky River. Hollyhocks were blooming in the yard. It was Mary Breckinridge's house, and home of the Frontier Nursing Service.

When Breckinridge came here in 1923, the U.S. maternal mortality rate was 870 per 100,000. And in these deep hollows, where people were cut off from medical treatment, women were even more likely to die in childbirth. Breckinridge changed that. In under a decade it would be safer to give birth in her corner of eastern Kentucky than in the best hospitals in New York. It was as pure an experiment as you could ask for: There were no rich women flying in to deliver, no hospitals to catch the most dangerous cases, just a group of midwives making improvements. What's more, the data were sterling: Breckinridge, a woman of great chutzpah, knew the world would doubt statistics generated by midwives in the mountains, so she recruited Dr. Louis Israel Dublin, vice president and statistician at the Metropolitan Life Insurance Company (now MetLife), to do the numbers.

The results, published in 1932, were astounding. The women the Frontier Nursing Service cared for, who were desperately poor and usually gave birth at home, were 10 times less likely to die in childbirth than the average American at the time. The nation would not reach the standard of care available in this corner of Appalachia until the 1950s, after the widespread acceptance of antiseptic and the discovery of antibiotics.

Breckinridge did not quite know what to make of these statistics. "The question that will arise in every thoughtful mind is why there should be this discrepancy between the Kentucky mountain woman and her city sister," she wrote. "Doubtless there is too much deliberate obstetrical interference in city hospitals but not so much, I am convinced, as people might think." Then, in what seems like an uncharacteristic lapse of reasoning, she laid out a theory that drew on eugenics: Rather than crediting her own work, she praised the racial stock and sturdy birth canals of the population she served. These explanations are no longer scientifically relevant, but even if the racial hypothesis had held up, it did not explain the radical improvement that had occurred among this population. Breckinridge had transformed one of the poorest parts of the country into a model for maternity care, and I wanted to know how she'd done it.

When I arrived a caretaker advised me to watch for snakes ("rattlers and copperheads"), and showed me where I'd stay until my meeting with Michael Claussen, the development coordinator for the Frontier Nursing Service. Just inside the house was a photograph of Breckinridge, who died in 1965. She stood before the camera among blooming rose bushes, a wooden cane in one hand, a pail of chickenfeed in the other, a white apron around her waist and, on her face, an expression of impish humor. The Breckinridge family was Southern aristocracy. Mary's grandfather had been James Buchanan's vice president and, later, the last secretary of war for the Confederacy. Mary Breckinridge remained nostalgic for the old South, outfitting her nurses in Confederate gray and giving her staff special dispensation to see the opening of *Gone with the Wind*. This Southern sympathy is inconvenient for most modern sensibilities, and it perhaps explains why her work has been largely forgotten.

Claussen arrived right on time, his hair buzz-cut, and his tie decorated with an eagle grasping an American flag. It became clear, as he walked through the grounds, that there was no miracle-working behind the drop in maternal deaths in rural Kentucky, unless it was a miracle of common sense.

During World War I, Breckinridge divorced her husband and reassumed her family name. After the war, she volunteered to serve as a nurse in France, where she assisted women and children. When she returned to the United States, the plight of Kentucky mothers stirred her noblesse oblige, and she resolved to muster a cavalry of midwives who could ride over the roadless terrain to reach homes that were days away from a hospital. She advertised in the United Kingdom, which had begun producing nurse-midwives (that is, midwives formally trained according to the current medical standards), with advertisements like the following, which appeared in the *Glasgow Times*.

ATTENTION! NURSE GRADUATES

With a sense of adventure!
Your own horse, your own dog, and a thousand miles
Of Kentucky mountains to serve.
Join my Nurses Brigade and help save children's lives!
Write to: M. Breckinridge, Hyden, Kentucky, USA

This excited a certain breed of daring woman, willing to work for next to nothing in exchange for freedom and a genuine opportunity to make the world a better place. One of these young women was Betty Lester, who left London on her own, crossed the Atlantic in a steamer, and then took the train until the rails ran out in Hazard, Kentucky. A nurse named Billy met Lester at the train station and told her to fill one saddle bag and leave the rest of her luggage behind.

"We rode straight up the mountain, and the rocks looked so big and the trail so bad that I wondered if I would topple over the horse's head," Lester wrote in a letter home. "We went straight down the other side and came to the river. I thought, 'Now what do we do?' Billy splashed right into the water so I did the same." She started work the next day and immediately lost her sense of direction on the branching horse trails. Eventually, however, she learned her way around the 700 square miles under the midwives' aegis. As promised, Lester was outfitted with a collie pup, which she named Ginger.

Lester also got the adventure she had hoped for. She and the other midwives would ride out into the mountains in snowstorms to deliver babies by candlelight. And, by virtue of being the closest medical providers available, they treated snakebites, fevers, and men shot in feuds. When attending births in mountain cabins, the midwives could not summon a surgeon or rely on the latest perinatal equipment, but what the Frontier Nursing Service lacked in heavy technology it more than made up for in care. The women made frequent house calls—18 prenatal visits and 12 postpartum checkups were standard for an uncomplicated pregnancy. They were also passionately committed: Betty Lester would spend most of her life in Hyden, and considered the people she served to be her family. (She was transformed by the work, from the dazed girl who had arrived with too much luggage, to a forceful presence who was nicknamed "The General.")

The Frontier Nursing Service slowly replaced the coterie of self-taught birth attendants who had lived in the mountains. The evidence suggests that some of these country grannies—as they were called—did not understand antisepsis, and they relied on superstitious techniques (like placing an axe under the bed to cut the pain of labor). The British form of nurse-midwifery that Breckinridge imported to Kentucky was, by contrast, a resolutely scientific form of medical technology. But it was also fundamentally different from the dominant obstetrical technology in America. British midwives learned that birth is a physical event, performed by the mother, while Americans learned that birth was a medical event performed on the mother. And it seems that this is where Breckinridge succeeded: At a time not too many years after it had been better to be gored by a bull than have Caesarean surgery, the Frontier Nursing Service nurse-midwives were able to simply support mothers while doing no harm.

The Frontier Nursing Service's low-tech armamentarium of time and attention was highly effective. When Louis Israel Dublin made his accounting in 1931, eastern Kentucky was suffering from a year-long drought and famine, and tuberculosis was running rampant. And, yet, maternal health was improving. Dublin concluded that if this style of maternity care became a model for the nation it would save a million lives within 15 years:

"If such a service were available to the women of the country generally, there would be a saving of 10,000 mothers' lives a year in the United States, there would be 30,000 less stillbirths and 30,000 more children alive at the end of the first month of life," Dublin wrote.

Dublin's vision never came to fruition. When we'd finished at the Breckinridge estate, I followed Claussen into town to the campus where the Frontier Nursing Service now runs a school, which sends some 200 nurse-midwives to work in underserved areas around the country. The midwives often work at the margins, where more technological care is unavailable. Rather than remaking obstetric practice in its image, the place of midwifery in the medical hierarchy hasn't changed much since 1925.

Ways of Seeing

As my research progressed, I became annoying: At a party I caught myself giving unsolicited advice to a pregnant pediatrician. She responded with a story of her own about a Bay Area midwife who had opted to treat a Group B streptococcus infection by stuffing the woman's vagina with garlic rather than using antibiotics. The baby contracted the bacteria during birth and developed permanent brain damage.

Beth put voice to my worst fears after I complained to her about a case that seemed to me a particularly egregious example of obstetrical ignorance. Beth frowned at me quizzically and said, "There are some really great OBs you know."

I quailed at the implication: In questioning the solid ground of medical orthodoxy, I had begun to sound irrational.

"Oh my God," I said. "I'm not one of those people, am I?"

"Of course not," she laughed, circling her arm around my waist.

But I was. Despite myself, I'd grown shrill. I was especially miffed by the fact that when I criticized the maddeningly unscientific practices I observed in obstetrics, I was the one who seemed irrational. The incident that made me complain to Beth occurred after I visited, in the same day, two Southern California hospitals with widely divergent practices. In the morning, I went to a hospital where a public relations agent proudly explained that they strictly followed the Friedman Curve for every birth; and in the afternoon I talked to the medical director at the other hospital, who explained that the Friedman Curve had been obsolete for decades. You could tell that one of the hospitals was missing something, even if you didn't know what the curve was (a graph developed by Emanuel Friedman in 1955, charting the progress of labor, which obstetricians used to determine when to intervene). It irked me that some doctors still swore by routine fetal heart monitoring, the obligatory episiotomy, and the separation of mothers from babies, despite the fact that the evidence supporting these practices was about as good as the evidence for curing infections with garlic. I wanted to know why these practices persisted while others, supported by better evidence, like the provision of emotional support throughout labor, were ignored. Why had the Frontier Nursing Service been all but forgotten, and the all-fours maneuver overlooked?

There were thousands of small answers to these questions, all wriggling off in different directions, like so many sardines. The one answer, however, that captured the whole school of fish had to do with the way American obstetricians see—or, as it were, refrain from seeing. An article in *Medical Anthropology Quarterly* describing this problem pointed out that in three influential trials weighing the risks of Caesarean surgery against vaginal birth, none had counted the Caesarean cut itself as an injury, though each diligently documented the other lacerations. For the mother who has to cope with the pain, it's obvious that the Caesarean wound, though perhaps lifesaving, is an injury. The researchers, on the other hand, who relied on the Caesarean as an instrument of healing, were blind to this fact. Claire Wendland, the author of this article, was herself an obstetrician, and she admitted that this "breathtaking move in the selection of evidence" had also been invisible to her until a midwife had called it to her attention. Unless doctors can recognize that incentives and ideologies are guiding them toward some data and away from others, Wendland wrote, they will be doomed "to the blindness in which, for example, we cannot see the pelvis-wide cesarean wound."

Wendland's point was that the obstetrical idea of birth was obscuring important information about the way birth really worked. The spire of medical science may be a powerful place from which to view birth, but certain parapets block key portions of the panorama. Another revealing example, Wendland wrote, was the fact that researchers considered operative laceration to be a major injury, and infection a minor injury. An accidental laceration is "major," sometimes requiring additional surgery. But abdominal infections sometimes require a woman to keep the wound open for weeks, during which time she must rely on her family or a nursing home staff to change dressings. "Scarring can be major, and recovery painful and prolonged, if predictable and uneventful from a clinician's perspective," Wendland wrote. The reason operative injury was classified above an infection was that the injury is almost always the result of surgical error, while an infection is not. The real morbidity in this example was the injury to the doctor's honor. Though the science was correct in its limited fashion, the perspective of the surgeon was so dominant that the mother—along with her pain and emotions—had been blocked from view. It's impossible to see what lies behind these obstructions—or even to be aware that they exist—unless you are capable of stepping back to observe your own position. For doctors unaware of their own subjectivity, papers on the all-fours maneuver might as well have been written in Swahili.

Just about everyone is complicit in ceding priority to the surgeon's perspective. America honors those who take swift, independent action more than those who empower someone else's agency. Even grammar bows to surgical authority: Surgery is performed *on*, not *with* the patient, though, of course, the patient must participate by healing the wounds the surgeon makes.

The obstetrical perspective also creates the blind spot I'd noticed while talking to Michelle Niska: Because doctors are responsible for—and more likely to be sued by—patients who experience an injury in their care, they may see only short-term consequences. One of the researchers studying this blind spot was Aaron Caughey, chair of obstetrics at the Oregon Health and Science University. Caughey's research clearly showed that the increase in surgeries was hurting women. When we met in his small, jumbled office (he was still teaching at the University of California, San Francisco, at the time), he initially lounged with one leg over the arm of a chair, but he couldn't sit still for long, bouncing up to find a paper or sketch a graph on the whiteboard. He was handsome—smiling Asian eyes, square American jaw, rugby-player's frame.

Everyone agrees, he said, that complications from Caesareans (like Michelle Niska's placenta accreta) crop up years down the road—there the science is clear. But it's hard for patients to weigh those dangers: When faced with a decision that requires the assessment of small risks and future trade-offs, people make bad choices.

"This is what economists call discounting," Caughey said. "We're really bad at it when we start looking into the distant future. It's almost like a glitch in the human brain." He added, "I get really into this sort of thing." Caughey was so captivated by behavioral economics that he ended up getting a PhD in the field after he became a medical doctor. Consider, he continued, the risk of a Caesarean to a baby: Many obstetricians think that C-sections increase risk for mothers, but decrease risk for infants. That seems logical, he said.

"I do feel like if you just did a C-section on everybody you might decrease this kind of acute neonatal morbidity and mortality. We don't know, but you might. We know that some babies are injured during the labor process, so it makes sense. But, *but*, there's a really nice paper by," he snapped his fingers, pulling the name out of the air, "Gordon Smith, out of Cambridge, that shows that a prior Caesarean increases the risk for fetal demise in subsequent births. So, if everyone has a C-section on their first baby, then you might see another 1,000 dead babies overall."

The risk of stillbirth at term is low, on the order of 5 per 10,000 births. Gordon Smith, a British obstetrician, had found Caesareans increase that risk to 11 per 10,000 births, presumably because the uterine scar can interfere with the attachment of the placenta.

To provide a similar comparison for maternal health, Caughey had built a statistical model, bundling all the risks associated with Caesareans, then letting it run projections for the future. If C-sections continue their current upward trend until 2020, he said, every year they will kill 50 more women than would otherwise die in childbirth.

"If you can stop the rate where it is, you'll still get more deaths because the Caesareans we did yesterday are going to cause some more maternal deaths. And then what if we turned it around? What if we were able to get it to go back down to where it was in the mid-nineties? Which should be really easy. Then we can start *preventing* maternal deaths."

When we'd finished, Caughey walked me out, and we continued talking as we rode the elevator down through the hospital. Released from the formal structure of the interview, I found myself spilling the story of my birth and confiding that when it came to making decisions about my own family I felt stranded in the no-man's-land between the idea that birth was a pathology and the idea that birth was an ecstatic, danger-free, natural event. He offered his commiseration, then asked me where I lived and, when it turned out to be on the way to his house, gave me a ride home.

ICARUS AND DAEDALUS

I hadn't realized it until I started blabbing to Caughey, but there was clearly another reason—the real reason—that I was miffed about the state of obstetric science: Beth was becoming more and more obviously pregnant, and I hadn't hit on any practical way of applying the information I was learning. I'd succeeded in making myself anxious, and not much else. We hadn't managed to pick a place to give birth, so by default we'd started prenatal visits at St. Luke's, a hospital a few blocks from our home, and it was there we had our first ultrasound.

According to my sources, which admittedly consisted almost entirely of Hollywood dramas, the ultrasound is supposed to be a mini-religious experience in which that grainy sonogram becomes a window to the chain of life stretching forward and back for eternity; then—as the father—I'm struck at once by my cosmic insignificance and newly interconnected importance, and I weep. Instead, I squirmed and silently repeated, "Is this absolutely necessary?" over and over, fighting to keep the words from coming out of my mouth.

It never occurs to most sane people (or cinematic characters) to fear an ultrasound. I shouldn't have worried either: I probably knew more about the risks and benefits than the ultrasound tech who was pressing the wand to my wife's belly, and I had come to the conclusion that there was almost no cause for concern. Which meant that I was not only anxious, I was annoyed at myself for being anxious.

The thing is, though the risks of an ultrasound are just about nil, so are the benefits. Studies comparing populations that got ultrasound screening with those that didn't found that the screened group was no healthier in the long run. Still, it seems obvious that you'd want to get in there and take a look to see if everything is all right. The question becomes, however, what happens if everything isn't all right? The doctors didn't bring this up. They'd simply told us we should come in on such and such a date. It had been up to me to ask what would happen if the ultrasound found something, and to start the hard conversation about what we'd do if the baby was missing organs or likely to develop Down syndrome. We'd grappled with that terrible prospect and finally decided that we wanted to know, so that ultimately we'd have the option of (gulp) ending the pregnancy. I'd loved the obstetricians we'd met with, but it bothered me that no one had uttered the word "abortion," or explained the cascade of tests and worries if an ultrasound found something, or acknowledged that every screening adds moral complexity to medical decision making. Instead, the ultrasound was treated as an automatic, risk-free (not to mention cost-free) part of pregnancy. And this initial one-size-fits-all assumption made me feel just a tiny bit like a widget on a conveyor belt, about to be incorporated into the system.

I also had a distressingly nonrational fear that the ultrasound would damage my baby's brain. After more than 20 years of regular use, and several long-term studies, no one has linked any deficiency in children to scans. Yet, in medical science there is no such thing as a sure thing. When fetal mice are exposed to more than half an hour of ultrasound, some are born with slightly malformed brains. And the mainstream consensus holds that the scans should be employed as infrequently—and at as low a power—as possible. I don't like to think of myself as the kind of person who becomes petrified at the slightest suggestion of risk, but I still wanted the scan to be over quickly.

Our ultrasound technician, a short woman in her fifties with a strong Eastern-European accent, babbled on in a mixture of cooing and medical jargon as she probed Beth's belly and produced a grainy image on a screen.

"Baby is anterior, see?"

She rattled the keyboard and zoomed in.

"This is heart. Cute. I will show you face. There. Cute."

This seemed to go on for a long time. I wondered if her accent wasn't a bit sinister, and immediately afterward added xenophobia to my growing list of reasons to hate myself. Was she providing a lingering tour for our benefit? Maybe I should ask her to keep it short? After our conversation with the doctor, I had thought it would be quick: Find the baby, check the heartbeat, measure the thickness of its neck, go home. But the tech clearly had other work to do. She punched notes into the computer and printed a chain of photos for us. Then she zoomed in, so that we were looking directly into the top of the baby's head.

"This. Brain. Left hemisphere, right hemisphere. We are looking down into brain."

The two halves of my own brain were locked in combat. My urge to interject was tackled by my desire not to sound like a crazy hippie, and was held down by an impulse of empathy for this blameless woman, who undoubtedly was following practice guidelines established by higher-ups. And so, as frequently happens when I enter a hospital, I sat there feeling nervous, abashed, and totally out of control.

I didn't want an industrial birth, but I also didn't want to slide all the way over to the other extreme. I'd found a few birthing centers in San Francisco: Jade Lotus, Rites of Passage, Sage Femme. But I'd nixed each of these, perhaps unfairly, because of their names. I was looking for something more like No Nonsense Evidence-Based Midwifery. I wanted to live in a world where the model midwife-led birth—the model pioneered by the Frontier Nursing Service—was the norm, but where women and babies who needed it could get the miraculous, high-tech treatment that, say, interventional radiology and neonatal intensive care can offer. I wanted the hippie midwives and numbers-driven doctors to exist, not in oppositional worlds, but together in the same space. As Beth and I were asking around about our local hospitals, I found myself thinking of the story of Daedalus's escape from Crete: I wanted to employ technology's wings, without suffering from their overuse.

There are organizations that have managed to make use of technology without overusing it. In 1999, Utah-based Intermountain

Healthcare, employing the same concept of quality improvement that Toyota used to rationalize its factories, began to review its labor and delivery practice. The conclusion of Intermountain's industrial audit was counterintuitive: Instead of calling for more medical surveillance or more mechanized labor, it recommended more "low tech, high touch" births. The statistics had shown what the human eye couldn't see: that the industrial logic had pushed past the point of diminishing returns.

At first, a successful new technology offers a massive bang for the buck: When the Frontier Nursing Service built a hospital and started making C-sections available to the women around Hyden, Kentucky, each surgery was likely to save a life. But, like Icarus's flight, the returns derived from the increasing reliance on technology often form an inverted parabola. Increasing use of an innovation is intoxicatingly profitable at first. Then the cost grows steeper—to save one life you must perform 100 Caesareans instead of one, then 500, then 1,000. The curve flattens out, then tips down. The wax begins to melt, and more vigorous flapping only damages the wings. Increase the Caesarean rate again, and the lives you lose start to outnumber those you save. The logical thing to do in this type of situation is to slow down, which is exactly what Intermountain did.

The hospital system made a few small changes, focusing first on reducing the number of women they induced into labor for no medical reason. The effects were wholly positive. Mothers were able to go home sooner. Complications and admissions to the neonatal intensive care unit decreased. But there was also a hitch: Because the hospitals were performing fewer treatments and keeping women for less time, revenues fell. The reforms were saving patients around $1 million a year, money that came directly out of Intermountain's bottom line.

"Intermountain is nonprofit and that makes it easier for us to take such steps," the company representative told me. "But the incentive for most organizations is to provide more care, not less."

St. Luke's, despite my misgivings after the ultrasound, turned out to be close enough to what we were looking for. Like Intermountain, it was owned by a nonprofit, and discouraged early inductions. Like the Frontier Nursing Service, the deliveries there were attended by nurse-midwives. The building was old and scuffed, but the policies were up to date. The midwives at St. Luke's, however, weren't going to stay with Beth for her entire labor, let alone juggle for her. They suggested hiring a doula if we wanted a professional there to manage the emotional elements of birth. Doulas, however, aren't cheap—most of the people we looked up charged between $1,000 and $3,000, or around $500 if they had very little experience. We interviewed three, and each meeting was a bit like an awkward first date: It's hard to determine, in 45 minutes, if someone will have the calm-in-crisis compatibility to make a grueling experience less, rather than more, stressful. We couldn't agree on anyone we both liked and eventually decided that my presence would be enough. But, in the end, I think our decision not to hire a doula came down to money—if the hospital had offered to have someone there to provide support as part of the package, we would have accepted without a second thought.

A week and a half after the 40-week due date, the baby showed no signs of budging, and we reluctantly went to the hospital to start labor artificially. Neither of us liked the idea of an induction, but there is a slight statistical increase in the risk of stillbirth for babies after 42 weeks of gestation. The risks were small, an increase of one in a thousand, but the risks of C-sections were even smaller and I couldn't very well use the statistics to argue against the latter while ignoring the data for the former. All the same, it felt wrong.

The night before the induction, Beth started crying. She wasn't worried about being induced to labor, she explained, but being induced into

the role of a patient, of firing her body as head manager and giving control
to a team of medical professionals. I commiserated—it certainly didn't
seem like there was anything wrong with her body, I said.

"My body has been awesome," Beth said, laughing through her tears.
"My body rocks."

She had had a radiant pregnancy. There had been minimal morning
sickness, she'd slept easily, and felt none of the aches and pains that
other women complained of. The baby was squirming vigorously and
making inverse footprints on her distended belly. The notion that there
was anything wrong with the pregnancy, that it was becoming dangerous, ran counter to intuition. For the induction, she'd have to be hooked
up to an IV drip of Pitocin and wear fetal heart monitors throughout. I
didn't want medical technology to transform my vibrantly healthy wife
into an invalid.

The midwives patiently talked us through the decision. If we wanted
to wait (to avoid an induction) we'd have to go to a hospital with a high-
level neonatal intensive care unit. St. Luke's, following a protocol developed by Aaron Caughey and other researchers, did slow inductions over
24 hours or more, which, unlike standard inductions, did not increase the
chances of a Caesarean. After that conversation, Beth was ready to move
forward, as was I—or at least the part of me that could be convinced by
data. Still, I was disappointed. I liked the idea of this improbable process
happening magically rather than mechanically. I'd imagined Beth and me
staying in our homey little apartment until the last possible minute, putting on music, dancing between contractions, making something good for
dinner, then catching a cab to the hospital when active labor began.

Instead, we walked to the hospital, carrying a mason jar of flowers
to brighten the room. After a night of fitful sleep, the contractions
started in earnest. Beth handled them with aplomb, but as the hours
ticked by she grew tired and tense. She was struggling, fighting each
contraction, and it twisted my insides to watch her. My efforts to soothe
were inevitably misguided, and my suggestions began to sound like

hectoring, even to my own ears. When night fell again, Beth took some morphine to help her sleep and was able to catnap between contractions. I remained wide awake. Somewhere in the haze of night she got up to go to the bathroom, but the cords from the fetal heart monitors had twisted around her arms to tangle with the surgical tubing attached to the intravenous needle in her wrist. She pulled at this snarl foggily, then indicated she would make do, and lay back again.

In those hours I began to sympathize with American obstetricians: The desire to do something, to help, was overwhelming. I could understand, for the first time, how alien it felt to submit to the frustratingly obtuse impulses of a body in labor. My mind buzzed frantically, generating one plan for action after another. Obstetricians are trained to save lives, to take charge, to turn tragedy into triumph, to perform miracles— it only makes sense that they deploy these skills when confronted with what felt like a problem. It must take nerves of steel for a doctor to sit on her hands, to stay out of the miracle's way, so to speak. At the same time, I resented the fact that Beth was literally bound by medical technology, and that the nurses were monitoring the fetal heartbeat so carefully while paying scant attention to guiding her (or perhaps it was me that needed guidance) through the psychological labyrinth of birth. I rehashed our decisions: The induction had been a mistake, I decided. In fact, we should have opted for a homebirth—and really all my research had been for naught. It had become clear in that my mother's postpartum hemorrhage, the emergency that had launched my investigation, really hadn't been so terrifying: I'd learned along the way that that particular complication is routine enough so that any well-trained midwife can resolve it. Perhaps I should have forgone all the facts and data and had faith in nature. Or perhaps my mistakes had started even earlier, and I should have married a woman who trusted her body enough to give birth outside a hospital. It was at this point that I realized I was going a little bit insane. My nerves too jangled to remain still, I found a nurse and confessed my anxiety. She nodded knowingly.

"Whenever there's uncertainty or discomfort, people tend to want to fix it," she said. "We have absolutely no tools in this culture for simply accepting, but that's what you have to do sometimes."

Somehow, this made me feel better. I returned to Beth's side calmer, and this jittery peace lasted through the night. Early in the morning Beth started pushing. I stood at her side, humbled and quiet, distrustful of my brain's power to produce anything useful in its shocked state. Beth didn't need my help. She simply slipped into the urgent current of birth. But then the nurse began having trouble finding the baby's pulse, and when she did find it the midwife muttered that they needed "to get this baby out, now" and my raw nerves began convulsing once again. Then I could see the baby's hair, and then another push and a face and shoulders and tiny flailing hands burst free, and—as she began to caterwaul, and I held her shocking warmth, and she suckled at my finger—my fear began to expand into something new. It wasn't that the terrifying uncertainty ended with the birth of my daughter, I think, but merely that I was coming to terms with the fact that this child was, and would always be, an engine of uncertainty: No matter how strenuously we worked to protect her during labor or afterward, sooner or later she would be hurt, she would suffer, and eventually she would die. Somewhere along the line I'd allowed myself to stop grasping and to simply tumble with a little more grace. Later, as I walked home, squinting in the early morning light, punch-drunk with exhaustion, my heart fluttering, I realized the frantic buzz of planning and organization—and had started when I'd first called my parents to ask about my own birth, which had reached its fever pitch during my vigil the night before—was gone. In its place was a buoyancy in my chest. I recognized this sensation. I'd felt the same dizzying mix of fear, elation, and hope before: when walking home once on a similar sunny, sleep-deprived morning as a teenager; again in college; and once more the morning after I'd first kissed Beth. Improbably, the acceptance of the suffering and uncertainty that comes with new life felt exactly like falling in love.

CHAPTER TWO

MICROBIAL FRENEMIES

THE IMMUNE SYSTEM

The basic split between those who favor nature, and those who favor technology, widens into a chasm when it reaches the field of baby-ology because in many ways an infant is a representative of nature—an unsocialized wild creature. For the rationally ordered household of muted color scheme, decorated with objets d'art, the undomesticated baby is a clear and present danger. No other form of wilderness poses a greater threat to order: Termites may be gassed, mildew bleached, mice poisoned, roving packs of wolves held at bay with a shotgun, but there is no defense against a baby. Even in the innermost sanctums of civilization, where nature has been refined away to the periphery, a baby forces the most primitive aspects of existence—rugged nudity, and excretion at its most savage—into the focal point of life. It's no wonder then that much of child-rearing literature is concerned with taming the baby and molding it to civilized norms as quickly as possible.

My parents, on the other hand, were determined to mold themselves to my desires. According to their assessment, my lack of socialization gave me special authority. I was like Rousseau's noble savage: small, chubby, and incontinent, but noble nonetheless. I ate whenever I wanted to eat, and—because I seemed happier in my parents' presence—slept on a pad next to my parents' bed (they moved their mattress to the floor so that I'd be within reach). I might have slept in the same bed, but Dad was against diapers, and Mom was against excretory surprises. So Dad used cotton rags to build a sort of fecal containment lagoon around my posterior when I slept, and he mopped up before handing me over to Mom at midnight mealtimes. He did this because, in masseuse Ida Rolf's book, he'd seen pictures of children supposedly turned bowlegged and pigeon-toed by the constant pressure of diapers on their developing bones—nature's perfection warped by technology.

The prejudice against diapers put my parents in the decided minority, even among granola crunchers. Actually, as a rule of thumb, you could guess on my parents' child-rearing choices by determining what most people would do in any given situation and then searching out its opposite. Most parents, for instance, like to have their child's paperwork squared away from the very beginning, so that the child is correctly recognized by the state. My parents opted not to obtain a birth certificate. Instead of worrying that I would be ineligible for school, they worried that someday the government would call up my number for dark purposes. Because I had been born at home, far from medical charts, physician signatures, and all other instruments of the regime's panopticon—they decided that it would be better to keep me out of sight and off the books.

When it came to protecting me from wild microbes, my parents likewise took the weedy path less traveled. When friends would point out that I was about to put something vile in my mouth Dad would wave off their concerns by saying: "I don't believe in germ theory. Johnsons don't get sick." Thus liberated from fear of contagion, I was allowed to roam as a free-range baby. In my earliest memory I sit beneath a towering old jade plant in the sunshine while Mom works in the raised beds of the front garden. I was probably going on three at that point, a round-faced boy with corn-silk hair, a serious countenance, and an utter contempt for pants—a fashion crusade that my little brother and I maintained for years, prompting one neighbor to refer to us as "the half-naked brats." There were unseen threats there all around me: poisonous vegetation, dog's droppings, spiders casting strands, parasites that would like nothing better than to squirm from the soil toward the undercarriage of some half-naked brat. But while others might have preferred to keep their progeny safely in a nursery nest—or armor them with an artificial exoskeleton of washable, antibacterial materials virginally free from the taint of biological origin—my parents preferred the germs, and spiders, and worms.

The garden sheltered great roving herds of these lower life forms, and it was only a matter of time before I encountered them. My sister remembers rounding the corner of the house one morning to find me hunting escargot on the hoof. The snails were large and plentiful, and I sat in the dirt contemplatively gumming them to viscous mush. My sister, whose opinion of the innate nutritive value of gastropods evidently differed from mine, ran into the house, screaming with such brio that Mom thought I must have been hit by a car. Nonetheless, she determined that I had simply been following my instincts, and was therefore in the right.

It wouldn't be fair for me to imply that my parents were antiscientific. If anything they went through life with eyes more open than most, refusing easy acceptance of what others generally assumed to be obvious. They were intoxicated by the scientific promise that there is knowledge to be found in observation of nature. Dad worked to pass on this sense of scientific wonder by taking me to the museums around the San Francisco Bay Area. I remember watching, entranced, in the blue darkness of the Steinhart Aquarium as rays and tuna, each larger than I, scythed past in their endless circular pool. I like to think that in prompting these excursions I was a moderating influence on my father. There is some superficial evidence for this: Dad carted me around the halls of science in a backpack, and he eventually cut his long, countercultural hair to frustrate my practice of pulling on his mane while shouting, "Go!" But I also have reason to suspect that these hours of observation complicated my father's feelings about the relative dangers of nature and technology. There's an entry in his journal from the day he first took me to the zoo, which mentions that I reached and squirmed in my backpack perch toward the bears.

"How can I teach you that the world is made up of teddies, rattlesnakes, and rattlesnakes that look like teddies?" Dad wrote. "How will you learn to foray through it with both boundless trust and a ready stick?"

THE WILDERNESS OF THE BODY

When I reflected on the results of my parents' alternative child-rearing theories, it was fairly easy to identify a few that deserved the stick. Despite my freedom from diapers, my pelvis today is asymmetrical: If I were to stand on the face of a clock my left foot would point toward the twelve and my right toward the two. My gait is inferior to the 90 percent of professional athletes who spent years bound in those downy vices. And as a new father I quickly appreciated the immense utility of diapers. It boggles the mind to imagine the amount of labor, both physical and social, my parents endured to support my free and breezy lifestyle—especially given that I spent a significant portion of my infancy on a porch that jutted out over the play area of Mom's day care. There, I must have been the equivalent of a giant, truculent pigeon, strafing from above.

My parents determined for themselves that their efforts to hide me from the state's eye were misguided, realizing it would limit my career choices to hunter-gatherer, criminal, and guy-under-bridge. Nonetheless, their 3-year delay in obtaining my certificate of birth was sufficient to confound the bureaucratic apparatus in ways they did not anticipate. Years later—when I tried to renew my passport in a newly paranoid, post–September 11 country—I found myself in the unusual position of having to prove my own existence to State Department clerks who knew better than to trust the breathing, meaty evidence who appeared before them.

I could not dispense so quickly, however, with the notion that babies should be exposed to germs. The more deeply I studied this idea, the more intriguing it became. I seem to have survived my parents' enthusiasm for congress with the snails and spores without permanent injury. In fact there's growing evidence that this welcoming of wild microorganisms into my infancy may have made me healthier. In 1989 David Strachan proposed what he called the "hygiene hypothesis," suggesting that excessive cleanliness was causing problems, and that certain infections might actually prevent allergic disease.

Some of the most interesting evidence in this area comes from the study of milk. For years, scientists had assumed that the antibodies present in mother's milk—IgA-type antibodies—served to disable and remove bacteria from the gut. But when they tested this assumption they found precisely the reverse was true. Germs were better able to adhere to human cells in the presence of IgA. The antibodies formed a framework on which the bacteria were able to build a continuous layer of slime—a biofilm. Breast milk, it seems, encourages bacterial infection in the baby's digestive system—which suggests that certain infections are desirable.

Milk has long served as a currency of interspecies exchange. Besides linking humans to microbes, of course, it links us to domestic mammals. The ancestor of the cow was the aurochs, *Bos primigenius*, which stood as high as six feet tall at the shoulder with dramatic sweeping horns. These beasts, as we can see in the art they inspired, must have kindled a kind of religious reverence in our forebears.* And yet somehow, perhaps through the connecting power of milk, these fearful animals were able to enter into the domestic world of *Homo sapiens*. The first aurochs that consented to domestication was agreeing—in essence—to convert

---

* This wasn't prehistoric: The last of the aurochs was killed in Poland in 1627.

grasses into a form of nutrition that humans could use, in return for protection. The ability to conclude this deal with milk, rather than meat, was enormously profitable to both sides. Evidence of this profit can be seen—on the human side—in dominance of a mutation allowing adults to digest lactose, the main sugar in milk. This mutation occurred some 10,000 years ago somewhere in Europe and spread through the region's population in the evolutionary blink of an eye. What this means is that the ability to digest lactose so enhanced the likelihood of survival that 95 percent of Northern Europeans are descendants of those first lactose-tolerant pioneers. Like breast milk, aurochs milk would have brought bacteria with it: Food historians have shown that the drinking of fresh, uncultured milk was a rare anomaly, found only where dairy could be kept cold. And food historian Anne Mendelson has noted that the vast majority of traditional dairy dishes eaten around the world are neither cooked, nor fresh, but fermented into yogurt, cheese, or some form of soured milk.

Most milk sold in stores, of course, is pasteurized—which generally means it's heated to 161°F for 15 seconds—and therefore has much less bacteria and a longer shelf life. Before the science began implying that exchange between species—both large and small—might contribute to human health, a small group of people had begun promoting raw, bacteria-laden milk as a cure-all. When my family moved to Nevada City, we found ourselves in a haven for raw milk. By the time I began investigating my parents' child-rearing practices in the early millennium, the town was in the throes of raw-milk fever: You could buy it at health-food stores, and people in the know were getting it straight from small-time farmers who kept a few nanny goats in the clearings where the pines and manzanita opened into meadows. These people didn't have good explanations for how the milk cure was supposed to work, and some spouted pseudoscience. But not all of their claims curdled under the light of examination. Instead they matured into something richly ambiguous, like a ripe cheese that evokes both desire and disgust.

Pasteurization—pioneered by Louis Pasteur in 1862—neutralizes potentially deadly bacteria like *Campylobacter jejuni*, *Listeria monocytogenes*, *Escherichia coli*, and salmonella. (Pasteur, it should be said, discovered pasteurization in the same, limited sense that Columbus discovered America: The Chinese had been pasteurizing alcoholic products since at least the 12th century.) Between 1919, when only a third of the milk in Massachusetts was pasteurized, and 1939, when almost all of it was, the number of milk-borne disease outbreaks fell by nearly 90 percent. Pasteurization is just a small piece of a security cordon assembled (with increasing desperation) over the last century: Water treatment plants, flush toilets, antibiotic soap, and Purell hand sanitizer all stand guard at the perimeter between nature and civilization. And though our zeal for sanitation has now entered its baroque stage, it's also clear that the initial efforts account for the most of the modern declines in sickness and increase in longevity.

Despite the risks, people have fought to drink raw milk ever since mandatory pasteurization became the norm. When the skirmishes broke into the news in the 1980s the *Los Angeles Times* called them "A Holy War Over Health." This was more than overheated newspaper rhetoric. The people wrapped up in this struggle, on both sides, were—and are—religious in their convictions. There's more than milk at stake here: In every heretical uprising the fulcrum of struggle—whether it's milk processing (heated versus raw), or prayer (standing versus kneeling)—is generally a stand-in for a larger system of beliefs. In this case, the revolutionary idea—the thing that gives the raw-milk heresy its vigor, that enrages public health officials, and that threatens the modern dairy industry—is the notion that the father of pasteurization was wrong.

Pasteur argued that germs cause the body to become diseased, while his friend and fellow scientist, Claude Bernard, argued the causal relationship was reversed: Bernard thought germs can only multiply when the *milieu intérieur*—the terrain of the body—is compromised. There's a story that Pasteur recanted the germ theory of disease on his deathbed, murmuring, "Bernard was right, the germ is nothing, the milieu is every-thing." The evidence that Pasteur actually said this is sketchy at best, but that hasn't stopped raw milk advocates from repeating it in their attempts to transform Bernard into their champion. Clearly the germ is *not* noth-ing, there are too many examples of diseases killing perfectly healthy people (think of the introduction of smallpox to the Americas) to take my father's quip about not believing in germ theory seriously. If you trace your genealogy back to your great-grandfather you will almost certainly find that he had a sibling who died of an infectious disease. Back then, germs were the enemy that crept in and carried off children in the night. But now that Pasteur's theory has helped us defeat smallpox, and measles, and scarlet fever, it's also clear that many of the remaining diseases (dia-betes, for instance, and heart disease) are caused by milieu—that is, our environment, both interior and exterior. Our germ-fighting medical sys-tem is poorly equipped to deal with these illnesses.

In the last few decades more and more people in developed countries have begun showing up at their doctors' offices with autoimmune disor-ders. In 30 years the rates of multiple sclerosis, type 1 diabetes, and Crohn's disease have doubled, tripled, even increased by an order of magnitude in some places. Between my first birthday and my freshman year of high school, U.S. childhood asthma rates increased 75 percent. Almost half the people in First World nations now suffer from a combi-nation of allergies, asthma, and eczema. In less developed nations, these afflictions are almost completely unknown. All of these illnesses are related to overactive immune systems. Perhaps, scientists have hypoth-esized, we've become too clean—without foes to attack, our inner defenses may be turning on our own cells. Because milk is such an effec-tive agent for interspecies exchange, it has become a symbol in this larger struggle over microbial security. The very thing that makes raw milk dangerous, its dirtiness, may be precisely what makes people healthier.

Selling raw milk for human consumption is illegal in Canada and in about half of the U.S. states. Nonetheless, thousands of raw milk enthusi-asts have set up black-market networks and every so often the authorities crack down. In October 2006 police destroyed a truckload of Richard Hebron's dairy products in Michigan. The month before, the Ohio Department of Agriculture had shut down Carol Schmitmeyer's dairy. In March 2006 cops moved in on Gary Oaks as he unloaded milk in the parking lot of St. Bernard's Church in Cincinnati. When bewildered Cincinnati residents gathered around, an official told them to step away from "the white liquid substance." In September of 2005, an undercover agent asked Amish dairyman Arlie Stutzman for a jug of milk. Stutzman refused payment, but when the agent offered to leave a donation, the farmer said he could give whatever he thought was fair. Busted.

Though my father had grown up drinking raw milk from the family livestock, I had not. It had simply never occurred to either my Mom or Dad. Nonetheless, I saw that the conflict over milk could serve as a referendum on my parents' theory that it was healthiest to befriend the wildlife in and around the body.

There were no easy answers. The facts presented by both sides were in a terrible muddle—a highway pileup created by the high-speed convergence of mysticism, dogma, and bureaucratic shallow thinking. Then, in the midst of my inquiries, the holy wars broke out again, this time in Canada. There, a farmer named Michael Schmidt had begun holding a series of dramatic protests after health authorities had seized his cheese-making equipment and cited him for selling raw milk. I called Schmidt, hoping to learn his story and to judge the threat on his farm for myself. If I could sort out this mess, I'd also be sorting out the welter of logic and rebellious illogic that made my father claim he didn't believe in germ theory.

The Making of a Milk Martyr

The agents had arrived before dawn and concealed their vehicles behind the trees on the road that runs past Michael Schmidt's farm in Durham, Ontario. There, they waited for the dairyman to make his move. It wasn't the first time they'd watched in the dark for Schmidt to pull up the driveway in his old blue bus. A team from the Ministry of Natural Resources had been following Schmidt for months, shadowing him on his weekly runs to Toronto. Two undercover agents had even worked their way into his inner circle and obtained samples of the product he was moving. The lab tests had been damning: It was milk, and it was raw. Now the time had come to take him down.

Schmidt had risen at 4 a.m. He milked the cows, loaded his wares, and fired up the bus. But before he reached the end of the driveway, two cars pulled out in front of him. A policeman stepped into the road and raised his hand. Another banged on the door. Others were close behind. Eventually 24 officers from five different agencies would search the farm. Many carried guns.

"The farm basically flooded—from everywhere came these people," said Schmidt in his lilting German accent. "It looked like the Russian army coming. All these men with earflap hats."

Schmidt showed the inspectors around, alternately annoyed and amused by the absurdity of the situation. And it was, by any rational standard, absurd. If, in the course of the undercover investigation, the government had done some surveillance on its own files, it would have found that Schmidt had written letters to regulators 12 years earlier, informing them that he was producing raw milk. But this information would have undermined the theatrical rules of a bust, which demand the exposure of something hidden.

Schmidt responded to the raid with theatrical élan. He immediately went on a hunger strike. For a month he consumed nothing but a glass of milk a day. He milked a cow on the lawn outside Ontario's provincial parliament. This was a fight, he said, for which he was prepared to lose his farm. He was ready to go to jail. Instead of being dispirited by the raid, he leapt into the fray with a kind of pent-up exuberance. Which made sense: He'd been waiting to be busted for more than a decade. For all that time, he told me, he'd carried a camera with him so he could take pictures when the authorities came to shut him down.

"You carried a camera for 11 years?" I asked.

"Twelve years," he said. "And I upgraded, you know, first it was still, then video, then digital came along."

Schmidt doesn't have the demeanor of a rabble rouser. In fact, his temperament is not unlike the cows he tends. A large man, he speaks softly, moves deliberately, and reacts placidly to provocation. He has thin blond hair, light blue eyes, and lightly pockmarked cheeks. Shaking his hand is difficult because it's so wide. His uniform consists of black jeans, a white shirt, and a black vest. In the summer he wears a broad-brimmed straw hat. In the winter he wears a black newsboy cap.

When Schmidt emigrated from Germany in 1983, he wanted to start a farm that would operate in a manner fundamentally different from that of the average industrial dairy. Instead of confining his cows to a manure-filled lot, he would give them capacious pastures. Instead of feeding them corn and silage, he'd give them grass. And instead of managing hundreds of anonymous animals to maximize the return on his investment, he would care for about 50 cows and maximize health and ecological harmony. He believed that if he kept the grasses and cows and pigs and all the components of the farm's ecosystem healthy, the bacterial ecosystem in the milk would also be healthy, and, by extension, his customers, too. Schmidt bought 600 acres 3 hours northwest of Toronto. There he built up a herd of Canadiennes, handsome brown-and-black animals with black tipped horns. Most cattle farmers burn off the horn buds—a guarantee against being gored—but Schmidt believed it was better to leave things in their natural state whenever possible. The dangers posed by the horns (like the dangers of drinking unpasteurized milk) weighed less heavily on him than the risk of disrupting some unknown element of nature's design.

He hadn't come to these ideas on his own. In Germany, Schmidt had studied both agriculture and classical music. He had seriously considered pursuing a career as a musician. (In Canada he periodically assembles chamber ensembles in his hayloft and conducts, his ham-hock hands floating with improbable grace.) But ultimately Schmidt was won over by the ideas of the mystic agronomist (and Waldorf school creator) Rudolf Steiner. Steiner, the founder of biodynamic farming, saw the farm itself as something of a musical opus—a decades-long process of cajoling the assembly of species on a plot of land into tune.

The farm flourished under Schmidt's hand. He set up a cow-share system where, instead of buying raw dairy, customers leased a cow and paid a "boarding fee" when they picked up their milk. The animals were still Schmidt's property for all practical purposes, but the scheme made defiance of the law less flagrant and health officials could look the other way. Then, in 1994, the Canadian Broadcasting Company made a documentary about Schmidt and his unpasteurized product. A few months later he was charged with endangering the public health.

It was during this time, when papers were quoting Schmidt on the superiority of raw milk, that strange things started happening around the farm. Vandals broke into his barn. Schmidt found two cows lying dead in the yard, apparently poisoned. Then an unmarked van ran his cousin's car off the road. Men leapt from the van, forced him inside, and held him for 2 hours. Schmidt hadn't been prepared for the struggle to take this turn. He sent his cousin back to Germany, agreed to plead guilty in court, and sold all but 100 acres of his farm to pay the government fines and cover lost income.

Schmidt is a man of Teutonic certainty, but as he walked into the field soon after he'd sold the land, he was filled with doubt. The morning sun had turned the sky red and mist hung around the legs of the cattle. While he twitched his stick at the bull, Xamos, to turn him away from the cows, Schmidt wondered whether his dream of farming with nature was just a miscalculated attempt to resurrect the past. If he started selling his milk at industrial prices, it would erode his meticulous style of farming. He would lose the direct connection to his customers. He'd have to push his cows to produce more milk. He'd be compelled to adopt the newest feed management strategies, herd-health supplements, and modern equipment.

Schmidt didn't see Xamos coming, just felt the explosion as the bull struck him. Even as he hit the ground the bull was on him, bellowing. The animal stabbed with one horn, then the other, tearing up the earth and ripping off Schmidt's clothes. One horn sank into Schmidt's gut, another ripped into his chest and shoulder, grazing a lung. Only when Schmidt's wife, Dorothea—flanked by snarling dogs—charged into the field, did Xamos retreat. Another man might have taken this attack as a clear sign, a demonstration of the folly of seeking harmony with nature. But as Schmidt lay there, stunned to be alive, and bleeding into the grass, he felt only humility. "Nature is dangerous, yes," he would tell me later. "But I can't control it, and I can't escape from it. I can only learn the best way to live with it."

By the time Schmidt could walk again, almost 6 weeks later, he'd decided to continue farming on his own terms. He announced his intentions publicly, but the regulators must have felt that they'd made their point. For years he continued farming quietly, as an outlaw, until the morning that government agents descended on his dairy. After the hunger strike and the other public acts of protest, Schmidt settled in for the long fight. He hired a top defense lawyer in hopes of overturning Ontario's raw-milk ban.

OUTBREAK

In the 35 years that Schmidt has operated his dairy no one has ever reported falling sick after drinking his milk. Yet suspected raw-milk illnesses do crop up. According to the U.S. Centers for Disease Control and Prevention, the United States averages a hundred cases of raw-dairy food poisoning each year out of approximately 9 million people drinking the stuff (CDC surveys showed that 3 percent of people said they'd had raw milk in the prior week). In the fall of 2006, for instance, California officials announced that raw milk tainted with E. coli was linked to a rash of illnesses. It is legal to sell unpasteurized dairy in California, and the suspected milk came from Organic Pastures, in Fresno, the largest of several farms that supply the state's health-food stores. Even as the state veterinarian ordered store managers to destroy the milk they had in stock, Organic Pastures customers rushed in to buy whatever they could. They brushed off concerns, saying that every time outbreaks occur, health workers have leapt to conclusions based less on evidence than on the assumption that unpasteurized milk is poisonous. When inspectors failed to find any of the E. coli that had allegedly sickened the children in Organic Pastures milk, it seemed these people might actually be right. When I called up Mark McAfee, the owner of Organic Pastures, he said the inspectors seemed to be acting less out of malicious intent than blundering Keystone Kops incompetence. They'd been out to his farm, clad in white biohazard suits, swabbing his cows' rectums, and had walked away with nothing to show for it, he said. "They haven't found a single pathogen anywhere on my farm," he told me, "let alone the milk."

By this point I'd heard some version of this same story from several dairymen who had been the subject of busts. The news-clippings I collected from around the country portrayed the people buying raw milk as poor benighted citizens who deserved what was coming to them for defying the orthodoxy. In these stories, reporters obediently repeated the official findings without hinting at the possibility of uncertainty. But tracing an illness to its source is sometimes more art than science, requiring investigators to filter out scores of possible leads (spinach, hamburger, eggs, sushi?) while zeroing in on the most likely sources. It was entirely possible that in some cases health officials had been blinded by their exasperation with the raw-milkers in their backyard. So I resolved to make an example of this case, to investigate it myself, and retrace the regulators' steps with an open mind.

When I got Tony Martin on the phone, he told me he had stood in the aisle of Sprouts, a heath-food store in Temecula, California, agonizing over the Organic Pastures bottle with the leering cartoon cow on the front. He knew that milk was pasteurized for a reason, but he'd also heard that raw milk might help his son's allergies. "There was a lot of picking it up off the shelf and putting it back," he said. In the end, he brought it home. Chris, his 7-year-old son, drank the Organic Pastures milk 3 days in a row over Labor Day weekend. On Tuesday he woke up pale and lethargic. On Thursday he had diarrhea and then started vomiting. Friday morning he had blood in his feces and the Martins rushed to the hospital. Shortly afterward, several other children checked into Southern California hospitals. They all had drunk Organic Pastures raw dairy products, and they all were infected with a virulent strain of *E. coli* known as O157:H7. Some of the children recovered rapidly, but two, Chris Martin and Lauren Herzog, were transferred from one hospital to another as they got progressively worse. The O157:H7 strain releases a jet of toxins when it comes into contact with antibiotics—which puts doctors in the position of making a terrible choice: Either wait for nature to take its course, or intervene and risk further damage. Chris's doctors administered antibiotics, Lauren's did not, yet both children's kidneys shut down. While Chris was on dialysis, his body became so swollen that his father said he wouldn't have recognized him if he passed him on the street. Chris was in the hospital 55 days. Lauren went home after a month but then relapsed and had to return. Both children eventually recovered, but may have suffered permanent kidney damage.

For Tony Martin and Lauren's mom, Melissa Herzog, it seemed like an open and shut case: They blamed the milk. But for Lauren's father, Pete Herzog, several facts stood in the way of that assessment. His girlfriend, Chelsea Higholt, had made the raw-milk smoothie Lauren had drunk. The odd thing was that Higholt and her two sons, aged three and five, drank the same smoothie from the same blender, and they didn't even get the runs. Higholt had turned the remains of her milk over to health workers (they dug the bottle out of the trash) and tests for *E. coli* came back negative. In San Diego, Kari Way, who had given raw colostrum (another Organic Pastures Dairy product) to an 8-year-old neighbor, was also scratching her head. The boy had had a 6-ounce glass and got sick (a minor bout of food poisoning). Her son had finished the rest of the carton and he was fine. Then health workers identified two more boys sick from E. coli with a DNA fingerprint that they said matched Lauren's bacteria. Both these boys happened to be from Nevada City. One had drunk the milk. The other said he hadn't.

These facts didn't seem to add up. McAfee, when he called to check on my progress, offered an alternative explanation: What if this talk of a DNA fingerprint (the patterns from "pulsed-field gel electrophoresis" to be precise) was just so much scientific mumbo jumbo designed to humble the laity and convince doubters they were out of their depth? After an outbreak, blamed on Clearview Dairy in Wisconsin, officials had claimed to have found the same DNA fingerprint in the milk and in the stool of the sick. But, the dairyman told me, when protesters called their bluff, the health department inspectors had refused to show the matching patterns. In any given week there are probably hundreds of people who show up to the hospital complaining of food poisoning, McAfee said. What if—on this particular week—a few of those people happened to mention that they'd had some of his milk?

It seemed implausible that the state would frame McAfee, but it was possible that health workers might have stopped asking the parents what the sick kids had eaten when they heard patients say the word "raw milk." Government employees might have been led astray by their assumptions. When state veterinarians came to search Organic Pastures for E. coli, they'd been surprised to see that the manure they pulled from the cows' rectums was watery, and that it contained fewer bacteria then usual. Patrick Kennelly, chief of the food safety section at the health department, confronted McAfee with these facts in an email, writing, "Not only is this unnatural, but it is consistent with the type of reactions an animal might have after being treated with high doses of antibiotics. . . . Why were your cows in this condition, Mark?"

McAfee does not use antibiotics on his organic farm. The state tests every shipment of his milk for antibiotic residue and has never found any. Allan Nation, a grazing expert, offered another explanation: The cows had been eating grass. Grass-fed cows carry a lower number of pathogens, he said. And for a few days in the spring and fall, when the weather changes and new grass sprouts, the cows "tend to squirt," as he put it. But grass feeding has become so rare that, to Kennelly and the veterinarians, it seemed unnatural. The norms of industrial dairying are so deeply ingrained that perhaps a regulator could jump to the conclusion that all milk is deadly until pasteurized.

PASTEURIZATION'S CONSEQUENCES

Around the time that Chicago passed the first pasteurization law in the United States, in 1908, many of the dairies that supplied cities had themselves become urban. They were crowded, grassless, and filthy. Unscrupulous proprietors added chalk and plaster of paris to extend the milk. Consumptive workers coughed into their pails, spreading tuberculosis; children contracted diseases like scarlet fever from dairy. Pasteurization was an easy solution. But pasteurization also gave farmers license to be dirty. They knew that if fecal bacteria got in the milk, the heating process would eventually take care of it. No one noticed, or paid less, when they drank the corpses of a few thousand pathogens. As a result, farmers who emphasized animal health and cleanliness were at a disadvantage to those who simply pushed for more milk. After a century of this, modern dairies, to put it bluntly, are drenched in excrement. Most have a viscous lagoon full of it. Cows lie in it. Wastewater is recycled to flush out the concrete alleys where the cows eat. Farmers do carefully dip cows' teats in iodine before milking, and strictly comply to the standards. But the standards mandate only that the number of germs swimming around their bulk tanks be below 100,000 per milliliter.

When I was working as a newspaper reporter in Cassia County, Idaho, a local dairyman, Brent Stoker, had wanted to raise thousands of calves on his farm and sell them to dairies as replacements for their worn-out cows. Stoker's neighbors, incensed by the idea of all that manure near their houses, stopped the project. Stoker wasn't an especially dirty farmer—on the contrary, dairy associations showed off his farm on tours. But to survive, dairies need to produce a lot of milk, which means producing a lot of feces. As I was tracking down sick kids and badgering the California Department of Health Services about my public records requests, I came across Stoker's number in my Rolodex and, on a whim, called to talk dairy and catch up. He was in the middle of another fight with the neighbors. This time he wanted to build a large organic dairy.

"I never took you for the organic type," I said.

"Pay me enough and I am," he said.

Organic, however, doesn't necessarily mean grass-fed. Stoker's cows can make a prodigious 80 pounds of milk per day. That's mostly because they are fed like Olympic athletes. They eat a carefully formulated mix of roughage and high-energy grains. "If you were to try to pasture them you'd lose production, down to about 40 pounds," Stoker said. "Of course, the cow would last a lot longer." Cows are designed to eat grass, not grain. Most mammals can't digest the cellulose in grass, but ruminants are able to access the solar energy locked in a green pasture by enlisting the aid of microbes. These bacteria are cellulose specialists that turn grass into the nutrient-building blocks that cud-chewing animals need. In return, cows provide a place for bacteria to live—the rumen—and a steady supply of roughage. This relationship shifts when a cow begins eating grain. The cellulose specialists lose their place to bacteria better suited to the new food supply, but not necessarily so well suited to the cow. The new bacteria give off acids, which in extreme conditions can send the animal into shock. Pushing too much high-energy feed through a cow can twist its stomach around other organs. Such a kink will back up the digestive flow to a trickle. The cow will stop eating, and sometimes you can see the knotted guts bulging under the skin. Other disorders also result from the combination of high-energy feeds and high production: abscessed liver, ulcerated rumen, rotten hooves, inflammation of the udders. It is in a farmer's interest to keep a cow healthy—but not too healthy: If a dairyman decreased the grain portion of a cow's rations to a level that eliminated health problems, he'd lose money. A balance must be struck between health and yield. It's not surprising then, that farmers end up sending grain-fed cows to the hamburger plant at a much younger age than their pastured counterparts. On average, dairy farmers slaughter a third of their herds each year. As Brent Stoker put it, "We're mining the cow."

There are other bacterial opportunists that move in when a cow's gastric environment is disturbed by a change in diet. Tired cows, crowded together, with ubiquitous feces, create conditions that are ideal for the transmission of pathogens. In a 2002 survey of American farms, the U.S. Department of Agriculture found dangerous strains of campylobacter in 98 percent of all dairies, and *E. coli* O157:H7 on more than half of farms with 500 or more cows. When the milk at these large farms was tested, the researchers discovered pathogens in a lot of bulk tanks. If that milk were shipped to supermarkets without pasteurization, many people would get sick.

I asked Stoker if he'd ever considered returning to a smaller, healthier style of farming.

"If I had a way to provide for my six kids and have a comparable standard of living I would do that," Stoker said. "The way it is now, I'm more stressed, the animals are more stressed, our crops are probably more stressed. There's nothing I would like more than to go back to that, but I'm too stupid to figure out how."

The problem isn't Stoker's intelligence, it's what he calls the "dishonesty of the market," the advertisers' promise that consumers can have the healthiest possible food from happy animals in idyllic settings, at low prices. It's a lie, but a convenient lie for consumers—one that most of us accept. As a result, people are periodically outraged at the realities of modern agriculture but never stop demanding cheaper food. Stoker doesn't mind playing the hand he's dealt. He's good at producing cheap food. But, he warned, "Cheap food makes for expensive healthcare."

Canadian Pastoral

After months of delays, the California Department of Health Services responded to my public records request. But instead of sending the DNA fingerprint patterns or redacted case histories, the state sent a packet of press releases—all easily available from its Web site. When I pointed out that there were several items missing, there was more foot-dragging. It might take another month, a representative told me. In the meantime, I visited Michael Schmidt in Ontario. I arrived at the farm in late February, an unflattering time of year. The trees were skeletal, and the wind bitterly cold. There was snow, melting into the dirt by day and freezing again each night. All the same, the farm was beautiful—the very image of pastoral harmony that I'd fallen in love with as a child while reading Laura Ingalls Wilder. Despite the snow and all the creatures moving about (cows, chickens, pigs, geese, and farmhands), the land was not muddy—instead the water filtered into a little creek, while trees held down the earth with their roots. The barn was a solid timber-framed structure—the beams linked with mortise-and-tenon joinery. Inside the hayloft Schmidt had hung great bunches of fragrant branches: During the summers, he'd noticed the cows browsing from the trees and bushes on the periphery of his field, so he took note of the species they chose and began cutting green boughs to put up for the winter. Just as my parents had faith that their baby was wiser than they, Schmidt trusted the cows to optimize their own nutrition. Through trial and error, he found a method like this one, of adding ground branches to the feed, that kept the herd healthy through the grassless season.

I'd risen with Schmidt at 4 a.m. to see how he milked the cows. Though it was below freezing outside, the barn was warm with animal heat. It smelled sweetly of alfalfa and excrement—not the overwhelming scent of a feedlot, but something like a pet store. The cows were waiting inside. Each had a white placard above her head bearing her name: "Anna," "Sofia," "Cantate," "Laura." They were glossy-coated and solid on their feet. Schmidt told me he hadn't had to have someone trim their hooves in 15 years. These matters were of more than aesthetic importance, he told me as he touched each animal and looked it over. The appearance of his farm was a by-product of his focus on the long view (the barn was built to last centuries for example), and the attention he paid to every part of the land: He believed that thriving trees, a thriving compost pile, and thriving frogs in the stream were just as crucial to his success as a thriving herd of cows. When organisms live together long enough, they adapt to each other. Tinker gently with a farm for a few decades, he said, and the resident species—the cows, plants, microbes, and humans—will sort out their differences.

Schmidt's logic ignores feed efficiency—the primary metric that determines the success of modern animal farms. His cows make only around 25 pounds of milk a day, one-third of the production of Brent Stoker's animals. But Schmidt can take advantage of some other efficiencies: He doesn't have to pay much for veterinary service. He doesn't have to slap haunches to roust exhausted animals from their beds. The life expectancy of a conventional dairy cow is a little under 5 years. Schmidt pointed out cows that were 8, 9, 12 years old—and healthy.

When Schmidt finished milking the first eight cows they trooped across the barn and out onto the snow. As he milked the next set, his apprentices brought hay and fresh bedding to the other animals in the barn: a sow and her litter of piglets, a cow with two calves, and a mountain-like bull named Leif. One of the apprentices picked up a piglet and stroked its crinkled snout. It promptly nibbled her finger. When the milking was finished and all the cows were outside, the farmhands shoveled out the manure, spread fresh beds of straw in the stalls, and piled mounds of hay in front.

"Watch this," Schmidt said, and pulled open the door. The cows came jogging in, each one peeling out of line to take her place under her own placard. They buried their heads in the hay. Schmidt beamed.

After the chores and breakfast, Schmidt loaded up his blue bus for his weekly delivery to town. We drove to a parking lot near the Toronto Waldorf school where Schmidt parked, started the charcoal stove in the back of the bus, and set up his counter at the rear. He'd installed wooden shelves where the seats had been, and they were packed with food. Nearest to the curved roof sat loaf after loaf of dense German bread. Below, along the windows, stood tubs of yogurt, jars of applesauce and honey, baskets full of cookies, rectangular pans of cakes, muffins, and brownies. Crates of eggs jammed up against baskets full of vegetables from a root cellar. As for the milk, Schmidt took the money and gave a sign to his assistant handling the product across the street, so as to avoid a direct exchange that regulators could classify as a sale.

I had thought that the customers would be young white hippies toting yoga mats: the next generation of people who, like my parents, had lost faith in the conventional wisdom on health. Instead, many were immigrants—a young father speaking to his daughter in Russian, an elderly German couple, a man from Romania, a man from the Middle East, and another from China. They'd grown up drinking raw milk and were convinced it made them healthier. When I told one man I had come to see if the province would enforce its cease-and-desist order, he inhaled sharply.

"Screw them! Screw them! It's a great thing Michael's doing." Then he laughed apologetically at his own outburst. "I'm Greek you know, I always want to kill people."

Then there was the lunatic fringe. Three different men cornered me at various points during the day to explain their raw-milk theories—at length. These monologues all followed the same pattern: They generally started with a story of raw milk curing cancer, veered (with disorienting lack of connection) into government conspiracy, then segued into a scattering of semi-scientific terms (enzymes, probiotics, long-chain fatty acids) cobbled together with the same level of reasoning someone might use to prove that pirates are superior to ninjas. If I hadn't figured out how to escape by that point, the lecture could leap to new topics—alien abduction or the benefits of enemas. I had expected this (one in ten conversations that occur in Nevada City seem to follow these parameters). What surprised me was how normal the rest of the customers appeared. They chatted warmly with one another as they waited in line, down the aisle of the bus.

"I suggested he have two cashiers," said a bearded man with an English accent, "but he won't do that on principle. He wants to see everyone himself."

"Hello, Paul," Schmidt greeted him. "Do you know this music?" He pointed toward the speakers in the rounded roof, transfixed for a moment. "Beethoven. *Fidelio*."

The next woman complained as Schmidt totaled her bill. "Don't forget to write in that Michael is the only businessman who will undercharge his customers," she told me.

"But she doesn't say that she always brings me soup," Schmidt replied, lifting the lid of the paper carton she had given him.

The winter sun fell and Schmidt lit tea candles on the emptied top shelves. It was cozy in there, in the near dark, with the stove radiating heat. A group of about six lingered, chatting. "This is my bodyguard," Schmidt said, winking at the man I'd been talking to, an Italian restaurateur. "He'll make sure they don't arrest me."

"Nah, there's no way they'll arrest him," the restaurateur said. "We're talking bureaucrats here. They'll just wait till the trial. Forget about it." He was a big guy who, though he carried his bulk comfortably, was certainly overweight, and it struck me that the 150 or so other people who'd come on the bus that day were all slim, despite their affection for fatty whole milk. The people who buy from Michael Schmidt believe Stoker's axiom about cheap food and expensive healthcare. They just reverse it. They pay a premium for food they believe will keep them healthy. So far, it's worked out. The microbes that end up in Schmidt's milk have been benign, perhaps even beneficial.

MACHINING GERMS

It turns out that black-market buyers aren't the only ones who think germ-infested milk is healthy. The yogurt giant Dannon has invested heavily in understanding the benefits of bacteria, and the company now sells dairy products stocked with healthy, or "probiotic," microbes: DanActive, "an ally for your body's defenses," which comes in a small vial-shaped bottle and provides a dose of an organism owned in full by Dannon called *L. casei immunitas;* Danimals, a more playfully packaged bacteria-infused drink, designed to appeal to children; and Activia, a yogurt containing a bacterium the company has named *Bifidus regularis,* which "is scientifically proven to help with slow intestinal transit"—though after a false advertising lawsuit Dannon toned it down, claiming only that it "helps regulate your digestive system."

Both Michael Schmidt and Dannon are working to reintroduce bacteria into the modern diet, but their methods are fundamentally different. Schmidt labors under a principle of persuasion. He tries to make his milk healthy by coaxing species to support each other. In contrast, Dannon's is a philosophy of mastery. Milk comes to Dannon's Fort Worth, Texas, processing plant in tanker trucks, arriving wild, full of its own diverse bacteria. It leaves the factory civilized and safe, in 4-ounce cups. It takes a lot of machinery to accomplish this domestication: miles of stainless-steel pipes, huge fermentation vats, and dozens of white-frocked, hairnet-wearing workers. Although the process is intricate, the concept is simple: Kill the bacteria, then add bacteria.

All yogurt is made when benign bacteria are mixed into milk. But Dannon also adds its special probiotic bacteria, and when I visited the plant this is what I asked to see. The Dannon employees looked at each other nervously. The bacterial strains are proprietary, and so are the methods surrounding their use. My public relations minder, Michael Neuwirth, exchanged a few words with J. Erskin, the friendly plant manager, then nodded.

"We can see the place where it's done," Neuwirth said.

The room was lined with freezers. Neuwirth opened one and frost billowed out. Inside were stacks of what looked like one-quart milk cartons, encrusted with ice. "This is for Activia, right?" Neuwirth asked.

"Yep," Erskin said. "Regularis."

The Dannon workers explained that each carton contained thousands of tiny pellets consisting of frozen milk and microbes. You can buy cartons of common bacteria for about $30 apiece. No one would tell me the price of these proprietary strains, but Erskin said, "When our little friends die, it's very costly."

Workers wait for the moment when the milk reaches the ideal temperature, then add the bacteria. *Lactobacillus bulgaricus* comes first, converting sugar to acid, preparing the chemistry for *Streptococcus thermophilus*. I would guess that the one or two proprietary strains are added at the end. Every bacterial move is choreographed.

Although the Dannon people wouldn't show me this process, they indulged my desire to wander through the bottling room next door where the same precise control was on display—though mechanical, rather than biological in form. Pipes ran overhead, carrying yogurt down to machines, which to my delight looked like something an ingenious 12-year-old might assemble if given a few hundred gears of different types and sizes. The most beautiful machine was the one filling little bottles with DanActive. The bottles came across the ceiling, propelled by compressed air along a metal track, halting, then scooting forward, like a line of penguins. An auger caught the bottles in its threads, sending them spinning in an endless path around gears and carousels. The machine cleansed the bottles with acid, punched out their caps, zapped them with bacteria-killing UV light, filled, sealed, boxed, and stacked them—*in scherzo*—at 460 containers per minute.

Erskin stood beside me, watching through the Plexiglas window.

"It's like a ballet," he said.

Michael Schmidt would love this machine, I thought, though it represents the polar opposite of what he does. Dannon and Schmidt are so similar in their goals that the differences in method stand out in sharp contrast. Both are fanatically attentive to detail, but completely different details: Dannon knows the habits of *L. casei*. Schmidt knows each of his cows as an individual. Dannon relies on clinical trials that have shown some slight health advantages in eating the few germs they happen to own. Schmidt relies on tradition and the unscientific observation that the dozens (hundreds?) of open-source species in his milk seem to make his customers healthier. Dannon's method is atomistic: It tries to separate the milk ecosystem into discrete parts so that it can identify, bottle, and sell the element that allegedly makes people healthier. Schmidt's method is holistic: He thinks of health as the result of an indivisible system. Dannon executes its anonymous bacterium with totalitarian efficiency. Schmidt is a microbial free-marketeer, creating an environment—in his fields, his feed, and his animals—that provides incentives to beneficial bacteria while discouraging pathogens. Schmidt is a big-picture guy: He doesn't care to know the exact biochemical composition of his milk, but he believes it's crucially important that he keep his creeks clean, his cows content, and his farm a place that makes you feel good when you are there. Dannon focuses intently on the small picture: It cordons off a tiny piece of the world—a cup of yogurt—and controls its content absolutely. It doesn't have to worry about the exterior environment—festering lagoons and antibiotic-resistant bacteria—as long as it can safely conduct these little pods of nutrition through a background swarming with unknown germs. And while the Dannon factory is beautiful and fascinating in its way, you wouldn't want to live there. Dannon favors the germ, Schmidt the milieu. Find a way to get the best of both and you'd have utopia.

FARMACOLOGY

The food industry's search for microbes that make people healthier—though it has generated more advertising gimmicks than effective formulas—has lent some credibility to the claims of bacterial necessity made by Schmidt and other raw-milk advocates. Albeit cautiously, scientists have also begun weighing in on whether such technologies as pasteurization have purged necessary microbes from our food. When I started talking to milk experts, several told me I needed to speak to Bruce German.

A food chemist at University of California, Davis, German has the rare ability to work on the tiniest details of science while still thinking creatively about how they might fit into grand overarching theories. When I first visited, German was hosting a reception in honor of Agilent, a company that had helped develop a machine able to analyze oligosaccharides, sugar polymers found in breast milk. As we walked across campus German brought me up to speed. He's a slight, energetic man with smile lines creased into his face, and his excitement for his work is infectious.

Oligosaccharides make up a big portion of human milk: They are about as abundant as proteins. The curious thing about them, German said, is that they are indigestible: Humans can't break them down. Which means, he said, one hand chopping the air, that they must be there to feed the bacteria living inside a baby's gut, rather than the baby. Only a few microbes eat this sugar, and one in particular thrived on it, *Bifidobacterium infantis.*

"So we asked, what is this bacteria?" German said. "Is it similar to others? And no, it turns out its genome is very different than others. There's a lot of evidence that we coevolved with this organism—it's really specialized to us and vice versa. Mothers basically recruit another life form to babysit their infants. So then—we can look at it and look at all the strange things it does and begin to ask, why does it do that—why do we need that?"

The more scientists looked at milk, the more compounds they found that were there not to feed the baby, but to create a specific microbial ecosystem: Lactoferrin, lysozyme, and lactoperoxidase all selectively weed out some microbes, while allowing others to prosper. Consider, German said, what it means that milk has evolved such a sophisticated chemical system catering to our microbial friends. It suggests, he said excitedly, that bacteria are tremendously important to us. So important that researchers studying the microbes living inside us say it's unclear where our human bodily functions leave off and their functions begin. In 2006 a team of scientists surveying human gut bacteria published a paper in the journal *Science,* writing, "Humans are superorganisms, whose metabolism represents an amalgamation of microbial and human attributes."

This world belongs to microbes. They were mastering the subtleties of evolution three billion years before the first multicellular animals appeared. They continue to evolve and adapt in a tiny fraction of the time it takes us to reproduce once. They flourish beneath ice caps, in boiling acid, and in toxic waste. We exist only because some of them find us useful. Ninety percent of the cells in our bodies belong to bacteria. The entirety of human evolution has taken place in an environment saturated with microbes, and humans are so firmly adapted to the routine of sheltering allies and rebuffing enemies, that the removal of either can destabilize our defense systems. Some of our immune cells—like those in the delightfully named "crypts of Lieberkühn" of our guts—simply won't develop if bacteria aren't present. A healthy immune system is buzzing with what scientists call "crosstalk," signaling back and forth between human and bacterial cells. It's a wonderfully complex contraption with cascading chain reactions and baroque feedback loops of checks and balances. It regulates itself and reacts to stimulus with something resembling consciousness. Take the microbes away and you sweep out dozens of pulleys and levers from the machine.

For the last century, however, we've done our best to do just that. People began to realize that there might be unforeseen consequences to walling ourselves off from germs after Erika von Mutius, a pediatrician in West Germany, published a set of counterintuitive findings. In the late 1980s von Mutius was studying the prevalence of asthma in Munich and wanted to contrast the rates with those in East Germany, where diesel fumes left a film of grime on every surface, and chemical effluence had turned the river Saale violet. When the Berlin Wall fell, she expanded her study, hoping to definitively tie asthma to pollution. Instead, she found that rates were lower in the dirtier east. After combing through the data, von Mutius found that kids with fewer microbial infections were more likely to have asthma.

As the years have passed, many studies have helped refine this proposal. It wasn't simply a matter of genetics: The children of Pakistanis who had emigrated to England were dramatically more likely to develop type 1 diabetes than their families in the home country. Moreover, scientists also found that hygiene itself wasn't a problem. People who never used antibacterial soap were just as likely to have asthma as those who bleached their walls. It seemed that what really mattered was the company of old friends—microbial companions that had accompanied us so unswervingly through our evolutionary journey that human genetics could have incorporated them, building immunological bulwarks on their backs. For this reason, Graham Rook, a medical microbiologist at University College London, has suggested the term *hygiene hypothesis* should be replaced with a new one: the *old-friends hypothesis*.

It appears that at least some of these old friends are associated with cows. In a 2006 study of thousands of children living on farms in Shropshire, England, David P. Strachan and another scientist, Michael Perkin, found that raw-milk drinkers were unlikely to have eczema or to react to allergens in skin-prick tests. "The protective effect of unpasteurized milk consumption was remarkably robust," Strachan and Perkin wrote. Then, in May of 2007, a group of scientists who surveyed almost 15,000 children around Europe reproduced this finding. Either there's something about industrial milk that's harmful, Perkin wrote, or there's something in raw milk that's beneficial.

None of these findings, however, mean that raw milk is safe. Every single study contains the caveat that raw milk often harbors pathogens. From an epidemiological perspective, Bruce German told me, advising the public to start drinking raw milk at this point "would be crazy."

Pasteurization is a sure thing—as far as it goes. But it is usually applied in service of the misguided Cartesian notion that health is achieved by separating people from the primordial muck. We are great walking bags of primordial muck: We contain multitudes. We are super-organisms. We cannot transcend our evolutionary alliances and feuds to live like gods in sterile stainless-steel spheres. Our attempts to make this separation have led to ever weaker immune systems inside the wall, and ever more fearsome germs on the outside.

THE ORGANIC PASTURES PARADOX

When I arrived home from Canada, there was an email waiting for me from the California Department of Health Services with images of the DNA fingerprints attached. I forwarded them on to a microbiologist friend and printed them out—two columns striped with fuzzy black and white lines. Presumably they represented the *E. coli* cultured from two different sick kids. If they matched it would mean that the *E. coli* came from the same immediate family. That, in turn, would mean that these patients were probably poisoned by the same food. If they didn't match, it would exonerate McAfee.

I'd also received the paperwork documenting the search for the source of the outbreak. Just as McAfee had claimed, the inspectors hadn't found any *E. coli* in his milk. But that didn't put him in the clear. In fact, now that I understood the ecology of milk a little better, I was slightly more inclined to believe the official story. I called McAfee, packed up these documents, and started the drive to Organic Pastures.

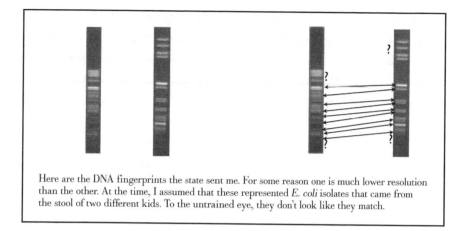

Here are the DNA fingerprints the state sent me. For some reason one is much lower resolution than the other. At the time, I assumed that these represented *E. coli* isolates that came from the stool of two different kids. To the untrained eye, they don't look like they match.

The events in California don't seem to add up when viewed through a lens focused on the germ: If it were simply a matter of a few bacteria breaking through the wall of sanitation, everyone who was exposed should have gotten sick. Inspectors should have found the germs in Chelsea Higholt's milk bottle, if not on the farm. But when I looked at those facts again, while focusing on the milieu, they made more sense: The selective bactericides we have in breast milk are also in cow's milk, as are friendly bacteria that thrive on lactic acid and crowd out other germs. Pathogens placed in raw milk tend to dwindle rather than multiply. The *E. coli* might have died off before regulators had a chance to test it, but not before people drank it. And when people did drink it, those whose internal ecosystems had not adapted to milk microbes would have been the only ones to get sick. The kids who became ill were trying raw milk for the first time. Back in 1987 the *Journal of the American Medical Association* published a study showing that several people living on dairy farms had developed an immunity to *Campylobacter jejuni*, and scientists were telling me, off the record, that they were sure the same thing was happening with *E. coli* O157:H7.

The Department of Food and Agriculture had also sent documents. They had found O157:H7 in the manure of McAfee's cows, though the *E. coli* was different from the strain that had infected the kids, and none of the cows that tested positive came from the milking herd. Nonetheless, it made me wonder about McAfee, who had claimed so loudly that—because they ate grass—his cows were pathogen free. Conventional wisdom held that O157:H7 lived only in grain-fed cows. The pathogen appeared in the early 1980s, so it made sense that it might have evolved acid resistance (needed to survive passage through human stomachs) in the newly acidic environments that formed in the rumens of grain-fed cattle. But reports were piling up, showing that O157:H7 could also be found in grass-fed cows. Maybe, scientists speculated, acid-resistant O157:H7 had been around forever, but we only started noticing this bug when we lost our immunity to it. In Brazil, scientists found that women have antibodies protecting them against O157:H7, and that they pass these antibodies to their children through the placenta and their breast milk. This suggests that Brazilians are so frequently exposed to similar germs that no one ever gets sick (there have been very few O157:H7 hospitalizations in Brazil). Perhaps the crucial change that had led to the O157:H7 outbreaks had occurred not in the cattle, but in us.

McAfee's dairy is made up of a few prefabricated double-wide trailers on 450 acres of pasture extending out into the hazy flatness of California's Central Valley. When I arrived, some 200 cows were chewing their cud on a shadeless plot of closely cropped grass. McAfee greeted me with a vice-like handshake and a mile-a-minute barker's banter that only slowed slightly when I interrupted. Years earlier he had been producing ultra-pasteurized organic milk for the giant conglomerate Dean Foods, when Janet Sheen (wife of the actor Martin) stopped in and asked if he'd sell her some raw milk. She paid him $300. That got him thinking, and with financing from his brother, who had made a fortune in biofuels, McAfee started Organic Pastures.

We walked through the fields. One cow sprawled out with her udders facing the sun. "Now you'd swear that cow was dead," McAfee said. "In a stall they can't relax like that." He whistled and the cow stood and ambled off. Other cows walked over to us. Because McAfee's cows live longer, he explained, he has to deal with a higher incidence of hoof problems—he pointed to one limping around and explained, "hairy heel wart." McAfee culls about 14 percent of his herd each year, far below the industry's average but higher than Schmidt's. When you have fewer than 50 cows, like Schmidt, it's different, McAfee said. "You have time to give each one a foot rub every night. You can do yoga with them every morning."

We sat down in McAfee's office and I showed him the DNA fingerprints. He scoffed. "These aren't the same. I've seen PGFE patterns before, they should line right up." He had a point. The two patterns didn't look the same to my untrained eye. But I pressed ahead—I explained that I'd tracked down and talked to all but one family of the sick kids (the 18-year-old in Nevada City had declined to speak with me—he'd claimed he hadn't drunk the milk, but it was in his fridge). I laid out the hypothesis I'd heard from scientists, that our lack of antibodies are as much to blame for *E. coli* outbreaks as food producers.

"It's an old story," McAfee said. "You see it again and again in the lists of outbreaks: City kids went to the country, drank raw milk and got sick, country kids didn't get sick."

But, I pointed out, that explanation still implicated Organic Pastures. McAfee shook his head. "Look, if I made four kids sick, I made four kids sick. But show me the 50,000 kids I made healthy. We don't guarantee zero risk. We aren't worried about the point-zero-zero-one percent chance that someone will get sick; we are worried about the 99 percent assurance that you are going to get sick if you eat a totally sterile, anonymous, homogenous diet."

The problem for McAfee is that the .001 percent is shocking and visible. A dying child will make people change their behavior. The problems caused by a lack of bacteria are much more subtle. They come on slowly. It's difficult to link cause and effect. Businesses that contribute to chronic disease often flourish. Businesses that contribute to acute disease get shut down. But McAfee was incensed now, and there was no stopping him.

"If my milk gets someone sick I deserve some blame, but not all of it. People have to take responsibility for maintaining their own immune systems. And we have to look at an environmental level, too. Where did these germs come from? *E. coli* O157:H7 evolved in grain-fed cattle. It's amazing to me that we've sat by as factory farmers feed more than half the antibiotics in the country to animals and breed these antibiotic-resistant bacteria. At the same time the food corporations are destroying our immune systems. I believe our forefathers would have grabbed their muskets and gone and shot someone over this."

Instead of grabbing his musket McAfee is expanding. He's shipping milk all over the world: to Australia, and to Kuala Lumpur, ostensibly as pet food. I asked what he'd do when regulators come again to shut that down.

"I have an email list of 8,000, ready for immediate revolutionary action," he said.

A Final Reckoning

On the drive home my microbiologist friend called me from his lab at University of California, Berkeley. Though one hundred times more cautiously, he told me essentially the same thing that McAfee had: The DNA fingerprints didn't match.

"There should be more patterns," he said. "Usually we do this twice, with two different enzymes to chop up the DNA, and make sure that pattern matches on both. So there should be two patterns for each sample. And didn't you say there were six kids?"

"Yeah, but they only found the bacteria in five of them."

"So they should have ten patterns," he said. "It doesn't make any sense that they sent you two."

When I inquired, a government technician explained that he'd sent me the same fingerprint, obtained using two different enzymes.

"So it's two pictures of the same bacteria?" I asked.

"Yeah, basically," he said.

"Okay. But aren't there five different samples of bacteria, from five different patients?"

"Yeah."

"So . . . Did you make patterns for those?"

"Yes."

"Okay. Can I see them?"

"Well, they all look the same. They are identical."

I reminded him that I'd asked for all the patterns, identical or not, and, amazingly, they appeared in my inbox the next day. There were ten patterns, two for each child, just as my friend had explained. And I could see for myself that they matched. The health department hadn't been deliberately evasive, it had just been so senselessly unresponsive that it had seemed deliberate. Now that I held the evidence in my hands I was convinced that each of these five children scattered around the state had been sickened by the same thing. It could have been something besides milk, another food that they'd all eaten, but the chances were vanishingly low.

McAfee was unfazed by this evidence. "Until you show me a matching pattern from my milk, it's meaningless," he said. But I had no doubt

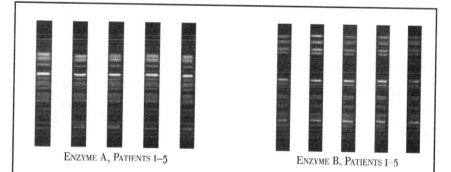

Enzyme A, Patients 1–5   Enzyme B, Patients 1–5

What we are looking at here is *E. coli* O157:H7 DNA taken from five sick children around the state, prepared using two different enzymes. *E. coli* mutates swiftly enough that O157:H7 that is not from the same recent lineage does not line up neatly. However, it's clear that these match perfectly.

that if such a finding ever appeared, he'd find it meaningless as well. Earlier McAfee had referred me to the case of Clearview Dairy, in Wisconsin, where health officials had supposedly never provided evidence of microbes from the outbreak existing in the milk. When I'd asked, the Wisconsin health department had sent me the DNA fingerprints without delay. The three samples of bacterial DNA isolated from the milk clearly matched samples found in 14 different sick people. When I asked McAfee and a representative from Clearview Dairy about this, they moved back the goalposts, saying that they'd need to see the same results from a non-government lab.

I'd been reading about earlier milk wars, and I'd started to notice a pattern in these denials. Back in the 1970s and 1980s, the owners of Alta Dena dairy—a raw-milk giant serving some 200,000 people in California alone—had shown that no evidence could convince them they were doing harm. At the time Alta Dena was the largest dairy in the United States. Its crowded feedlots contained 18,000 cows in eastern Los Angeles County. Between 1977 and 1983, private and government laboratories had found salmonella in Alta Dena milk 191 times. The dairy was responsible for at least 22 deaths, according to a paper in the *British Medical Journal*. And a 1986 study, which Alta Dena itself had financed, concluded that the milk was hazardous to people with compromised immune systems.

The owners of the dairy reacted to each of these findings by going on the offensive. They even condemned a study that they had paid for, and blamed a profit-driven cabal of politicians and competitors for their troubles. Alta Dena founder Harold Stueve told that paper, "What we are talking about is a conspiracy of state bureaucrats who want to put us out of business."

But there were also bureaucrats supporting the dairy. Alta Dena was the sole farm regulated by Los Angeles County Milk Commission, a body that—in turn—was funded entirely by the dairy. Alta Dena also had the chairman of the commission—pediatrician Paul Fleiss (the father of Hollywood madam Heidi Fleiss)—on payroll as a consultant.

And in Sacramento, the dairy had Republican politicians fighting mightily—and for years successfully—for its interests, while groups like Ralph Nader's Public Citizen Health Resource Group pushed for regulation. In 1992, after a California judge required the dairy to place a warning on its raw milk, the Stueve family sold Alta Dena.

We shouldn't forget, despite the conclusive momentum of this saga, that drinking unpasteurized milk is probably safer than driving for most people. Just about everyone injured by milk has been a child or an immune-compromised adult. Amid the furor over Alta Dena, Joshua Fierer, an infectious disease specialist campaigning for tighter controls over the sale of raw milk, noted that the risk for otherwise healthy adults was "almost nil." This story, and that of Organic Pastures, are parables on the folly of combining all-natural ideology with industrial economics. It's perilous to thrust wild bacteria into the invisible (and blind) hand of the market. When the microbial cultures in milk are mediated by the attention of human culture the moral may be different. The fact that Schmidt insists on seeing each of his customers in person means that he can tell them each about the health of the cows and offer a few words of advice to someone trying raw dairy for the first time (explaining, for instance, how they might culture the milk with heifer microbes that would competitively inhibit pathogens during the initial adjustment period). A smaller farmer in McAfee's position might have made adjustments that week before the outbreak, when summer temperatures peaked and dairy cows up and down the Central Valley died in the heat. A smaller farmer might have shifted the milk of heat-stressed cows to butter (bacteria can't survive in concentrated fat) or kefir (where the addition of other microbes can crowd out pathogens).

After the outbreak in 2006, Organic Pastures products were recalled on suspicion of containing *Listeria monocytogenes* or various species of campylobacter twice in 2007, and once in 2008. Between August and October of 2011, five more children were sickened by *E. coli* O157:H7 with matching DNA. Three were hospitalized. All had been exposed to

Organic Pastures dairy. Once again, investigators did not find the germ in the milk, though they did find it in McAfee's calving pen.

For many unpasteurized promoters, there is almost no evidence that would convince them that raw dairy, even coming from an industrial giant like Alta Dena, could be harmful. This devotion stems from personal experience: They notice that, while their friends complain about ragweed, they can enjoy the spring air; they notice that while everyone else sacrifices a day of vacation, they never have traveler's diarrhea; most of all, they notice that years of drinking raw milk has never made them sick—despite the assurances from the medical mainstream that it will. After you've lost faith in the orthodoxy, it's unlikely that you will be convinced by further appeals to science.

The other side can be just as obstinate. It's hard to unemotionally weigh the trade-offs after hearing about kids like Lauren Herzog and Chris Martin, but for most people the risk of food poisoning from unpasteurized milk is something like the risk of food poisoning from sushi. The current one-size-fits-all regulatory approach to milk does not differentiate between industrial and pastoral, between immune-suppressed infants and strapping adults.

For a while after my journey into the heart of the raw milk heresy, I saw no reason to drink it myself. It was only when Beth became pregnant that I remembered the studies of the women in Brazil, which showed that it was possible to pass immunity to E. coli strains to an infant. Perhaps if we found some good raw milk, we might be able to pass on some forms of immunity, or allergy resistance, inoculating our child against Claritin, inhalers, and insulin pumps. I found a farmer I trusted, and Beth only started drinking the milk a bit at a time, after the baby was born. The idea was that organisms in the milk might trigger maternal antibodies in Beth that she might pass on through her breast milk—while she served as a buffer between milk and baby to screen out anything nasty. I felt a little sheepish about the way this line of logic piled speculative theory upon preliminary science.

But there was also a larger reason I felt drawn to this milk: The farm where my milk came from was a pretty place—though not quite as idyllic as Schmidt's—and I thought of it every time I lifted a glass to my lips. If I had the power to reshape the world for my children, I'd want it to look more like Schmidt's farm and less like an industrial feedlot. Of course the world was moving in the opposite direction. Dairies were growing bigger and germier, and consumers were demanding lower prices even as they demanded more protection for increasingly delicate immune systems. Pasteurization seemed to be the solution. We now pasteurize almonds, and there is a movement afoot to irradiate vegetables and sterilize eggs. The time may come when we react with disgust when anyone mentions that they ate raw spinach. As we wall ourselves off from nature's perils we also cut ourselves off from beauty and deliciousness.

When I asked Bruce German how large of a role bacteria play in our lives, he mentioned the finding that people with certain strains of gut bacteria were more likely to be obese. "We'd only thought of infection as something that affects the immune system," he said. "Well, now we know that an infection could affect the *metabolic* system. Well what else? Sensation? The olfactory system? Jesus, maybe the bacteria are affecting sense of smell. I think we ought to go sequence Mozart's gut bacteria—see where that great music was really coming from."

It's only a matter of time, he said, before someone shows that bacteria can make us crave certain types of food. Perhaps they even can affect our emotions. All this is playful conjecture, but nonetheless, it's food for thought. What else disappears if we succeed in closing ourselves off from interspecies exchange with our old friends?

A pasteurized world makes it easier for business to operate efficiently: It allows for economics of scale and greater centralization, fewer redundancies. Michael Schmidt is one of those redundancies, but I like having him around nonetheless, as a diplomat of human microbial peace. If there's any hope to build a cooperative relationship with our germs, rather than a purely combative one, we'll need stewards like him.

A judge eventually decided in Schmidt's favor—a surprising ruling given that he fired his lawyer and began representing himself. The state then appealed to a higher court, which reversed the ruling. Schmidt went on hunger strike yet again. The struggle will no doubt continue, in court and out, for years to come. Someday science may provide us with more guidance, but until then we will have to conduct our own calculations to determine how to mend relations with our microbial frenemies. When I sat at Schmidt's breakfast table on the first day of my visit, I picked up my glass of milk and turned it slowly. I understood the possible consequences of my choice. All the competing science was there, along with the stories of epic sickness I'd heard. And I have to confess, the thought crossed my mind that if I got sick it would make a hell of a story. But when it comes down to it, here's why I drank the raw milk. The sun had just come up, and we'd already finished three hours of work in the barn. I was filled with a righteous hunger. The table was laden with eggs from the chickens, salami from the pigs, jarred fruit, steaming porridge, cheese, and yogurt. Although dairy isn't for everyone, I come from the people of the udder: For all recorded history, and perhaps back to the time of the aurochs, my forefathers had sat down to meals like this after the morning milking. I am the first generation that did not grow up with livestock to milk. It felt unambiguously right. This, of course, is the very definition of prejudice: the conflation of what feels right with what is scientifically correct. But as it was, I could only hope that that sense of natural goodness was rooted in something more than nostalgia. Perhaps it was. The way a place feels won't tell you anything about whether bacteria have breached the wall of sanitation, but it does reveal something about the overall health of an ecosystem. Humans have relied on such impressions to assess the quality of their food for most of history. Without scientific certainty, I'd have to rely on my gut. I drained my cup and poured thick clabbered milk and apple syrup on my porridge. If any bacteria disagreed with my body, the conflict was too small to detect.

CHAPTER THREE

FIXING DINNER

NUTRITION

U p until the age of 5—until, specifically, the day my family attended a potluck at a lake near our house—I'd had unswerving faith in my parents. I needed it, because without faith it would have been hard to remain cheerful on my family's diet. I knew, from the moment I was old enough to begin exercising some judgment over what I put in my mouth, that we took food more seriously than most families take religion. We believed wholeheartedly in the old aphorism "you are what you eat," which—if you think about it—puts an awful lot of pressure on the eater. It encumbers every forkload with the possibility of salvation or damnation. By choosing the right things to put in your body, you could transform your life, become smarter, happier, and more energetic—or by making the wrong choices you could grow ugly and sick. Though this idea seems self-evident (if you eat fat you get fat, right?), I've come to feel that it is fundamentally misleading. In some ways, dietary health is more akin to Calvinist predestination. At the age of 5, however, I'm sure I must have been thinking about all this on a far more basic level. I was only dimly conscious that the question of what to eat was fraught with terrible consequence. Doubt had yet to stir.

For most Americans there was nothing particularly traumatic about the summer of 1983, but for me it was The Time of Unceasing Zucchini. Though Mom had refused the beasty-yeasties, she was forever discovering new dietary theories, each of which would inevitably lead to a purging of the pantry. During these food-culture revolutions, undesirable elements disappeared from our already meager menu until we were surviving like Chinese peasants. My little brother, Tim, had grown—from a jolly baby built like the Michelin Man—into a sort of nutritional censor, unwittingly redacting foods from the table. When he'd first gotten a rash, which wrapped around his torso, my parents had taken him to a naturopath, who suggested that they take the family back in time to a Paleolithic diet. This meant no foods of the agricultural revolution—no wheat and no dairy (which in the United States eliminates pretty much everything). Meat and tubers were permitted, along with vegetables (which meant cartloads of zucchini), and brown rice, though I doubt cavemen often snacked on grasses, let alone made them a staple. There was always brown rice, typically with a few overcooked kernels of tooth-chipping toughness. Tim and I scooped at it dutifully: It was this or the snails. And even the snails were hard to come by in our new home in the California foothills.

Dad said that he'd known it was time to leave Berkeley when my little brother and I started falling on the sidewalks and scuffing our knees. It was yet more proof that civilization could damage young bodies—children weren't meant to learn to walk on concrete, he said. That was when we moved to Nevada City, the little town tucked in a hollow between the knees of the Sierra Nevada Mountains. The sun-fired rocky soil of our new home was hardly more forgiving than concrete, and in the next few years I'd mix my blood with that red earth—with pine sap, river water, and blackberry juice. But these were injuries my parents believed in.

The problem with moving back to the land is that, paradoxically, you leave behind many of the people who like the idea of moving back to the land. Romantic liberals, despite their passion for nature, tend to stay in coastal cities, relinquishing the country to conservatives and acolytes of technological progress. My parents had picked our little town because other San Francisco Bay Area hippies had already colonized it. There were yoga classes, communes out among the hills, and a spiritual community that ran a health-food store in town. Still, the majority of our new neighbors were Republican businessmen who went to church regularly, red-necked loggers who converted dead cars into chicken coops, or grizzled marijuana-growing libertarians who panned for gold in the rivers. The children of these types would be my classmates when I started school, and would show me alternatives to my sackcloth-and-squash existence.

At the age of 5, however, I still assumed my diet was perfectly normal. I lacked means of comparison. We had no TV and, though we read, families tend to dissolve into the background in children's literature. Kids cannot become heroes if they have parents standing in their way, so authors kill off the adults or separate them from their children or simply dress them in dark floral prints and force them to sit in matching armchairs. It wasn't that I had no contact with the outside world; Mom had moved her day-care center up to Nevada City, and every day adults delivered a throng of companions to the door. But the parents who felt comfortable leaving their children at my house had to have been at least somewhat like-minded. And while there, the other kids ate like me. I was unaware of the Oreo cookie. I had not deduced the theoretical possibility of Cadbury Cream Eggs. So when we went to that potluck at the lake just outside of town, I was innocent to any possibility that others might see my way of life as strange.

It was a warm summer evening. Casseroles and salads were spread out along the tables by the water. Adults batted at mosquitoes. Children ran up and down the lakeshore in screaming waves. On a platform floating offshore kids were playing king of the hill, forming alliances, betraying them, and splashing into the water in glorious defeat. Lake Vera is a miserable little algae farm, but at that moment it looked marvelous. I stripped down and crashed though the shallows, my pudgy little brother hard at my heels. When I reached the platform, I flopped aboard then pivoted, bracing myself to take all comers. But instead of rushing me, everyone stopped. It was only then that I noticed that—in stark contrast to me—every other child was wearing a swimsuit.

We've all experienced what I experienced next. You show up at school or work, and realize two things in quick succession—first, that you are naked, and second, that this is highly, excruciatingly, inappropriate. The difference is that most people undergo this trial while dreaming. I got to live the dream. Nakedness had always been a part of our household. My father believed it was better to sleep naked, for one thing.

"Gives your balls a chance to breathe," he'd say.

When sleeping naked I certainly wasn't going to bother with clothes each time I went to the bathroom, got a glass of water or even, for that matter, when I wandered into the dining room for breakfast.

My brother was struggling onto the floating platform when a treble voice shrieked, "They're naked! They're naked!" It was like a scene from a 1950s monster movie in which a horrific crustacean-thing emerges from the depths and wanders into a beach party. Kids swarmed off the other side of the raft and porpoised for shore. I tried to savor having this little kingdom to myself. I pushed my brother off the platform a few times, but there was no satisfaction in it. We swam in and put on our clothes. I felt an odd sort of shyness the rest of the evening and stayed close behind my mother's legs. It was the first time I understood that the things I had assumed to be self-evident might be wrong.

My parents believed that they were raising a new generation of Tarzan-like power children by liberating us from the nudity taboo and enforcing strict food rules. But I began to suspect that their techniques were actually doing us harm. Within a few years I had been over to the houses of some of my classmates and had seen the refrigerators full of Capri Suns (those silver space-pods of juice), wondrous Creamsicles, and spreadable cheese food. Instead of being dens of disease, these houses had luminous white carpets, pastel furniture, and glass coffee tables where magazines spread in perfect fans. These families went to church on Sundays, the girls took ballet, the boys were star pitchers, and nobody was *ever* naked. It seemed unlikely, on my diet of nudity and zucchini, that I would ever become an athlete, or a cheerleader's boyfriend, or any sort of clean, crew-cut hero, like the boys in the books.

At school, my family's strangeness became inescapable, and nowhere were these quirks more starkly pronounced than in the lunchroom. The trip to the cafeteria was like my own personal version of Marco Polo's first expedition to China: It was an encounter with a more advanced civilization, which each day reasserted its dominance through the display of the Lunchable triumphs it had crafted. My friends would lift the tamper-evident plastic veils to reveal their meals, pristine at the moment of consumption. Surely there could be no greater contrast to these wonders of food technology than my bruised and oozing pear, my sweaty Lebanon baloney, my translucent lettuce, my grubby stub of carrot.

Some basic inclination had reversed itself since my toddlerhood. Instead of yearning for crawly things to put in my mouth, I'd developed a fear of foods that were too close to their living, organic state. I was especially apprehensive of the pilafs and stir-fries my parents sometimes made, with their multitudinous unidentifiable components. When I bit into something anonymous, large, and crunchy, I would stiffen as a vivid image of the giant rhinoceros beetle I had seen in *National Geographic* magazine lit up in a high-traffic sector of my brain. Naturally, I was envious of my friends' lunches. The refined perfection of prepackaged food spoke to me. "Observe, my healthful symmetry," it said. "These perfect disks of meat, these Doric breadsticks. I was shaped not by fungus, nor mealworm, nor inner-backpack compression, but by the principles of Euclid. Three thousand years of culture have transubstantiated me. Take this cracker, the body of Pythagoras. Take this juicebox, the bathwater of Archimedes."

There's a fundamental divide here, not just between my parents and my 6-year-old self, but also between two ways that we think about food: the conviction that foods closest to the earth are the healthiest, versus the conviction that foods most firmly under technological control are the healthiest. For some the fish lifted moments ago from a lake is more wholesome than anything you could buy in a grocery store. For others it is suspect, unknown, unsanctioned by food-safety authorities. Better to reduce this fish down to pure nutrient parts—to protein, and vitamins, and omega-3 fatty acids—and count out precisely the right number of each into a rationally formulated, fortified, health-enhanced fish stick. If you subscribe to the view that you are what you eat, isn't it then crucial to know exactly what you are eating, down to the molecule?

The implications of dessert, in particular, shook my faith in eating naturally. My parents forbade the consumption of anything containing refined sugar, and for that I craved sweetness even more. I pondered it: What if my parents were fundamentally wrong? What if I could be more like my cooler, more popular, Vans-and-Jams-clad friends if only I were allowed to eat Oreos? What evidence existed to back up my parents' conviction that sugar was a dangerous substance?

DIETARY BEFUDDLEMENT

I'd thought my project would be a simple one: I'd spend a few days in the library, talk to a few scientists, and determine who was right. What I found was much more complex, and much more interesting. Americans never seem to tire of books and articles telling them how to eat scientifically, yet our knowledge of these topics is shallow. Once my research took me beyond the bromides regularly printed in health magazines, I was dumbstruck by how little science there was to support even the basic nutritional advice I had assumed was certain. We generally think we know which types of fats and cholesterol are good and which are bad, but the jury is still very much out. The evidence for the health benefits of monounsaturated fat and the ill effects of saturated fat is contradictory and startlingly incomplete. Even the distinction between "good" and "bad" cholesterol turns out to be a crude oversimplification. People tend to think that sugar (which I'll deal with later) is harmful for a variety of reasons—most of which are false: Studies fail to show that sugar makes kids hyper, or that it weakens the immune system. The only firmly established reason I could find to avoid sugar was its association with cavities, but there wasn't enough evidence for scientists to come right out and say that high-sugar diets *cause* tooth decay. It's revealing that the diet-related diseases (obesity, type 2 diabetes, and most forms of heart disease) are only prevalent in those cultures advanced enough to have— or to think they have—an understanding of food science.

When it comes to nutrition, our knowledge is so limited that, if someone claims they know how to eat scientifically, it's a fairly reliable indicator that they are actually selling pseudoscience. America's grand tradition of nutritional pseudoscience goes back to John Harvey Kellogg, who, around 1900, began alerting people to the dangers of protein, masturbation, and toxic bacteria, while promoting enemas and cornflakes. His influence may be measured both by the degree to which his family name is now synonymous with cereal, and by the degree to which later health gurus have copied his techniques.

Nutrition is an oddly public science. It shows off its first drafts. It's almost irresistible for the various factions—raw foodists, high-tech pill poppers, animal protein enthusiasts, low fat hardliners—to take up the provisional science and, like Kellogg, extrapolate to form a complete (that is, marketable) dietary theory. In most other fields, basic research is of interest only to those scientists following the various competing hypotheses. But in nutrition, each contradictory finding makes headlines and produces radical changes in the way people live. One day we are carbo-loading, the next we are asking for our hamburgers without the bun. The humble omelet shifts from a heart attack on a plate to a health food. I read a handful of the most respectable diet books I could find: One advised shunning protein, another warned against fat, and a third pointed the finger at carbohydrates. That left nothing free from suspicion, which shouldn't have surprised me, given that we generally think of calories (simply a measure of how much energy—or life force—is contained in a food) as something to be avoided.

After a few false starts in parsing the science from the pseudoscience, I called Bruce German, the food chemist at University of California, Davis. I remembered that his fascination with bacteria was the natural outgrowth of his larger project on nutrition. It wasn't until I called that I learned how large his project really is: He has devoted himself to linking an understanding of food metabolism on the microscopic level to a holistic understanding of how foods (the whole fish) affect health (the whole person). It's uncharted territory, and when we spoke, he didn't hold back. There was a good reason I was confused, he said.

"What people are beginning to realize to their horror," German told me, "is that we actually don't know much about diet and health."

For nearly two centuries nutrition scientists have been saying just the opposite: that we've figured out everything we need to know about nutrition. Michael Pollan has acidly etched this history of scientific arrogance in his book *In Defense of Food*, starting with Justus von Liebig who, in 1842, proposed that humans only needed potassium, phosphorus, and nitrogen to thrive—along with fat, protein, and carbohydrates. Liebig was obviously missing a few things (vitamins, for example), but no one knew that at the time and many doctors suggested that babies should be exclusively fed on Liebig's formula—which, they presumed, was superior to breast milk.* It was assumed that Liebig had closed the book on nutrition.

In the 1950s, German said, conventional wisdom yet again held that scientists had solved the problem of diet. This overconfidence sprang

---

* Liebig, though a brilliant chemist, wasn't so good when it came to food: He also claimed that searing a piece of meat seals its juices inside, but this actually does just the opposite, drying and caramelizing the outer layer, and to this day cooks sacrifice steaks to Liebig's confusion. Harold McGee has pointed out that you can achieve the same effect without drying out the meat by searing it at the end of the cooking process rather than the beginning.

from a decision to approach nutrition not as the study of foods, but as the study of their molecules. Going molecular was wonderfully enabling: Scientists were able to see what happened when they removed one chemical at a time from the kibble they were feeding to rats. If that nutrient was important, the animals would get sick. Methodically, researchers worked their way down the list of chemicals.

"In about 40 years, scientists were able to identify every single nutrient molecule that animals need to survive and reproduce," German said. "There was the feeling that all the work was done. We assumed that all we needed to do was fortify the heck out of the food supply with essential nutrients. It was a great idea, but we will probably end up looking back at it as one of the greatest scientific goofs of all time."

The view at the molecular level fostered confidence by exposing the details of a small vista with perfect clarity—but it also left vast areas shrouded in darkness. The rapid accumulation of this sort of microscopic knowledge, German said, left three crippling assumptions embedded deep within nutrition science. First, the pinhole focus on minutiae left the impression that the big picture, the food itself, was unimportant. Under this assumption, it shouldn't matter whether sugars were latticed through a slice of bread or molded into a lollipop. Second, the cataloguing of essential nutrients didn't account for human diversity, and nutrition science treated everyone—Inuits, Bushmen, distance runners, and couch potatoes—as if they required the same diet. Third, given the focus on deficiencies, the best solution seemed to be the supplementation of nutrients to the national food supply. This final assumption had the consequence of putting large institutions, rather than individuals, in control of nutrition, because it was easy for governments and corporations to simply fortify salt, bread, and milk, with more than enough essential nutrients to everyone.

"We didn't teach people what iodine is," German said (it's an element, commonly found in seawater and soil, necessary to make hormones in the thyroid). "We just iodized salt."

As a result we are profoundly ignorant about diet and health. What little information did filter down into schools—like the food pyramid—was simplified to the point of nonsensicality.

These three assumptions—that molecules matter while the food itself is irrelevant, that everyone is the same, and that institutions rather than individuals should be trusted to control nutrition—are to a large extent responsible for the epidemics in heart disease, obesity, type 2 diabetes, and osteoporosis, German said. More than a third of U.S. citizens are clinically obese. Demographers estimate that one of every three children who were born in the year 2000 will develop type 2 diabetes during their lives. Today's children are expected to be the first generation in 200 years to die younger than their parents. And the epidemic reaches far beyond the United States. Countries rapidly modernizing are suffering the heaviest brunt of diet-related illnesses. Walk into clinics in China and you will find doctors overwhelmed by diabetes and heart disease. The results of our experiment in eating scientifically haven't been good.

THE GREAT WHITE HOPE

The problem with doing science that attempts to look, not just through the microscope, but also at the big picture, is that the work becomes exponentially more complex each time you zoom out. In a lab you can control variables so that only one element changes at a time: When you take all the salt out of the kibble and the rats sicken, it's fairly safe to infer that they needed salt. If you've done the experiment carefully there shouldn't be any other causes—no confounding factors, as they are called—to muddle the results. But if you want to ask how diet affects people's health in a larger context, then you must wade through truckloads of confounding factors: Was it the fat that caused my (hypothetical) heart disease, or the sugar? Or could it be the fact that my grandmother passed me a susceptible gene, or that I didn't exercise, or could it be because that my sleep was interrupted several times each night by police sirens? Nutrition research had been, all too often, focused on a field either so broad as to render the results nearly meaningless, or so specific that it was hard to find applicability outside the lab. The challenge for researchers was to find some new angle from which to study their subject, some new way of seeing that could break open the scientific logjam by providing microscopic accuracy and macroscopic applicability. That's exactly what German did.

He began by asking what a food would look like if it was precisely designed to make us healthy. Such a food would be a Rosetta stone with which to crack the code for dietary health. No plant would do as a model because evolutionary pressure tends to favor plants that can avoid being eaten, and plants have honed their expertise in defending themselves by building poisons. The model food would have to be just the opposite: something that wanted to be a meal, that gained evolutionary success by being eaten, something shaped by constant Darwinian pressure to satisfy all the needs of mammals. That ur-food, of course, was milk.

"In milk you have the Darwinian engine of your dreams," German said. "You've got a mother who is literally dissolving her tissues to make milk whatever is going into it is costing her—so if it's not helping the infant, evolution should weed it out. But if she creates something that enhances the infant's chance of survival, that provides a tremendous boost to the chances of it spreading. You let this engine run for a few million years and you end up with this complex, almost magical substance. It's a spectacular gold mine for science."

When I asked German to show me what the research looked like he took me to a room that one of his colleagues had set up. This room looks a lot like your high school chemistry lab might have, only more so: more pipes and cables swooping up past hanging fluorescent lights, more battered machines cluttering the faux-wood lab benches, more substances that could blaze or boom, along with stern prohibitions against blazing and booming taped to the walls. One, in a red font, read:

DANGER INVISIBLE LASER RADIATION AVOID EYE CONTACT OR SKIN
EXPOSURE TO DIRECT OR SCATTERED RADIATION. Acronyms and arrows
crowded a blackboard, stuffing leaked from an old chair, and a dozen
lab coats burdened a coat tree. Grad students drifted in and out. A
mass-spectrometry machine, which looked as if it might have come
from the engine room of a steamship, dominated a quarter of the lab,
shrouded in hissing ice clouds. A wooden sign hung above, carved with
the words SPECTROMETRY FOR THE MASSES. The machine was essentially a scale, but a scale so precise that it could determine the type and
number of atoms in a milk molecule by weighing it. "It's like weighing
a battleship to see if there is a fly on the deck," German said, shaking his
head in admiration for his colleague who had built it. "Carlos Lebrilla:
He's an absolute wizard."

On the other side of the room was a freezer containing hundreds of
tubes, beakers, and vials of milk. Milk from humans, gorillas, mice, and
seals scabbed like white lichen to the glass. The milk research is still in
its infancy, but already these samples have shown German and the scientists working with him just how far astray our nutritional assumptions
have taken us. The reason this excites German—"Sometimes this stuff
gets me so excited I can't sleep at night"—is that this failure of dietary
theory presents the opportunity for a Copernican revolution in nutrition, an opportunity for a better theory that changes our conception of
how the universe works.

ASSUMPTION 1: MOLECULES MATTER, FOOD IS IRRELEVANT

It's relatively easy for scientists to measure the type and number of molecules of any nutrient (using mass spectrometry for instance) but infuriat-
ingly hard to see how they fit together to form actual food. This is a
common problem for science—categorizing and counting the parts of a
system is simple (or at least feasible) but understanding the relationships
between the parts is difficult. So for a long time many scientists simply

assumed that the structure of food was irrelevant. When the early nutritionists thought about food structure at all, it was to plot its destruction. The molecular nutritionists, remember, had won their fame in identifying the nutrients needed to prevent deficiencies, so they favored simple foods that digestive tracts could easily absorb. For years, therefore, scientists encouraged processing the complexity out of foods. The results were products like Wonderbread—vehicles for vitamins and minerals that barely required chewing.

"They're rocket fuel," German said. "The nutrients have just been atomized—they go into the bloodstream like they've been injected."

Milk suggests that perhaps we should be striving for the exact opposite: calories bound up in complex structures that break down bit by bit. Milk doesn't start out in complex chunks; in order to pass through a narrow aperture—the nipple—it has to be fluid. But once through, enzymes in the baby's stomach trigger a transformation of milk proteins and, like a ship unfolding in a bottle, they open and link together, forming large curds. Put another way, evolutionary trial and error has fixed it so that babies drink milk, but digest cheese.* Next, of course, the baby must break down this cheese to extract the nutrients. Evolution would not tolerate the expense of knitting together this complex structure then breaking it down again if it had no benefit. But according to the dominant dietary theory, which holds that food is simply independent molecules, there is no benefit: Chunky milk and fluid milk are nutritionally identical.

It's unequivocally apparent to German that the structure of foods matters. A simple restacking of identical nutrients was so important, so advantageous in the sink-or-swim test of natural selection, that it made it worth solving the devilish engineering problem of getting cheese through a nipple. The implications are enormous: It means that

---

* If we are to give credit where credit is due, the honor for the invention of cheese belongs to babies. We still employ the enzyme, rennet, from the stomach of a baby goat, or sheep, to perform this magic trick. It's likely the first man-made cheese was a happy accident that occurred when someone used a bag made from a calf's stomach to carry milk.

a nutrient that's good for you in one food may be bad for you in another. And that makes the nutritional information boxes required on all food packaging almost completely irrelevant: The same type of fat may have different consequences if it arrives in a slice of coconut, a steak, or a scoop of gelato.

ASSUMPTION 2: EVERYONE IS THE SAME

There's a page from *Sports Illustrated* magazine that German sometimes uses in lectures with photographs of Olympic athletes in their underwear: Some bulge like comic book characters; some are planed down to willowy smoothness; some are birdlike, gracile; some hulk as if they'd been wrapped for shipping. It's ridiculous to suggest that each of these people would be better off eating the same diet. And yet for years the nutritionists have advised just that.

Mother's milk, on the other hand, is personalized for each infant. It contains antibodies specialized to protect against local germs. Its balance of fats and sugars shifts depending on the baby's size, hunger, and energy expenditure. When a baby is more active and burning more calories, its movements—butting and jiggling the breast—cause the fat content of the milk to increase. And—at least among rhesus macaques, which produce milk similar to human milk—the breast produces a different mix of nutrients depending on whether the baby is male or female (the boys get fattier milk, while the girls get a greater volume of thinner milk—the upshot is that males feed less frequently and explore more, while females feed more often and perhaps learn more from their mothers). Milk changes continuously, providing age-appropriate levels of nutrients for different stages of development.

The major components of milk, however, remain the same, even as their amounts shift relative to one another. The way that fats are assembled, in particular, are consistent. "The most well-conserved gene set across all mammals is the set that creates fats in milk," German told me. "It's one of the great treasures in the genome." The bulk of the fats in breast milk are saturated, which are suspect under the nutritional orthodoxy because they are associated with cholesterol. If breast milk were sold in grocery stores, it would be considered a dangerously high-cholesterol food. Yet researchers found that cholesterol levels in breast milk couldn't be budged by putting mothers on diets. Scientists also noticed that the more cholesterol neonates drank in their milk, the less they produced in their livers, which led to the hypothesis that mothers were programming their babies—tuning their bodies to produce no more and no less cholesterol than they uniquely needed. This discovery contributed to science showing that people can have high cholesterol for different reasons: Some are eating too much of it, some are producing too much, and some aren't efficiently eliminating it from the bloodstream.[*] The study of milk, in other words, has suggested that the meaning of "high cholesterol" depends utterly on context.

"The thing that bothers me most about the industrial, authoritarian model of nutrition," German said, "is that it is in diametric opposition with human evolution."

Homo sapiens has evolved a remarkable elasticity when it comes to diet: We have both shearing teeth and grinding molars, and our digestive system is that of a generalist. If you look deeper, beyond the tissue and bone, it becomes clear that the human genome contains multitudes: Most people in the world—aside from those with ancestors from the Eurasian cow belt, and a few cattle-rich spots in Africa—lack the genetic mutation required to digest dairy after infancy. Similarly, descendants of grain-growing cultures have genetics to manufacture more salivary amylase—an enzyme that breaks down starches—than hunter-gatherers. Furthermore, people routinely overcome these genetic predispositions, recruiting gut bacteria to help them digest lactose, for instance.

---

[*] It's possible to zero in on these issues by looking at different molecules in the blood: One (phytosterol) can show you are taking too much cholesterol in, another (mevalonate) can reveal if your liver is the problem, and a third (7-α-hydroxy-4-cholesten-3-one) can indicate that you aren't eliminating enough cholesterol by converting it to bile. Each condition demands a different treatment. But these tests aren't routinely performed before doctors make a prescription to control cholesterol.

"We are at the platinum level of freedom," German continued, "and yet nutritional dogma says we are all supposed to eat the same way?"

Humans have been molded to eat diets as diverse as humanity itself. To cater to the wondrous diversity of humankind, German thinks that nutrition science must follow the example of milk, and tailor recommendations for each individual. Which brings us to the third assumption.

ASSUMPTION 3: INSTITUTIONS, NOT INDIVIDUALS, SHOULD BE IN CHARGE OF DIET

It would be impossible for institutions to fabricate and furnish tailor-made diets for every individual on a national, or industrial, scale. To accomplish this, people would have to devise guidelines for themselves, which seemed like a recipe for disaster to early nutritionists. The example of milk, however, shows that people are capable of learning and adapting to personalized dietary guidelines by the time they are six months old.

Breast milk, as it shapes itself to the needs of the baby, is also shaping the infant to its surroundings. Long before babies are capable of speech, mothers communicate with them through flavors and scents to provide a personalized education in nutrition. This education starts in the womb, where babies begin to imprint on volatile compounds they inhale with amniotic fluid, and continues through the breast as they drink milk. Scents are transmitted from foods into milk (a phenomenon that the dairy industry studied extensively since cows that eat wild onions or garlic can dramatically alter the flavor of dairy products). Researchers sniffing breast milk have successfully detected the smell of garlic, alcohol, vanilla, and carrots after mothers had ingested the same. And babies are more likely to welcome foods the moms have regularly eaten during pregnancy and breastfeeding. It seems that a mother tunes her children's tastes, using the knowledge she has accumulated over her lifetime about what foods best satisfy the needs of her genotype, along with the cultural knowledge built up over several lifetimes about what combinations of foods best meet the needs of someone living in the local climate, among the local of plants and animals, and within the local economic system.

"You see this not just in humans, but in all mammals," said Julie Mennella, a scientist at the Monell Chemical Senses Center who is responsible for many of the discoveries on the development of flavor preferences. "Information about what plants to avoid, what plants to eat occasionally, and when plants are at their peak nutritional content is not innate knowledge, it's learned. And it's learned through the amniotic fluid and milk. These are the biological mechanisms on which culture acts when it comes to food."

Cultures place great importance on food traditions and these established food preferences tend to outlast language when people immigrate to new countries. "When a cuisine disappears, that's when a culture is truly dead," Mennella said. And not only is the cuisine of every culture different, each mother offers her own twist, eating only what works for her and imbuing the infancy of her children with powerful flavor memories— be they of Parisian madeleines or brown rice. "When we think of the emotional potency of these flavor-based memories, those that take us to our past, those that trigger the reward centers in our brains, they all originate early in life," she said.

The early nutritionists eschewed this complexity. They understood that everyone needed slightly different amounts of nutrients, but figured it wouldn't hurt to provide double and triple doses in some cases. So they made food companies the stewards of our health by asking them to fortify the food supply. When it came to curing deficiencies, this strategy was wonderfully successful. Salt companies added a few drops of iodine to their crystals, and within a decade, goiters disappeared from America. Bakers cut rates of neural tube defects at least 25 percent by mixing folic acid in flour. Adjusting the nutrients at the national level led to the near eradication of pellagra, beriberi, and rickets. The great triumph of the uniform, top-down approach to nutrition was in providing an abundance of cheap nutrients. Rather than trusting individuals with the tools to solve our dietary problems, nutritionists simply drowned those problems in a flood of calories. By now, however, it has become clear that in attacking the nutrient-deficiency problem we created a super-sufficiency problem.

The education an infant receives through breast milk, of course, is only as good as the knowledge of the mother. And today, after years of misinformation have convinced people to mistrust the dietary evidence they observe in their own bodies, the lessons babies are learning from breast milk are not the result of years of optimizing and experimentation by the mother, but instead the dictates of the industry.

—◦—

I'd gone to nutrition science hoping to find a prescription for how to eat, or at least hard-and-fast rules that would allow me to judge my parents' dietary proclivities. But the problem with eating scientifically is that it's not supported by science. The microscopic view of nutrition has provided enough information to tell people how to avoid getting goiters and scurvy, but not enough to tell a healthy person how to be healthier. Instead, it reveals just enough to enable hordes of well-meaning (or profit-driven) reformers, each selling a diet book. I'd been thinking that eating scientifically was the opposite of eating naturally, but the more I learned, the more they looked like two sides of the same coin. Both ideas extend beyond the reach of real evidence. Both produce pseudoscientific gurus who claim certainty where, in fact, there is complexity.

German has great ideas for tackling this complexity: He talks about biomarkers, metabolomics, and a moon-shot investment in dietary science. Most of all, he talks about education. Rather than teaching nutrition as a set of laws delivered from on high to be memorized and obeyed (no matter how wrong they are in context), German wants to candidly explain the limits of our knowledge to students, then set them loose on the mystery.

"We need a new generation to solve this," he said. "I have a set of pre-assumptions that I'm not even aware of, and it's dictating what I'm thinking. We need these young minds when they're not stuck."

The greatest contribution of the milk science seemed to be the excavation of nutritional nonsense—it defined the negative space in our understanding and explained our dietary confusion. It couldn't provide the kind of evidence I would have wanted as a kid—the kind that would have convinced my parents that there was really nothing wrong with processed sugar. It did, however, offer some indication of how to proceed, because the revelations brought by milk suggest that nutritional truth is contingent upon its surroundings. It seemed appropriate, therefore, to broaden my perspective, so that I was looking not just at the chemistry, but also the context that alters the fate of any given nutrient. If the relationship between nutrients is important, surely the way a food is constructed and consumed is as well, which then makes it important to understand the history and economics—in short the culture—of a food. When I'd gone looking for precise science to tell me whether sugar was good or evil I'd come up empty-handed. But it deserved another look, I thought, with this broader lens.

FEAR OF SUGAR

Of all my family's dietary restrictions, the sugar ban had the most staying power. Usually, my mother would relax her strictures over time, allowing tofu, perhaps, or whole-wheat bread back into the rotation. But the sugar ban remained stubbornly in place. This made sweetness a novelty, and even more exciting. For me, sugar was the taste of a better life. When I was lucky enough to get my fingers into something sweet, it provided a moment of pleasure, but not relief. Instead, the taste just made me drool for more. Looking back, I can see that while the discovery of the nudity taboo had sent subterranean shockwaves through my developing id, the discovery of sugar reordered my conscious world: Sweetness became the definitive proof that I was missing out on the party. It became a representation of all the hallmarks of the mainstream American life I yearned for, a life foreign enough from my own that I didn't recognize the signs that it had never existed outside a television screen.

When people like my parents talk about the evils of sugar, they are usually not implying that all forms of sugar are bad. They're not worried about sugar in milk (lactose), in fruit (fructose), or the complex sugars in whole grains. What bothers them is refined sugar (sucrose—which is 50 percent fructose and 50 percent glucose), and high fructose corn syrup (which is usually 55 percent fructose and 45 percent glucose). The liver can transform all of these sugars into glucose, which is necessary for survival.* The brain requires a steady stream of glucose, and if you're running low it will send out panicked messages to drop everything and eat—preferably something sweet and therefore not too many metabolic steps away from glucose. The urgency of the resulting impulse is tantamount. This helped to explain my rapturously feral feeding on sweet things when I had the chance, but it didn't explain why I felt this impulse even when I was full and in no danger of glucose depletion.

To see if I could understand what had led so many young parents to deny sugar to their children (which of course continues in some circles to this day) I went looking for documents expressing the sugar angst of the time. At the zenith of this canon is William Dufty's 1975 book *Sugar Blues*, a swashbuckling account of the author's own battle with sucrose addiction. The book tickled the concerns of the day about new chemicals in foods, and Dufty, who knew his audience, grasped the trope of sugar as a dangerous technology and carried it to the point of absurdity. "After all, heroin is nothing but a chemical," he wrote. "They take the juice of the poppy and they refine it into opium and then they refine it into morphine and finally heroin. Sugar is nothing but a chemical. They take the

---

* Though glucose is necessary for survival, you don't have to eat sugar to get it: The liver can synthesize glucose from amino acids. But it is a more elaborate process, and the amino acids usually come from breaking down muscle.

juice of a cane or a beet and they refine it to molasses and then they refine it to brown sugar and finally to strange white crystals."

Dufty blamed sugar for the plague, depression, hallucinations, and traffic accidents. His critique must have strained the faith of even the most credulous readers when he claimed that people who don't eat sugar won't be sunburned or bitten by insects. These claims were easily falsifiable for a sunburned, itchy, and sugar-free kid like me. Still, where he lacked for evidence, Dufty made up for it with a turn of phrase. He was a master of the false analogy: "Just as spilled sugar in our kitchens attracts ants and insects," he wrote, "so does sugar in our bloodstreams attract mosquitoes."

Sugar Blues was obviously not written as a logical argument to convince the skeptical, but as a sermon to affirm a fear already present in the cultural imagination. Clearly there was, even at that time, alarm about sugar—but not the science to justify it. The details of Dufty's book were pure malarkey, but the force behind it, the sense that there was something fundamentally wrong with the amount of sugar we were eating, made sense. It was people, not ants or mosquitoes, who were swarming to sugar. Throughout the era, consumption of sugars steadily rose. Americans went from eating 15 pounds of sugars a year in 1830, to 105 pounds in 2005. Now, the average American tips back more than half a cup a day. Dufty had exposed a deep vein of sugarphobia, and yet our fears have seemed only to stimulate our appetite for sweetness.

THE SUGAR HYPOTHESIS REBORN

In 2009, the proposition that there was something fundamentally noxious about sugar roared back to life with new scientific vigor. The University of California, San Francisco, pediatrician Richard Lustig stirred my hopes for a simple, scientific explanation of America's dietary woes by pointing the finger at the nutritional scoundrel of my youth. The sugar we ate, he said, whether in crystalline or liquid form, was killing us.

"High fructose corn syrup and sucrose are exactly the same, they are both equally bad," he said. "They are both dangerous. They are both poison, 'kay? I said it. Poison."

It was an unusually blunt statement for a doctor of Lustig's stature, and as someone starved for information about what to eat, I was transfixed. Apparently there were others like me. Soon after it was posted on the Internet, the video of his lecture, "Sugar: The Bitter Truth," went viral. In a few months half a million of us had watched the full hour and a half. It's probably safe to say that it is the most watched 90-minute biochemistry lecture ever.

Fructose is what's really doing the damage, Lustig said (fructose is the principal sugar in fruit, but context is crucial—the fiber that comes with an apple mitigates the effect of the sugar, he said). When people are fed fructose, 30 percent of it is turned into fat, compared to almost none when they are fed glucose. Fructose does not suppress ghrelin (the hunger hormone from the stomach), nor does it stimulate leptin (the fullness hormone produced by fat cells). Furthermore, Lustig showed that the chemical reactions required to break down fructose in the liver triggered a cascade of other problems: the formation of new fat cells; inflammation and hypertension, which has implications for heart disease; insulin resistance, which has implications for diabetes; and leptin resistance, which has the effect of leaving the body's starvation-distress beacon stuck in the on position.

For this lecture, Lustig wore a navy blazer, a light-blue shirt, and a shiny silver tie with a fat knot. He looked more like a politician than a medical-school professor. He sounded like a politician too: "We've had our food supply adulterated, contaminated, poisoned, tainted," he said, adding: "on purpose." That last shot was a sharp elbow in the side of soft-drink makers, which are responsible for most of the sugar added to our food since 1970. Many sodas are formulated to make you thirstier as you drink, he said, because they contain both caffeine—which makes people urinate—and salt: "Fifty-five milligrams per can. It's like drinking a pizza." The mixture produces dehydration, and the urge to keep drinking. "They know what they're doing," Lustig said darkly: "They know."

This was stirring stuff—Lustig's ability to command such a large audience came, no doubt, from his willingness to name a villain in no uncertain terms. And yet, given our record of demonizing single nutrients while ignoring the big picture, I couldn't swallow this new sugar hypothesis without a spoonful of caution. The narrow focus on fructose smacked of the old nutrition myopia, uninformed by the revelations that people like Bruce German were bringing to the field with milk science. To be clear, I was completely convinced by Lustig's biochemistry. The evidence did suggest, as he claimed, that fructose was a poison, but it's the dose that makes the poison—even the healthiest of substances (water, for instance) becomes poisonous if consumed at sufficient quantities. The real question wasn't "Is sugar toxic?" but "What impels people to eat so much sugar that it becomes toxic?"

Lustig, a pediatrician who works with obese children from around the Bay Area, allowed that small amounts of sugar are no more toxic than water. The problem is that massive consumption has become the norm. "The science is important," he said when I called him, "but it's not enough. There has to be a cultural element. I can't do individual therapy without societal control." To illustrate the point, he told me a story about an appointment he'd had a few months earlier. Lustig had explained to his patient that he was on track to become obese and diabetic. The solution was simple, he told the boy: Stop drinking sodas.

"Inevitably, he returns a month later and admits that he hasn't stopped drinking sodas," Lustig said. "So I ask why, and do you know what he says? 'Water doesn't taste good.' And I look at the mom, who is also obese, and ask, 'Surely you didn't drink soda as a kid?' and she says, 'We drank Kool-Aid.' And I go, okay, I get it. I get it."

The problem, Lustig said, has nothing to do with the fact that all children prefer sweetness, but everything to do with our learned flavor

preferences, with the food traditions passed from generation to generation, and with the fact that it's cheap to quench the brain's thirst for sugar
from a carbonated two-liter bottle. It may seem strange to the wealthy
that people who can barely afford food are drinking soda, but this isn't
the first time that the poor have found that it makes economic sense to
buy unhealthy luxury foods. Ever since the 18th century the use of sugar
as a primary source of calories has been more a symptom of desperation
than indulgence. Back then, the Victorian poor drank tea rather than
soda, and the social historian, David Davies, observed "Tea drinking is
not the cause, but the consequence of the distresses of the poor."

As the milk science suggested, the context of a nutrient—in any particular food, or in any particular person—was of the utmost importance.
And sugar, in particular, is entangled with its economic context.

SUGARCANE CAPITALISM

The strange thing about the world's sweet tooth is that it didn't really
exist before 1700. During the Renaissance, sugar was a rare spice, and it
spread slowly in the following centuries. Then, between 1700 and 1900,
British sugar consumption increased 2,250 percent, until it made up a
fifth of all calories in the national diet.

Clearly people are attracted to the taste of sugar, but that isn't enough
to explain this sudden and titanic shift in food culture, argues sociologist
Sydney Mintz, in *Sweetness and Power,* his book on the history of sugar.
Furthermore, a liking for sweetness certainly doesn't explain why the
poor eat immense quantities of sugar while those with money eat less.
Mintz's explanation is that sugar served as midwife at the birth of modern
consumerism, and as this particular form of economy grew, sugar thrived
as a new calorie source for commoners. Historian Fernando Ortiz called
plantations "the favored child of capitalism," and Mintz shows how the
sugarcane farms of the Caribbean in the 1700s provided a test case for
global markets and financial speculation. They were so successful that

they became "one of the massive demographic forces in world history," moving hundreds of millions of enslaved Africans to the New World.

This economic system enriched even the poorest Englishman in that it put luxury imports—like tea and sugar—within his reach, but it did not change his position within society. "Slave and proletarian together powered the imperial economic system that kept the one supplied with manacles and the other with sugar and rum; but neither had more than minimal influence over it," Mintz observed. "The growing freedom of the consumer to choose was one kind of freedom, but not another."

And even this freedom, the freedom to shop, proved illusory as consumer choice was increasingly constrained to sugar in various guises. Food historian John Burnett wrote that, in the 18th century, white bread and sugared tea were transformed from luxuries of the rich to, "the irreducible minimum beyond which lay only starvation." The newly urban poor no longer could supplement their meals with parsnips from the garden, or milk from the family cow, and in the newly commodified economy where time was money, there simply weren't enough hours to make vegetable broth or porridge. English commoners found that their new factory jobs also demanded a new diet—food they could prepare quickly between shifts, that prevented them from nodding off at the loom. Sugar—usually mixed with tea—met both criteria. "Sugar was taken up just as work schedules were quickening," Mintz writes, "as the movement from countryside to city was accelerating, and as the factory system was taking shape and spreading. Such changes more and more affected eating habits."

Around this time, sugar began to spread under subterfuge, by infiltrating other foods and driving down their costs. Mix enough sugar with fruit and you get preserves that will not rot, and therefore may be mass-produced and distributed cheaply. By 1905, preserves made with Jamaican sugar were less expensive than butter from British cows. The cheapest midday meal came to consist almost wholly of simple carbohydrates: bread slathered with jam or treacle (sugar syrup), and tea with the requisite two lumps. While some reformers were aghast to see sugared tea push its way into the center of the diet, teetotalers welcomed the beverage, which was replacing beer as the refreshment of choice among the poor. The arrangement also pleased industrialists, who found that employees worked more efficiently when they exchanged alcohol for a diet of stimulants.

Historical circumstance had led to the rise of sugar, and businessmen began campaigning to ensure that circumstances remained favorable. Politicians started working to influence governments for the promotion of sugar. This was a novel development: An inanimate commodity had gained a seat at the table of power, trumping allegiance to king and country.

Early attempts to influence nutrition science on the behalf of sugar began around this time as well. Mintz identifies a Dr. Frederick Slare as the chief nutritional propagandist in the 1700s. Something of an anti-Dufty, Slare recommended sugar for curing ailments of the eye, as a hand lotion for healing cuts, as a snuff substitute for snorting, and even as a form of toothpaste. In response to evidence associating sugar with diabetes mellitus, Slare wrote an outraged rebuttal, bemoaning the damage that would be done if the world were denied the curative powers of this panacea should its reputation be wounded by a mere hypothesis.

SUGAR'S POWER TODAY

These initial efforts to influence politics and nutrition science were refined over the centuries as sugar flexed gracefully into the postcolonial world, insinuating itself into more countries, more foods, and more adipose tissue. Slare and his kind were replaced by more formidable entities like the Washington, DC–based International Life Sciences Institute, ILSI. The organization's stated mission is "to improve the well-being of the general public through the advancement of science," and it produces enough legitimate science that many have assumed that the organization is focused purely on the public interest. But it's been shown, through internal memos made public during litigation against tobacco companies, that a major part of ILSI's true mission is to serve its members: food, agribusiness, and drug corporations.

In the 1990s, ILSI was run by Alex Malaspina, who also happened to be vice president of Coca-Cola. Geoffrey Cannon, who in 1992 was a British delegate to a World Health Organization (WHO) conclave on nutrition, said that Malaspina comported himself as if he were in charge of the WHO. "I can still see him striding at the head of a phalanx of rent-a-profs, dispatching two to talk to this national delegation, two to the next," Cannon said. During that particular meeting, these scientists-for-hire succeeded in fomenting enough disagreement over details that the participants eventually agreed to refrain from mentioning sugar at all.

In 1997 ILSI was even more successful, sponsoring an "Expert Consultation on Carbohydrates" in which the WHO concluded there was no upper limit on sugar in a healthy diet. "Good news for kids: Experts see no harm in sugar," read one press release.

These techniques of guiding the scientific conversation and spreading doubt were pioneered by the tobacco industry when working to deny the connection between smoking and lung cancer, and the use of the same tactics in the debate over sugar was not coincidental. In 2001 a WHO investigation found that "ILSI was used by certain tobacco companies to thwart tobacco control policies." It was later banned from participation in WHO decisions on food or water standards.

Sugar has also employed more direct tactics. In 2004, after the WHO recommended that added sugars should account for no more than 10 percent of a diet (a widely accepted proposition already enshrined in the U.S. food pyramid) the emissaries of sugar appealed to the U.S. government. President George W. Bush's administration responded to the call, denouncing the WHO's recommendation and threatening to pull U.S. funding from the organization. This time, the WHO, to its credit, stood firm.

This access to presidential power hasn't been restricted to Republicans. Monica Lewinsky's testimony revealed that President Bill Clinton interrupted one of their oval-office interludes to take a call from a member of the Fanjul family—one of the handful of Florida cane growers receiving government sanction to ship in Caribbean workers and pay them less than minimum wage. South Florida columnist Carl Hiaasen, who watched the Fanjul family power grow, told *Vanity Fair,* "The most telling thing about Alfy Fanjul is that he can get the president of the United States on the telephone in the middle of a blow job. That tells you all you need to know about their influence."

Perhaps the most important factor in sugar's success, however, has not been the aid of the rich and powerful, but the way it affects the minds of the people who eat it. It wasn't just the convenience of sugar that endeared it to the Dickensian poor, but it was also the way it made them feel. It provided a bit of a fix to keep them going, just a hint of the luxury they were generating. "Sugar seems to satisfy a particular desire (it also seems, in so doing, to awaken that desire anew)," Mintz wrote.

THE CULTURE OF DESIRE

It's possible to get an idea of the collective experience of sweetness by looking at the meanings of the word we use to describe the sensation. The word *sweet* has been used in thousands of different contexts over the course of the last millennium, and this spectrum of connotations shifted with the spread of sugar—there was a semantic devaluation corresponding with the declining value of sweet foods. In the Middle Ages "sweet" was used in settings that ranged from approval to religious ecstasy; from the 16th to 19th centuries the synonyms downgraded slightly—from "pleasant" to "delightful"; in the 20th century "sweet" was nice or pleasant, and was often used in faint praise that implied a lack of substance, as in, "sweet nothings," or "she's a sweet woman." Despite these changes, however, one meaning has withstood the wear of centuries. John Lydgate's usage of "swetness" in the 15th century, to describe how siren songs could "Brineth a man to confusioun," would still be perfectly apt if used today (albeit with spellcheck). A confusion of siren-like temptation with the actual experience of pleasure seems to be the enduring hallmark of sweetness.

Joan Ann Teitz has recorded these meanings in *A Thousand Years of Sweet,* and as I leafed through this book I was struck by how infrequently sweet has implied fulfillment—there were pages of desire but hardly a note of satiation. Sweetness is associated with "satisfaction" only when used to describe victory or revenge—which is a peculiar species of satisfaction, unrelated to contentment. And, while spiritual comfort and contentment were sweet during the Middle Ages, this usage faded by the 15th century. Particularly interesting is the fact that the Indo-European word *swad* was the root of both "sweet" and "persuade." These meanings rejoin in modern idioms like *sweet-talking* and *honeyed speech.* The insight captured in this confluence of meaning is that sweetness is advertisement: It implies pursuit of pleasure rather than pleasure itself.

This is a subtle distinction, but one that neuroscientists would make independently. For years, scientists studying pleasure confused *wanting* with *liking.* Experiments were rigged for rats so that they would spark an electrode implanted in their brains by pressing a lever. If the zap was unpleasant the rats would stop. But if the rodents started hitting the lever like crazy, the scientists thought, "Aha! The electrode must be in a pleasure center." When rats were willing to work for reward, these areas, which are located in the mesolimbic brain, were flooded with the chemical dopamine. So the whole pleasure system was named the mesolimbic dopamine reward system.

This went on until 1989, when the psychologist Kent Berridge set out to confirm that dopamine was in fact related to pleasure. Berridge took rats and wiped out their ability to produce dopamine. Then he gave them sugar. He expected that they'd be totally uninterested because, without dopamine, the sugar wouldn't give them pleasure. But the rats enthusiastically licked their lips, which is what rats do when they like a taste.

Without dopamine, rats were not as driven to work for sugar, but they still enjoyed it.

"It was just a little study," Berridge said. "We thought we just did something wrong."

So they did it again. But they kept getting the same result. It was clear that the rats were experiencing pleasure. Then Berridge went back and read old experiments, in which electrodes had been put into human brains. Unlike the rats, these people could describe the sensations they experienced, and they didn't sound all that great.

Berridge recounts the travails of "B-19," a young man undergoing treatment for depression, epilepsy, and—this was the early '60s—for being gay. Robert Heath, who led Tulane University's psychiatric research at the time, implanted an electrode running through the ostensible pleasure centers in B-19's brain. While showing the man heterosexual pornography, Heath would press the button to trigger the electric pulse. The idea was to kick-start B-19's pleasure centers while he was looking at naked women, and turn him into a heterosexual.

"The stimulation evoked strong sexual arousal and interest," Berridge wrote. "But it did not produce pleasurable sexual orgasm, not even after a thousand consecutive stimulations, unless B-19 was allowed to simultaneously masturbate (or to copulate with a prostitute who was persuaded to provide 'therapy' on one occasion, in what must be one of the most astounding accounts ever published in scientific literature)."

Heath thought he'd found not just a method for converting gay people to a more wholesome lifestyle of prostitutes and porn, but also the ultimate source of human pleasure. Berridge was unconvinced: "There were no exclamations of delight reported, not even a 'Oh—that feels nice!' Instead the stimulation seemed to fail to provide the particular sensory pleasure it made him most eager to pursue." B-19 would mash the button over a thousand times, and when it was taken away he would, Heath wrote, plead "to self-stimulate just a few more times."

When I first read the description of this joyless compulsion to click a button over and again, I happened to have my own finger on a computer mouse, and I felt a shiver of recognition. The sensations of another patient, a woman given a brain electrode in hope that it would ease her chronic pain, were even more hauntingly familiar: "At its most frequent, the patient self-stimulated throughout the day, neglecting personal hygiene and family commitments. . . . At times, she implored her family to limit her access to the stimulator, each time demanding its return after a short hiatus." She reported a vaguely erotic urge, a goading undercurrent of anxiety, the desire to eat or drink without hunger or thirst, listless inactivity, and most of all, a driving compulsion chanting, "More." For me, as a child, that had been the voice of sugar. I have an early memory of pilfering a forbidden cask of candied popcorn, and watching myself with growing horror as I methodically, joylessly, worked my way to the bottom.

Compulsion without pleasure, whether provoked by sugar consumption or B-19's electrode, seems to be related to a flood of the neurotransmitter dopamine into the middle of the brain, where the mesolimbic dopamine reward system lies. The same neural trigger also fires in the brains of drug abusers and gambling addicts. This mechanism must have evolved as a crude neural-override switch, to lock attention on the pursuit. The power dopamine has over us reflects the evolutionary importance of its mission: It's there to keep us from starving and insure that we reproduce. It is activated as parents bond to their infants (it's no coincidence, I think, that Beth and I exclaim "Oh, she's so sweet!" with something like pained dismay at the feeling of rapacious attraction we feel for our baby daughter). This system, in other words, is normally vital, allowing the perseverance and focus required for all achievements. But when abused or damaged, it can produce manic, destructive behavior. Anyone who has been unable to tear themselves away from inane Web clicking, or compulsively mined a pint of ice cream for bits of cookie dough long after they have stopped enjoying it, or promised themselves they'd play "just one more level" (this is my particular demon), has felt the grip of dopamine. Interestingly, animal studies show that the brain reacts to sweetness, not by switching off this seeking mechanism, but by further heightening the reaction. In a world where sweetness is rare, it's logical for sugar to trigger focused seeking. It makes some sense, for instance, for the taste of one ripe berry to elicit gorging before this ephemeral sweetness disappears. But when these sorts of binges are routine—as they can be in a sucrose-drenched world—they cause changes in the brain structure similar to those found in brains altered by heroin.[*]

Complicating all this is the fact that wanting and liking are tangled. Liking seems to be related to endorphins as opposed to dopamine, but almost everything that activates the endorphin-linked pleasure centers also activates the mesolimbic dopamine system. The key difference is that it's harder to provoke liking than wanting. The liking centers in the brain are much smaller, each about a cubic centimeter, "an archipelago of interacting islands," Berridge wrote. These islands must be triggered simultaneously to create a feeling of pleasure. Desire is robust. Pleasure is fragile and fleeting. The first taste of sugar provokes genuine pleasure, but the desire to eat more only grows as satisfaction fades. Of course we are talking about the simplest form of pleasure here, associated with sweetness. I would expect that the pleasure that comes from a symphony, or a skyline, or a smile, is even more ephemeral.

Food companies have learned to manipulate this neurochemistry, argues former FDA commissioner David Kessler, in his book, *The End of Overeating*. Of course, it's not just sugar that jukes our wanting system into overdrive: Fat and salt can also cue dopamine, and it's the combination of all three (fat, salt, and sweetness) that triggers the most intense yearning. An overeater, in Kessler's vision, is like a Manchurian

---

[*] Dufty was partially right to compare sugar to heroin. But his larger point, that sugar is categorically evil because it is a pure chemical, is totally nuts. Salt (sodium chloride) and water (sometimes called by the playful and scientifically correct name dihydrogen monoxide) are examples of the hundreds of pure chemicals we need to live.

candidate who, instead of killing, has been conditioned to respond to a surge of dopamine with a strong hand-to-mouth reflex.

According to Kessler, food makers—oblivious to the extent that they are controlling their customer's minds—are simply responding to market pressure to design foods that sell. Kessler describes speaking to a group of executives from some of the world's largest food corporations. He laid out the science, explaining how their products exploited brain chemistry. When he finished, he wrote, "there was complete silence in the room. Then one executive spoke up. 'Everything that has made us successful as a company is the problem,' he said."

It's not just the food industry. Marketers and advertising agencies working in all sectors of the economy have cobbled together an empirical understanding of what makes our brains flinch with desire. They might not realize they are practicing neuroscience, but they have developed a Madison Avenue folk knowledge for juicing the mesolimbic reward system. Central to this knowledge is the deliberate confusion of desire and pleasure, so that the thrill of the purchase becomes an end unto itself. Plants invented this form of dopamine marketing in fruit—offering sugar as an advertisement to the tongue, a loss-leader given away in exchange for seed distribution. Capitalism perfected this innovation by stripping the satiating bulk and fiber that came with fruit, and offering pure *swad*—that alluring sweetness that when consumed only cues greater yearning. The success of this strategy has made it pervasive. We now live in an empty-calorie world, where sugar's equivalents flash their for-sale phosphorescence from highway signs, smartphones, and television screens. The world for sale is a world reduced to lust and hunger—endless oceans of wanting interrupted by brief atolls of contentment.

While it's too much to blame sugar for everything wrong with consumerism, it is a fair symbol for our excesses, given its role in the creation of the culture of desire. And because its consumption awakens further desire, sugar is especially well suited as a metaphor that demonstrates the connection between superficial rewards and manic striving—whether that striving is pushing a lever in a lab or pushing paper in an office. The neurologist Robert Sapolsky, speaking about the mesolimbic-reward system, has said, "Dopamine is not about pleasure, it's about the anticipation of pleasure. It's about the pursuit of happiness rather than happiness itself. If you block that rise of dopamine from occurring you don't get the work." As Sydney Mintz wrote, sugar's success in at once creating a market among workers, and keeping them attentively at their stations, "made visible, perhaps for the first time in history, a critical connection between the will to work and the will to consume."

Work hard, and you'll someday have not just a house with a car out front, but also a designer range in the kitchen, a pool, and a second car, a second house, a second spouse, a yacht, a modest Mediterranean island. . . . This is the American dream in cancerous metastasis, growth unchecked by reason, consumption divorced from pleasure. Of course the people of the culture of desire are fat. It would be astonishing if we were not.

I could see why people like my parents worried about sugar. Sugar easily represents all the despicably materialistic elements of our culture. But it would be a mistake, and distraction from the larger problem, to get too hung up on the debate over whether it's evil, or poisonous. Everyone, except perhaps for a few industry-funded hacks, agrees that Americans consume way too much. We could eat a lot of sugar, heck, we could all eat a quarter cup every day (that's about the government-recommended maximum) and that would still be less than half as much as we are eating now. What really makes sugar bad are those corrosive elements of our culture that induce some people to guzzle truly heroic quantities of the stuff.

THE SWEET LIFE

What I'd thought was a small question—how does a rational person achieve the health my parents sought through diet?—had produced an impossible answer: You must end the culture of consumption and the inequity it breeds. I was looking for tools I could apply in the kitchen, not grand political theories. I didn't want to start researching tax policy or tactics for revolution. There was, however, one glimmer of hope for a more domestic solution because, in uncovering this dementedly complex tangle, I'd also uncovered a simple, but perhaps powerful, tool with which to extricate myself.

The sales pitch that promises everything and delivers nothing—that tickles our wanting neurons while making sure we can't get no satisfaction—relies wholly on confusing pleasure with desire. Perhaps it could be defeated by simply learning to distinguish the one from the other. For food, this would mean learning to truly taste—slowing down enough to take pleasure in the flavors and textures in each bite. Food corporations have learned to cater to what they call "the lazy American palate," which basically means lots of sugar, fat, and salt. They don't waste subtle flavors on us because, in the grip of a dopamine-driven desire, people stop tasting. When I ate this way I was trying to muffle craving, not produce pleasure. The problem of gluttony is not too much love of food, but too little.

Taking pleasure in food also meant taking pleasure in sweetness, for while I'd uncovered any number of reasons to be concerned about the spread of sweetness, at the end of it I was still an unabashed lover of sugar. This, I decided, was no more contradictory than drinking wine while abhorring alcoholism. The trick, at least for me, was cultivating my attention to sweetness, so that I noticed, and was able to stop, when pleasure subsided.

It seemed radical, and maybe foolhardy, to champion an individual's own sensation over the calorie-counting abstractions of conventional wisdom. Surely telling people to "eat what you enjoy" would be catastrophic for those with a suite of metabolic conditions, and laughable for those without a penny to spare. I absolutely wanted the reductive science curing goiters and pushing innovation forward, I just didn't want to place so much faith in our limited knowledge that I stopped trusting my own senses. As food research progresses it should produce solutions that work in concert with the senses, rather than insisting—as the old nutrition orthodoxy did—that our bodies are leading us astray.

In fact, the nutritional assumptions that Bruce German was doing his best to debunk had all served to help industrialized uniformity triumph over sensation and the taste preferences passed down from mother to child. The assumption that structure did not matter allowed technologists to rebuild foods—mostly by removing fiber while adding sugar, salt, and fat—to increase shelf life and withstand the rigors of long-distance transportation. The assumption that everyone should eat the same diet facilitated mass production. And the assumption that industry was better situated than individuals to control nutrition put a healthy halo over processed foods, while making traditional foods look bad. As early as the 1930s, the food writer M.F.K. Fisher was already able to observe that we were losing flavor in this victory of industry over tradition: "The foundation of all French cookery is butter," she wrote, "as that of the Italian is olive oil, German lard, and Russian sour cream. In the same way, water or drippings may be designated, unfortunately, as the basis of the English cuisine, and perhaps the flavor of innumerable tin cans, of American!"

Despite the current hegemony of industrial nutrition, however, food culture persists. There are pockets of resistance—delicious traditions—in every family. The way to fix dinner and find our way back from obesity could be lurking in these recipes—and in the deep flavor memories from infancy. There is raw emotional power in those memories: The Chinese writer Lin Yutang gauged their potential energy when he asked, "What is patriotism but the love of food one ate as a child?" Perhaps we could reclaim our dietary homelands if we remembered how to distinguish between Kessler's dopamine-driven craving and genuine satisfaction—if we found a way to take, not guilty pleasure, but a kind of holy joy in every mouthful.

It seemed to work for Beth and me. The more we learned about food the more we appreciated it. And this appreciation steadily changed the foods that took form in our kitchen. We began spending a little more money to receive a box of produce directly from a farm, first twice a month, then every week. Next we added six eggs—pastel shells and bright orange yolks—to our order. Then, a half-gallon of milk. I experimented in the kitchen, basing my creations on bits of overheard advice, inspiration from food writers, and snatches of half-remembered culinary science. Some attempts were disastrous (my high-density whole-wheat bread), some traumatic (my wrestling match with elastic fish guts), some simply disgusting (my sour, alcoholic kefir made from the cauliflower-like microbial spores, which a stranger had handed me in an alley behind the TransAmerica building). But my failures were occasionally interrupted by modest successes, and our lives grew steadily more delicious. With much more grace, Beth also built up a repertoire of dishes, and a library of cookbooks. I have to admit that I frequently fell off the wagon: I wolfed down my food unthinkingly, and amid the deliciousness there was (and is) a fair share of bland brown rice with bitter greens—those are my flavor memories after all. But we were also eating marbled meats, triple-cream cheeses, and molten-chocolate pudding. We chose these foods not because we craved them, but because they truly made life richer. And though most of our food was arriving without a nutrition-facts panel, we managed to maintain our good health. More and more frequently our table was crowded with friends. Life grew sweeter, but not sweet in the diminutive, or yearning senses commonly evoked by the word in English—this was sweetness as the Italians must experience it in order to produce a phrase like *la dolce vita*, the sweetness of fulfillment. Changing a culture, it seems, isn't so hard when it begins at home. And if people were able to stop striving and fighting long enough to find contentment in good food, lovingly prepared, with a small group of friends, in universal solidarity that can be found around the table—well, perhaps that really could change the world.

CHAPTER FOUR

VEGETABLES AND VACCINES

TOXINS

At the age when most boys start filling out, I was shrinking. One afternoon, as I was mixing sprouts and spinach for an after-school snack, Dad laid a tentative hand on my shoulder and suggested that I eat something more substantial.

"Your collar bones are sticking out," he joshed. Then his tone became tender. "I'm a little worried about you."

Teenagers have at their disposal a special kind of scorn, which is born in the discovery that conventional wisdom can be wrong and buoyed by the certainty that adults are incapable of seeing past convention. I made a show of mustering the last reserves of my patience and explained, as one would to a toddler or a particularly bright cocker spaniel, that I still had plenty of fat—it was just secreted amid my muscles rather than beneath my skin. It's a testament to Dad's parenting skills that he didn't try to argue with me. He just repeated that he was worried, and added, "You know, one of the signs of anorexia is believing you're fat when, by all reasonable measures, you are unhealthily skinny."

"Dad," I scoffed. "I don't have an eating disorder."

The real problem was that I was failing to live up to my own standards, not for body image, but for speed on the track. I'd gone to a practice with the high school team my freshman year mostly because "long-distance running" sounded unimaginably awful. I was growing up and I wanted to learn what my grown-up self was made of. In my first race I set a minor record, and this gave me hope that, if I pushed hard enough, the man I was becoming would turn out to be some species of righteous badass.

On workout days we'd run grueling sprints around the track, and on rest days we'd do slow-loping 10-mile jogs through the pines. I felt as if I was part of something on that track team, a fellow in a league of higher mortals. The daily workouts were made bearable by this fellowship: Teenage boys aren't natural talkers, but on these runs there was nothing else to do but talk, and so we would joke, confide, commiserate, and make up offensive nicknames for each other. Mine, Nature, was totally innocuous, though it changed to something more sinister when I started looking skeletal.

I had one year of greatness. Then I started running in varsity races, and stopped winning. I trained harder, pushing past the point of diminishing returns. I stumbled through school in bleary exhaustion. I contracted colds that ebbed and surged for months. Training on its own, it became clear, wasn't going to make me an all-American.

Mom told her chiropractor about my problems, and he suggested I come in for a checkup. He listened to my breathing, massaged the outlines of my organs through my abdomen, and photographed my eyeballs in search of imperfections that might indicate deficiencies elsewhere. Afterward he gave me some advice having to do with my liver but, to his credit, told me that the real problem was in my expectations. There was no way I could train harder, continue studying, and stay healthy, he said. Instead of listening to him I picked up one of Mom's diet books when I got home, and finished it the next day. It was a rapturous read. Unlike the chiropractor, it told me exactly what I wanted to hear: My limitless potential had been muted, and there was a simple way for me to remove this handicap. The book explained that I was chronically fatigued (yes), disease prone (yes!), and lacking in energy (that's me!), because my body was low on enzymes. In my imagination these tiny enzymes buzzed with electricity, galvanizing everything they touched. As I read, a tantalizing idea began to take shape in my mind. What if my parents had simply not gone far enough in their embrace of natural foods? Cooking is a form of food processing after all, and I was learning that it melted—or denatured—enzymes, while also charring nutrients into toxins. It seemed obvious that I had smothered my potential with dead food. With a raw diet, I would run like the wind.

My road to recovery was paved in sprouts. I sprouted whatever I could get my hands on: beans, almonds, radish seeds, lentils. They strained up toward the light from within old almond-butter and pickle jars. As soon as I eliminated dead foods from my diet I felt pure, fresh, and vigorous. I ran one second shy of my personal record in the 800-meter dash. It was working.

The problems started almost immediately. First, there was the fact that the sprouts were not delicious. Nibbled, they tasted great—the watery crunch of the bean sprouts, the cool burn of the radishes—but chewed in volume they amalgamated into a stringy, astringent mush. The lentils, especially, seemed wrong. The taste of springtime in the flavor—that hint of young grass bitten at the white—which is so appealing in the warmth of cooked lentils, had an overpowering pungency in their sprouts.

I cultivated that peculiar frustration that results from the union of hunger and nausea. When I was sickened by my seeds I might gnaw at a head of broccoli or bolt down handfuls of raw almonds. But when that failed to provide more then a bloaty bulk, I'd turn back, with ascetic wretchedness, to the spinach and sprouts.

My diet also took up a lot of space. I was growing more than an inch a year during high school, running hard every day, and eating a prodigious amount of food. Due to caloric demand, the sheer volume of my meals was overwhelming. It was like feeding an elephant. My windowsill gardens became a part-time hydroponics operation. I spent hours coaxing juice apart from vegetable fiber, and then hours more scrubbing the fiber from the filter of our juicing machine. The resulting drinks were watery brown and struck at the back of the tongue with a bitter wallop.

I lost weight. The other distance runners, who were not exactly chubby themselves, changed my nickname from Nature to Auschwitz. My race times, moreover, were getting worse. Boys who lived on Twinkies and soft serve were beating me. Before long, empirical evidence began to erode my newfound ideology.

As I became aware of my wretchedness, my thoughts returned to Dad's concerns. I didn't have an eating disorder in the clinical sense, but what else could I call the state of mind that made me swallow only food that made me miserable? After three weeks of negative results I decided that to keep expecting things to get better as they got progressively worse really would be a form of mental illness.

There were a lot of borderline-crazy people around Nevada City, folks who were meticulously dismissive of facts from mainstream institutions—like universities, the government, or the mass media—and blithely trusting of information from self-taught theorists, newsletter writers, and angelic-healing instructors. I didn't want to be like them. I knew from hard experience not to cough in front of these people unless I was prepared to receive a diagnosis and lecture on how burdock-root tincture could purify the kidneys. But after the three weeks, my justifications for staying on a live-food diet (e.g., "I feel rotten because I'm flushing latent toxins") were starting to sound dangerously familiar. I quietly accepted defeat and began eating cooked foods again. Mom and Dad, bless them, said nothing.

The obvious alternative would have been to intensify my regimen. I'd seen people—the parents of friends—fall into this spiral in their quest for better health, which led from one expensive alternative treatment to another, until they were swallowing handfuls of herbal supplements. These people, though they monitored their health constantly, didn't seem healthy: They seemed haunted and delicate.

If you buy the idea that you can become healthier, stronger, and faster by returning to a more primitive type of subsistence, you also have to accept its flipside: that the modern world is making you sicker, weaker, and slower. The worst part of my raw-food diet was that it made me anxious. The world had filled with new threats: Chicken drumsticks, for example, which had seemed safe by virtue of their presence in Dad's cooking repertoire, suddenly bristled with toxins. This only got worse when I started rationalizing my lack of new superpowers. Was I failing to break records because of diesel fumes I'd inhaled? Or was it the remnants of laundry detergent seeping through my skin? Instead of charging me with vitality, my diet made me fragile. I'd become an invalid, stricken by my expectation of perfect health. I was a lot happier when all those putative toxins had just tasted like chicken.

Our best tool for gauging the threats of environmental poisons and toxic chemicals, for separating real and imagined risks, and for dealing with the unknown in general is, of course, science. But science alone is woefully inadequate. In the United States, about 700 new chemicals are introduced to the market every year, most without any testing for health effects. Studying any one of these substances can consume a decade—in the last 35 years the United States has only enough assembled evidence to ban 5 chemicals. Somehow we have to make decisions with incomplete information. Vigilance is important—it's no good to be oblivious to threats. But there's a real danger in becoming blindly fearful of every supposed impurity. The real question is, to quote the farmer-poet Wendell Berry, "How does one act well—sensitively, compassionately, without irreparable damage—on the basis of *partial* knowledge?"

Though I know I'm succumbing to my native romanticism, I'll often answer that question by simply siding with whatever seems most natural. I'm more likely to worry about a supposed poison if it's the product of human meddling. I'm suspicious of chemical pesticides, phthalates (plasticizers in everyday products), and petrochemicals, but I'll happily try a wild mushroom that, if misidentified, would leave me gravely ill. To put this reflexive reaction to the test, I decided to research the toxins that occur in two very different sources: vegetables and vaccines. Both are supposed to make us healthy, but both contain trace amounts of poisons. My hope is to come up with a way of acting on partial knowledge that can assess the risk of either, rather than giving arbitrary preference to the natural or the technological.

Vaccines set off all the alarms for my people. They are manufactured by large corporations, their use has increased dramatically in recent years, and they are composed of bits of pathogens. The making of vaccines has sometimes required genetic engineering, and it has at times been a murky, trial-and-error process, requiring scientists to grow viruses in exotic tissues. Mouse lungs, chopped fetal arm tissue, and monkey kidneys have all been used, prompting one virologist to quip that the witches in Macbeth were the first to give the instructions for attenuating viruses. First: "Round the cauldron go, in the poison'd entrails throw," add "Finger of birth-strangled babe" and "Cool it with a baboon's blood." It is clear that vaccines helped stamp out diseases that used to be commonplace, but many parents—by and large intelligent, well-educated parents—no longer trust the orthodoxy on shots, and 40 percent of Americans now refuse or delay at least one immunization. So who is being blinded by their ideology: those who trust the technology, or those who fear it?

On the other side of the spectrum, nothing appears more natural and ·intuitively healthful than vegetables. But you can't trust the wisdom of plants. They may be wise, but they aren't trustworthy. While animals are masters of movement, plants are masters of chemistry. Most animals can only process the chemicals they need to survive—this is called *primary metabolism*. Plants have *secondary metabolism*—they manufacture substances that have little to do with their basic vitality. When it suits them, plants build chemicals to nourish and heal; other times, they forge toxins.

In eating so many raw vegetables I'd been dosing myself with a poisoner's pharmacopoeia: canavanine in alfalfa sprouts, oxalic acid in Swiss chard, phytohaemagglutinin in beans, glucosinolates in broccoli, and solanine in potatoes. And the fuzzy-leafed comfrey, which we'd planted outside my bedroom door and used to make poultices for sports injuries, was packed with pyrrolizidine alkaloids. In other words, the food I'd forced down in an attempt to cleanse my body was full with toxins. Okay, maybe "full" is too strong. As far as we know, most of the poisons in vegetables are so diffuse that they are completely insignificant. But we have not identified, let alone studied, most of the plant chemicals we are eating. And research from the South Pacific island Guam implies that if I had been poisoned by plants I might not know it until decades later, when accumulation of toxins began to corrode my brain. The story of this research interested me because it demonstrated the power of narrative. Stripped of narrative, the evidence from Guam pointed to an absolutely genuine and exciting avenue for research on neurodegeneration, but not a threat that should make anyone stop eating plants. In the context of a story, however, the evidence also hinted that some forms of Parkinson's, Alzheimer's, and Lou Gehrig's disease—the brain-eaters of old age—could be caused by the accumulation of vegetable poisons over a lifetime. It was only a whiff of danger, but that was sufficient for my purposes. After all, I've avoided suspected synthetic chemicals on the basis of even sketchier evidence and a well-told tale. Should I react similarly to a story about natural toxins? And if not, why not?

DANGEROUS VEGETABLES

Guam is fascinating to scientists because it is the home to something evil. Rates of Lou Gehrig's disease (known there as *lytico,* as in *paralytico*) and

Parkinson's, along with associated dementia (known there as *bodig*), are the highest on the planet. No one knows why we get these diseases as we grow old, but part of the answer must reside somewhere on this 30-mile span of coralline limestone and volcanic rock in the South Pacific.

"Guam is the one area in the world that sticks out like a sore thumb," an epidemiologist told a group of scientists assembled at the National Institutes of Health (NIH) in Bethesda, Maryland, in 1962. "In general, the rates on Guam, both as regards incidence and prevalence and death statistics, are on the order of 100 times that of any place in the world."

In the 1950s one in five of the native Chamorro people was dying of Lytico-bodig. When doctors asked the Chamorros about the cause of the disease, they related a story about forbidden fruit: Around 1815, a priest had cursed a family for stealing mangos from his tree. To this day, the story went, descendants of this family were selling the fruit at the market, and everyone who ate enough of them became ill. It seemed unlikely to scientists that mangos were the cause—people eat mangos all over the world—but as NIH epidemiologist Leonard Kurland mused, "I wonder whether, in the intervening 150 years, there may not be confusion over the type of tree." In 1954 Kurland asked Marjorie Whiting—an anthropological nutritionist who happened to be passing through Guam on her way home from a 2-year assignment on the island Pohnpei—to stay for a while, and find out what the affected families were eating.

When Whiting first set foot on Guam she had only planned to stay long enough to catch a ship headed for the United States, but she was captivated by the island's mystery. It would hold her for the rest of her life and launch an international adventure in medical research that has continued beyond her death. Whiting spent 8 months on Guam, living with a family in Umatac, a town of about 600 where neurological diseases had been causing 50 percent of villagers' deaths. She spent days sitting on front porches with old-timers, listening to their stories while sniffing for clues. In the evenings she would type her notes on index cards, recording even the most mundane details about the people who had died from Lytico-bodig. On one index card she wrote, in a phrase that must have preserved her informant's syntax, "Luisa was a mean old woman living at the end of the village, chasing children from her yard." Who knew what seemingly irrelevant recollections might later prove germane?

Whiting could charm her way into any kitchen, and she would often stay up all night preparing communal feasts alongside village women, while picking up both recipes and gossip. Increasingly, she became interested in the *fadang* flour the locals used to make tortillas. Unlike tins of sugar and wheat, which were impossible to protect from the island's abundant insects, this flour was never infested. It was made, Whiting learned, from the seed of a cycad—a palmlike plant that had persisted since the Mesozoic era—and (most interesting of all) it was poisonous unless properly processed. The people chopped up the seeds and soaked them in pails for days, changing the water every few hours. Chickens that drank this water died, villagers told Whiting. Perhaps, she guessed, her hosts were not removing all the poisons. In 1963 she published a paper showing an association between cycad eating and brain degeneration on Guam.

Of course, there were other probable causes of neurological disease besides cycad eating. But if scientists were able to identify a cycad toxin, they could then watch it as it attacked neurons, and learn the mechanics of neurodegeneration. If they were able to show how a chemical caused the neural tangles in the people on Guam, it would help them identify the remaining missing pieces of the puzzle for diseases like Parkinson's because it occurred elsewhere in the world.

Researchers had begun experimenting on cycads even before Whiting's paper was published. At the NIH conference in 1962, one scientist presented his work showing that lab animals fed cycad flour developed tumors throughout their bodies, while another explained how his team had isolated a potent toxin from the seeds. Cycads knit poison into their sugars, forming a Trojan-horse compound the scientists named *cycasin*. Cycasin is benign until something—such as digestion—breaks down the sugar and releases its payload. This was the first vegetable carcinogen ever discovered.

Those early days were heady ones for the scientists. Medical doctors powwowed with biochemists and anthropologists. Veterinarians reported that livestock grazing on cycads developed "the staggers," movements that resembled those of people with motor-neuron disease. Pathologists shared their photos of dissected brains with geneticists searching for hereditary patterns, and botanists familiar with cycad history explained that the ancient organism may have evolved poisons to fend off dinosaurs. Scientists, caught up in this creative momentum, felt free to speculate: "Maybe," one offered, "if cycads have had cycasin all this time, that is why they have survived, because there may not have been many creatures that could eat it and live." It was, in other words, the sort of investigation full of the dramatic potential that makes children fall in love with science in the first place—a wonderfully unfettered ping-ponging of ideas across disciplines that opens new vistas from which to look afresh on life's grand mysteries.

This flare of excitement, however, burned out under its own heat. Lab animals, although they developed tumors after eating cycasin, did not have the telltale tangles of ruined neurons found in human victims of neurodegeneration. And then scientists found two other clusters of brain disease in places without any known cycads: the Kii peninsula of Japan and western New Guinea. Any compelling theory would have to identify a cause of illness that existed in all of these places. Scientists working on the project packed up their notes for long-term storage.

There was one young scientist, however, who—when he examined the very facts that were causing researchers to abandon the idea—saw something compelling. Peter Spencer, a toxicologist then at the Albert Einstein Medical College, understood better than most that ostensibly healthful vegetables could lay siege to the central nervous system: He had shown that the paralytic disease lathyrism was caused by a poison in the grass pea. Similarly, when Spencer had started his lathyrism research, scientists had all but abandoned this line of inquiry because no one could re-create the disease in lab rats. The problem, Spencer demonstrated, was in the vast differences between the minds of mice and men. When he'd given grass-pea toxins to monkeys rather than rats, they'd developed lathyrism. And his grass-pea poison was nearly identical to a chemical scientists had found in cycads—one with a name (beta-N-methylamino-levoalanine) so impossibly multisyllabic that people referred to it by its acronym—BMAA.

Spencer recruited Peter Nunn, a chemist who had isolated BMAA, to try feeding it to monkeys. They lived in Spencer's house, worked late at the lab, and cooked meals together while talking through the evidence. Unlike the rats, the monkeys developed symptoms of brain degeneration within a month. Autopsies showed that the toxin had damaged the motor neurons. The monkey brains, in other words, resembled the brains of people who had died from Lou Gehrig's disease. If Spencer and Nunn had pulled off this feat 20 years earlier, they would have been heroes at the next NIH conference. But it was 1986 by the time the paper was published and, as Spencer said, "nobody but nobody had heard about this cycad idea. It had all but been forgotten, and my career was very much on the line."

When Spencer presented his research at a conference in Vancouver, scientists were dubious. Even if there were some connection between the Guam diseases and cycads, they asked, how could he explain the disease clusters in New Guinea and Japan? Spencer suggested that the people in those places might also be exposed to cycads. At that, the Nobel laureate Carlton Gajdusek rose to his feet and gave Spencer a dressing down, as if he were a schoolboy claiming that his science-fair project had invalidated the theory of relativity. Gajdusek said he didn't know about Guam, but he had received his Nobel Prize for his study of human prions, which were causing some (though not all) of the brain disease in New Guinea, and he was certain that there were no cycads there.

So Spencer went to New Guinea with his colleague Valerie Palmer, who spoke Afrikaans and could understand some of the Dutch-influenced pidgin. They took a long canoe with an outboard motor up the Ia River, toward the center of a disease cluster discovered by Gajdusek. "As we went farther up the river it also seemed we were traveling through time," Spencer said. "One village had technology from the 1950s, but by the time we got to the next we were back to the turn of the century, until we reached the Stone Age." When they arrived at a village deep in the forest, Palmer showed a group of elderly women a cycad seed. They reacted with obvious recognition and led her through the jungle to a tall tree. The villagers showed how they made a compress from the pith, which served as an antibiotic to quell infected wounds and speed healing, but (unbeknownst to them) also introduced poisons into the bloodstream. A 29-year-old with Lou Gehrig's disease explained that he had treated an open sore on his ankle with this technique for a full month, and revealed that his mother, who had taught him how to make the poultice, had had the same paralytic disease.

Shortly thereafter, Spencer received an invitation to speak in Japan. He accepted and scheduled a side trip to the Kii peninsula, again with Palmer. The Japanese scientists politely assured them that they would not find cycads, but arranged for Masayuki Ohta, a neuropathologist, to go along as a guide and interpreter. They traveled by train to Kii, a forested land east of Osaka. At their first stop, Spencer halted halfway across the parking lot, transfixed by a plant growing amid the landscaped shrubs. It was, he told Ohta, a cycad.

Ohta nodded tactfully. These plants are common, he said, but unlike the Guam cycads, they did not bear seeds. Spencer, however, was already groping among the fronds, and he triumphantly produced a strand of bright red seeds. Ohta apologized, and explained that the Japanese must not know—let alone eat—this particular plant. But when they walked into a pharmacy they found a jar of seeds prominently displayed. When Spencer went to a healer to ask about his abdominal discomfort, he received a prescription for cycad—one seed per day. And when he showed the seeds to the mother of a woman who had died from Lou Gehrig's disease, she nodded: Her daughter had taken that medicine regularly as a girl.

Spencer had silenced his doubters. *Science* magazine published his results. It was a grand success, but while he had proved the *association* of cycads and all three neurodegenerative clusters, proving *causation* in chronic disease is always devilishly hard, and the work slowed once again. The idea that small amounts of a poison could act slowly, over decades, was difficult for some scientists to accept, and there was still no way to explain how a Parkinson's patient in Montreal might be linked to this tropical plant.

Then, in 2003, scientists found a source of BMAA that was far more prevalent than cycads: blue-green algae. Blue-green algae exists just about everywhere there's water. It lives in salty oceans and freshwater ponds, in damp soil, and throughout the fur of certain animals. It springs to life when the rare desert gully-washer leaves ephemeral puddles. It blooms in reservoirs, spiking water supplies with its chemicals. And, incidentally, during my raw foods experiment, it could be found in my diet: In health stores and juice bars it's marketed as a superfood and I'd dusted it over my sprout-mash, mixed it in smoothies, and scooped it into gelatin capsules for my school lunches. It's still sold to this day, though, of course, every manufacturer claims that their blue-green algae is BMAA free.

BMAA is just one in the Scrabble deck of poisonous acronyms in cycads. Spencer estimates that there may be hundreds of such chemicals.[*] Scientists have examined about five. Every plant, including the ones we eat, contains a similar profusion of unstudied chemicals. It's only logical that, if we start looking for toxins, we will also find them in the vegetables on our plates.

---

[*] Spencer now suspects that cycasin, not BMAA, is more likely to be responsible for the Guam diseases and he continues to publish findings as the science progresses.

"Plants are not here for our good," Spencer told me when we first spoke. "They have developed chemical weapons of such sophistication they would make the men in the department of defense drool."

You could argue that because we have evolved alongside plant foods they have adapted to us, and we to them. We know that coevolution has reduced the toxins in some of our staples. But what about a slow poison? A poison that didn't cause any noticeable harm until humans reached the age of 65 or 70—after the reproductive years and, for much of history, after most people died of other causes? Coevolution wouldn't exert much leverage on something like that.

It's possible that those of us who feel our healthful glow increase when forking down vegetables are instead chewing our way into their ranks, increasing with every bite the concentration of the neurotoxin marinade sloshing around our brainpans. This is entirely speculative, but it is also relevant in light of the aversion many feel to the equally speculative dangers of manufactured food additives, genetically modified organisms, and hormone-juiced dairy cows. Of course, even without this layer of speculation, the cycad hypothesis has its doubters.

"I think it's plausible, but a lot of people, including me, don't think it's the explanation [for the neurodegeneration]," says Bruce Miller, who studies Alzheimer's and dementia at University of California, San Francisco. Miller has great respect for Spencer but thinks there just aren't enough cycad poisons in food to cause the disease. Nonetheless, even skeptics are drawn to Guam in hopes of finding clues, and Miller, whose work focuses on genetic causes of neurodegenerative disease, visited the island in 2011. He was struck by the fact that the prevalence of disease had dramatically decreased since the 1950s. This reinforced scientists' suspicion that a disappearing environmental factor was spreading the illnesses.

"There's really only two explanations. A genetic shift, i.e., carriers of the genes are less likely to reproduce, or there's an environmental factor—there has to be an environmental factor. But it seems to be disappearing, and we may not figure it out before it's too late."

In some ways this idea—that there probably is something out there trying to eat our brains, but we have no clue what it is—is even more frightening than the hypothesis that one or two toxins found in cycads are causing dementia. The problem is an utter lack of certainty. We have very little understanding of how any given compound, whether organic or synthetic, affects the human body over the course of a lifetime. Spencer has proposed that a worthy goal for science would be the identification and removal of all harmful toxins from our diet (by the invention of synthetic foods if necessary), but that's a project decades, if not centuries, from completion. And I can't wait that long for dinner.

The Yolngu Solution

All this brought me back to my original dilemma: How does a reasonable person make choices when forced to act without certainty? If nature is trying to poison me should I be eating some ultraprocessed pabulum instead of sprouts? When I asked Spencer how he handled this problem, he chuckled.

"I eat fairly normally," he said. "I enjoy my vegetables." He paused considering, then cleared his throat lightly. "Look, there's no point running away until we know in which direction we should be running."

Instead of fomenting panic, Spencer would like to see his work spur a search to find where the specific cycad chemicals shown to cause neurodegeneration occur. These chemicals may be found not just in vegetables, he said, but in any number of environmental sources. Identifying these sources could be the key to a dramatic reduction in Alzheimer's dementia and Lou Gehrig's disease. As for the larger threat of poisonous unknowns in vegetables, Spencer said, it would be irresponsible to advise people to change their lifestyles based on such limited information. Though we are surrounded by poisons of all sorts, for the most part humans have evolved to cope with them.

These words became a source of comfort. When a headline proclaiming the toxicity of some previously unremarkable chemical beckoned me toward anxiety, I remembered that humans are tough: We evolved surrounded by poisons, and not just the accidental toxins we manufacture today, but poisons honed over millions of years by plants to sabotage the cellular machinery of their tormentors.

Spencer suggested that if I was interested in the problem of making decisions without clear scientific guidance, the example of the Australian Aborigines might be enlightening. He had flown to Groot Island off northern Australia when he had heard that there were cycads and a few cases of unusual neurological diseases there. But he'd been disappointed: Unlike Lou Gehrig's disease, this particular form of disease was entirely hereditary, and unrelated to the cycads. In Australia, at least, the people were able to eat cycads while avoiding its neurotoxins.

The people native to northern Australia have long relied on cycads for starch, but rather than simply soaking seeds, like the Chamorros of Guam, the Australians employ more precise methods. One procedure requires people to shell the seeds, crush them, then soak them in running water for a week. They next grind the seeds into a paste, wrap this in paperbark, and roast it in the coals of a fire for about an hour. Archeologist Wendy Beck observed that the Yolngu group, in northern Australia, are able to sense the presence of poisons. Only the respected elderly women are allowed to touch the cycads. They gather fallen seeds (the Yolngu call these older seeds *munbuwa*), shake them next to their ears, crack them open, sniff them, and crumble the kernels between their fingers. They reject about half the seeds they gather, and eat the rest. Assays of the rejected seeds found significant levels of the poison cycasin, while those selected contained none. Beck wrote, "it is clear that *munbuwa* preparation requires considerable intellectual 'know how,' together with the necessary skills of discrimination of the toxic factors. These discriminatory powers are extremely important and may well prove to have a genetic basis."

All this is somewhat mystical given that scientists are just now beginning to identify cycad poisons in our environment. It is also tantalizing for someone like me, searching for a better way to separate the healthful and harmful. How could a Stone Age culture learn to remove poisons from its food hundreds of years before Western scientists even knew it existed? When I put that question to John Bradley, an anthropologist who works with Australian Aborigines, he said, "They would tell you that they learned it in the Dreaming."

I wondered aloud what he meant.

"Well, that's tricky," he said. "From the point of view of a Western academic like me, that probably refers to the knowledge that accumulates when a group of people has been living with a community of plants and animals since the Pleistocene. But the people I work with in northern Australia might say that it is knowledge the cycad communicated directly to the people."

Some scholars have suggested that this communication with plants is made possible by their ingestion during shamanic rituals. These are plants—like the Australian desert shrub pituri—that do not kill, but poison just enough to allow people to enter a zone between life and death, a twilight zone of recoverable toxicity, or intoxication. The notion that intoxicated humans have access to a vault of knowledge off-limits to the waking mind dates back at least to the oracles at Delphi. It's an idea buttressed by the fact that almost every religion seeks knowledge through some form of altered consciousness—whether that altered consciousness is delivered by the grace of pharmacology or meditation. Within our own scientific tradition there are many famous examples of breakthroughs occurring when the conscious mind is stilled: Dmitry Mendeleyev saw the arrangement of the periodic table in a dream, August Kekulé realized the structure of a benzene ring after seeing the image of a snake biting its own tail in his fire, Otto Loewi dreamed his experiment for verifying the chemical transmission of nerve impulses, and several of Albert Einstein's revelations came in the form of visions rather than words or numbers. But perhaps the emphasis should not be on intoxication, but instead simply on a changed frame of mind. Aborigines rely on dance and art for their sorcery more than on pituri, and even that contains nothing more powerful than nicotine. And the insights delivered on the wings of dreams or drugs are creative rearrangements of information already present in the mind rather than the introduction of new information delivered via plant-crafted chemicals.

If the understanding of how to detoxify cycads is empirical, it wouldn't be surprising that it was passed down in the language of the supernatural, rather than the scientific metaphors we are used to. The hard line between bodily and spiritual health, after all, is an invention of the Western imagination, and a recent one at that. When the Hebrews divined the dangers of porcine trichinosis and the benefits of hand washing, they enshrined the resulting rules alongside the Ten Commandments, never thinking to separate the laws that guard against physical and moral dangers.

The ability to detect cycad poisons, however it was derived, has required a continuity of culture to persist. For the Yolngu, the concept of Dreaming is related to the Dreamtime, a heroic era of distant past, whence come their traditions. The health of the people, they say, depends on the maintenance of relations with this history. The Chamorros in Guam, by contrast, have only the most tenuous of links to their ancestral past. The Spanish, during their colonial rule of the island, eradicated Chamorro culture with systematic gusto. Between 1670 and 1710, soldiers extinguished 99 percent of the natives. Those who remained were turned over to the missionaries, who plowed under the old gods and traditions to prepare a fruitful harvest for Christ. But in burying the old ways, the Spanish were also burying a repository of knowledge. Perhaps the tradition of cycad eating persisted, while the nuances of preparation were lost.

In fact, every culture has developed some version of Yolngu poison control, better known as cooking. And though this common detoxification procedure we see practiced every day does not seem so astonishing, it deserves a measure of veneration. In addition to transforming the dull into the delicious, the culinary arts are often sophisticated techniques for coaxing nourishment from what is otherwise inedible, or deadly. The simple act of heating food kills bacteria, tenderizes fibers, and—most interestingly for my purposes—breaks down many vegetable poisons.

Cooking is a human universal. Although almost every cultural group eats raw foods on occasion, no one has ever documented a case of a people with an exclusively raw diet (aside from the modern enthusiasts). The Inuit in the Arctic eat raw whale blubber (*muktuk*) and occasionally raw fish, but they usually prefer seal stew or roasted caribou. Even chimpanzees, when given both raw and cooked food at the same time, prefer the cooked.

Compared to the great apes, humans have small mouths and dainty teeth. We have relatively small stomachs and shorter large intestines. These are all features one would expect to see in a species that had evolved eating a soft, high-energy cuisine. Our bodies have been molded on the armature of processed foods. We are also missing the massive muscles that wrapped from the crests on top of our ancestors' skulls down to their jaws, which would have allowed for better rending of raw foods. As brains expanded, these muscles—and the skull crests to which they attached—disappeared. It's unclear if these two changes are connected: Some scientists have suggested that the skull had to be released from this muscular vise in order to allow brain growth, but there are problems with the hypothesis. What is clear, however, is that as our forebears evolved they grew larger brains, became literally less meat-headed, and learned to process food while mastering those first Promethean flames.

According to the myth, Zeus had given Prometheus and his brother Epimetheus the clay to make humans and animals, plus a lot of exciting features: claws and prehensile tails, armored shells, venomous stingers, and, of course, big crushing jaws. Epimetheus, enthralled by the challenge of designing creatures with these features, used them all up before Prometheus even finished the delicate task of molding humans. And that's why Prometheus, feeling sorry for his defenseless creations, stole us some embers from the divine fires. We may not have the fancy hardware, but we can cook.

Cooking, argues primatologist Richard Wrangham in his book, *Catching Fire,* is the crucial innovation that separated our ancestors from the apes, and made us human. Considered in that light, the old flickering light of savanna campfires, food processing looks utterly natural. If, as a teenager, I had thought of cooking not as a corruption of nature but as an ancient tradition, I would never have become a sproutarian. And, as Wrangham points out, if I'd cooked my lentil sprouts, my body would have been able to unlock a far greater percentage of their energy. (Of course, easy access to caloric energy is the opposite of what most people need these days, which is why raw-food diets, though by no means natural, are such a brilliant corrective for many.)

Frustratingly, none of this changed my tendency to turn toward nature whenever I entered a grocery store: When I held two jars of peanut butter next to each other there was no clear way to determine which might be harmful. Sure, I could look at the ingredients and nutrition facts, but the more I learned about nutrition, the less meaningful those numbers became. And in this particular case the only difference between the peanut butters was that one contained palm oil[*] and the other didn't—was the oil separation a sign of virtue? I'd like to be able to take a product off the shelf, shake it, sniff it like a Yolngu elder, and be able to determine if it was good for me. I still tended to trust those products with a certain natural aura emanating from the jar. I suspected that this aura (like all auras probably) was actually the sum of a collection of signs—marketing, in other words. Was there some common element in the labels and product design of cod-liver oil, artisan-baked bread, echinacea powder, Dr. Bronner's Soap, and Tom's of Maine, sending me subliminal assurances?

---

[*] You may have heard something about palm oil being unhealthy, or healthy. We really don't know. It has got a lot of saturated fat, but less than butter. And though conventional wisdom holds that saturated fat is evil, this is still a hazy area of science.

FREE-RANGE ORGANIC TOXINS

As I was wrestling with this, a friend gave me an article from the *New England Journal of Medicine,* published in 2007, that helped crystallize the paradox. The paper described the findings of a group of scientists who had taken it upon themselves to track down the toxins that were causing pre-pubescent boys (between the ages of 4 and 10) to develop breasts. All these boys, the scientists discovered, had been exposed to chemicals found in cosmetics and personal-care products, which appeared to disrupt the endocrine system, interfering with normal sex-hormone signaling. What surprised me was that these chemicals were not some synthetic stew formed through the amalgamation of antiperspirants, shampoo, and body wash. They came instead from lavender and tea-tree oils. When the researchers exposed breast-tissue cells to these oils in the lab, it stimulated the cells' estrogen receptors and inhibited the androgen receptors. As soon as the boys' parents stopped rubbing these ointments on their chests, the breasts melted away.

I consider both lavender and tea-tree oil to be natural products. I never imagined that they could also be toxic endocrine disruptors. The first bottle of essential oil I turned up (conveniently located in my own medicine cabinet, near my lavender soap), was made of brown glass and had a purple label bearing a sunburst in the even geometry of a quilt pattern. On the label, the words TEA TREE OIL were printed in a font reminiscent of Japanese calligraphy. It looked like a tincture Laura Ingalls Wilder might have used, with a splash of new—agey Asian sauce. The product design assured me that it was made by a small company, staffed (I imagined) by friendly people, and located in the next county over.

My affinity for this rustic aesthetic didn't come from a desire to do away with modernity but a distrust of things made in ways I did not understand, by people I did not know, employed by profit-driven corporations. In some ways, I was more disconnected from cultural knowledge than the Chamorros. I was cut off, not by genocide, but by the span of international transportation and the pace of technological change, which has outstripped the speed of cultural adaptation. My environment was filled with things I didn't understand. There was very little knowledge passed down from my parents that could tell me if lavender oil, or Chinese-made baby formula, or the chemicals in my shampoo were going to hurt me. All I could do was look for products reminiscent of a simpler time.

Humans have always been technological beings, but until the last few centuries most forms of technology came with a set of cultural regulations that had been discovered through trial and error and passed on to the next generation. When my father taught me to chop wood, for example, a lot of his instruction had to do with protecting myself from the axe. Now that children teach their parents how to use technology rather than vice versa, we turn to science (or pseudoscience) for answers. And science can't keep up with the questions it raises.

In this fast-evolving age, where few technologies come with cultural knowledge, I sometimes feel like an old man who no longer fully comprehends his surroundings. Usually I'm resigned and compliant, doing as I am told even if I don't understand why, but sometimes I become frightened and unruly, lashing out blindly. For the most part, people employ the former mode to deal with being surrounded by unknowns. We hope that the experts in charge are capable, and cross our fingers. But when people of a curious frame of mind begin to poke around a little bit—enough to discover cases in which the authorities didn't know what they were doing, or were motivated by greed—they can easily shift to the latter mode. We become suspicious of the establishment, prone to conspiracy theories, and if we aren't careful, we start hanging around health-food stores and offering unsolicited advice.

Surely there must be a better way, some method of assessing the healthfulness of the world around us without either blind acceptance of official dicta, or descent into paranoia. Exhaustive research—understanding the details of exactly what we do and do not know—certainly helps, but even those writing books on the subject don't have the leisure to delve into the intricacies of every dilemma. If we are to take the Yolngu solution the question becomes, how do we construct the cultural tools to handle the pace of change?

THE GREAT VACCINE FREAK-OUT

There's probably nothing that more efficiently divides the blindly com-pliant and the blindly fearful than vaccination. Like cycads, vaccines have the potential to both sustain life and end it. Their utility depends utterly on the skill of the people who prepare them, and their acceptance depends on how completely the public trusts those people.

Vaccines entered Western medicine in 1796, when a country doctor in Berkeley, England, named Edward Jenner began deliberately infecting people with cowpox. Jenner was convinced by the folklore of rural Eng-land, which held that those who were exposed to cowpox by working with livestock could not contract smallpox. This belief followed from the readily visible evidence—the phrase "milkmaid complexion" alludes not to milky-white skin, but to cheeks unscarred by the lesions of smallpox. Vaccines train an immune system by exposing it to a small amount of weakened or dead microbes (in Jenner's case the cowpox worked like an attenuated version of smallpox). The immune system learns to recognize and attack the viruses, and it retains this memory for many years— sometimes a lifetime. For much of history the choice to vaccinate was an easy one, because the diseases they prevented were so common and so debilitating. In 1952 there were 21,000 cases of paralytic polio. After Jonas Salk created the first polio vaccine in 1955, infections dropped precipitously. Now vaccination is a victim of its own success: There have been no documented cases of polio in the United States since 1993, and to some the risk of the immunization has begun to look greater than the risk of the disease.

My parents didn't make a deliberate decision to have us kids inoc-ulated because opting out just never occurred to them. Though the vaccination controversy had flourished in Nevada City for some time, I only began to pay attention as an adult, around 2004, when stories about the immunization fight were regularly making news. I was drawn to the idea that, by avoiding once-routine diseases like chicken pox, humans were messing with the natural order of things. Then *Rolling Stone* published a piece by Robert F. Kennedy Jr. making the case that thimerosal, a mercury preservative in vaccines, was causing autism. I didn't know much about Kennedy, but I respected him: I knew he was an environmentalist with a track record of legitimate public policy work. He seemed like the kind of guy who understood science, but not someone with his face so close to the petri dish that he missed the big picture. Kennedy's smoking gun was a study by Tom Verstraeten, an epidemiologist at the U.S. Centers for Disease Control and Prevention, who had analyzed the medical records of 100,000 children. It showed thimerosal, Kennedy wrote, "to be responsible for a dramatic increase in autism and a host of other neurological disorders among children." According to Kennedy, Verstraeten then cited "the staggering number of earlier studies that indicate a link between thimerosal and speech delays, attention-deficit disorder, hyperactivity and autism."

The problem seemed to be that, while individual vaccines were safe, no one had stopped to ask what their cumulative affect would be as their numbers increased. Only recently had anyone noticed that the amount of mercury children received via injections was higher than the Environmental Protection Agency's (EPA) maximum recommended exposure via ingestion. The EPA guidelines referred specifically to methylmercury, and the ethylmercury in thimerosal was thought to be less toxic, but no one really knew.

Around the same time I read that the *Lancet,* probably the second most prestigious medical journal in the world after the *New England Journal of Medicine,* had withdrawn the seminal paper linking autism and vaccines. That paper, by London gastroenterologist Andrew Wakefield, had hypothesized that the measles, mumps, and rubella, or MMR, vaccine led to inflammatory bowel disease, which in turn led to autism. Ten of Wakefield's 12 coauthors had repudiated the work, saying that because the paper hadn't actually presented adequate evidence of a vaccine–autism link, they shouldn't have proposed a hypothesis that could scare people away from immunization. I didn't agree with this repudiation: I thought scientists should be free to discuss ideas and publish new hypotheses without fear of the consequences.

Then I forgot about the issue until a friend from Nevada City, Thea Chroman, asked me for help in researching immunizations for her baby. I didn't get to know Thea until we'd both left Nevada City. She was a young reporter, recruited to KALW, the public radio station in San Francisco where I was working. She'd show up in cat's-eye glasses and retro thrift-store outfits, always brushing a stray bit of brown hair out of her face. She had a gentle manner and an easy smile, but also possessed that essential quality for journalists: the innate tendency to convert frustration into steely determination. She was pretty, with large, slightly wide-set eyes that gave her—in certain lights—an uncanny resemblance to the elfish puppet in the film *The Dark Crystal,* an image that she self-mockingly used as her Facebook avatar.

Thea had grown up on the Ridge—the local appellation for a smattering of homesteads, communes, marijuana farms, and spiritual communities in the hills and hollows around the San Juan Ridge, about a half hour drive from Nevada City on winding roads. The area's truly committed back-to-the-landers settled on the Ridge, and while I sometimes accused my parents of taking half measures, Thea's family was the real deal. They lived completely off the grid, relying on a propane tank for heat, a pair of solar panels for intermittent electricity, and an outhouse for sewage. In the summers, Thea would ride her pony, Silver Pearl, four miles to Mother Truckers, the Ridge's general store, for Popsicles. The family only ate meat that they had killed, and Thea's mom sometimes hunted their neighbor's (annoyingly loud) peacocks with a bow and arrow. As part of their all-natural program, the family opted to trust the old process of acquiring immunity by weathering disease, rather than by vaccinating their children.

Like me (and like all children, I suppose), Thea became skeptical of her parents' philosophy as she grew older, especially after she was diagnosed with Hodgkin's lymphoma in 2003, at the age of 21. At the Stanford University hospital Thea received radiation, chemotherapy, and an abiding respect for the curative facility of conventional medicine. The doctors told her that no one died of Hodgkin's anymore, but the experience shook her already teetering confidence in natural living.

"I mean, I got cancer when I was 21," she told me. "What did my mom think she had protected me from?" Then she checked herself. "That's not entirely rational, but I was mad."

By 2009, Thea and her partner Ocean were living above Lake Merritt in Oakland, and ready to have a baby (it was a committed relationship of the why-continue-senseless-patriarchal-tradition-of-marriage? subtype). When she got pregnant, she started thinking about vaccinations right away. "I wanted to be informed, but I was pretty open," she said. "I kind of assumed it would be a fun little research project and the variables would all make sense and the answers would be clear."

At her first prenatal visit with a pediatrician Thea asked him to tell her about the arguments for and against the various vaccines, but the doctor balked. He muttered something about professional rules limiting what he could tell her. "What I'm supposed to say is that the baby should get them all," he said. "But you're the parent so you can do whatever you want." This was less than satisfying.

Thea had the opposite problem when she turned to the Internet. Instead of laboring to wring out droplets of information, she found herself submerged in a flood of inexpert opinion. There were blogs dominated by picayune, bile-fueled rants; slick, corporate-looking sites, which glibly dismissed concerns about vaccines; and dozens of forums full of worried people and misinformation.

To make matters worse, there were stories in the news every week about how the swine flu was killing pregnant women and their babies. In the first 4 months of the outbreak, 28 pregnant women had died. These stories were terrifying, and even Thea's mom (who had ardently opposed vaccination at the outset) began to quaver. Thea didn't want to make a decision based on anecdotes, but there didn't seem to be any clear way of weighing the risks. After agonizing for weeks, she made up her mind. When her doctor received a delivery of the swine-flu vaccine, she went in for a shot. It was easy: the businesslike nurse, the alcohol swab, the jab. So little after all that. But then, immediately afterward the nurse picked up another syringe and asked, "You want the regular flu shot too?"

Thea considered. She hadn't thought about getting a second shot. Before she responded, the nurse buried the needle in her arm.

Failure to gain consent is no great crime if you assume that vaccination is harmless, and even Thea had laughed bemusedly when telling me the story the next day. But she was also annoyed. The episode seemed like an extension of a campaign to bully, coerce, and scare her into toeing the line. There will always be a certain percentage of people who react poorly when told to stop asking questions and follow orders. If someone would just trust her with objective information, she'd make a reasoned decision, Thea said, exasperated.

We met at a café to talk and start trying to figure out who was right in this debate. By that time, Thea was 8 months pregnant and big enough that every trip to the counter through the cozily spaced tables required a rearrangement of furniture. We pulled a table up to her belly, and opened our laptops. What Thea really wanted to know was how risky the vaccines actually were. She wasn't so concerned about thimerosal, because childhood vaccines no longer contained it—all except some flu shots, and she could just ask for the mercury-free one. We started by looking at what the authorities had to say.

The CDC Web site on vaccines plainly stated that immunizations were not risk free: Sometimes serious, even deadly, side effects occurred.

But these risks were also contextualized with data from the randomized clinical trials used to test vaccines. A child's risk of brain inflammation after receiving the MMR vaccine was 1 in 1,000,000. The risk of death after catching measles itself, by comparison, was 1 in 500. The risk of death was 1 in 1,500 for a child who contracted pertussis, 1 in 20 for diphtheria, 1 in 5 for tetanus. On the vaccine side, there had been no reported deaths after the diphtheria, tetanus, and acellular pertussis shot. And the risk of brain damage after this TDaP injection was less than 1 in 2,000,000. A child is 200 times more likely to be struck by lightning. Furthermore, the suspicious injuries counted after vaccination could have been caused by something else; for instance, the odds are greater that a infant will be the victim of a homicide two weeks after a shot.

Despite this reassurance, it still seemed likely to me that the CDC officials were missing something, or failing to count subtle side effects. It seemed, moreover, unnecessarily violent to give babies so many shots. Kids sometimes receive five vaccines in a single appointment, and a total of 26 inoculations before the age of 2. When we looked up the recommended vaccination schedule, I was frankly shocked. My own immunization card had slots for seven vaccines. Thea's son's card would have 16 slots.

"So for instance this," Thea said pointing at the schedule, "Why is hepatitis B recommended at birth?"

Hepatitis B is usually transmitted via unprotected sex and dirty syringes. It also seemed strange that there was a vaccine for chicken pox, a disease that I thought of as an inevitable part of childhood. When I asked Thea what she was worried about, she shrugged. Not autism necessarily—she'd read about Wakefield being debunked—but she'd heard maybe there was some association between immunizations and allergies. Or something about overloading the immune system with antigens. Really, she didn't have anything specific, just a nebulous, free-floating fear that she wanted to pin down and assess. We weren't the only ones with reservations—a 2011 survey found that 77 percent of parents had some concerns about vaccination.

THE ROOTS OF SUSPICION

Two vaccine scandals in two decades had launched a cycle of suspicion. The first, in 1982, was triggered by a television documentary called *Vaccine Roulette*. The documentary was an example of sensationalist excess, but it also correctly identified a problem: A small number of children screamed uncontrollably for hours, or had seizures, after receiving the pertussis (also called whooping cough) shot. This vaccine was made with the whole bacterial cell, and it caused more adverse reactions than any other shot. There were allegations of children suffering brain damage, even dying after the immunization. The vaccine was a good one—it had helped reduced the incidence of pertussis by a factor of 157 since the 1930s. And there was scant evidence that the vaccine had caused the more severe brain injuries, but the rumor altered the nation's psychic weather enough to allow the flowering of fear. The public concern forced a response.

After some foot-dragging, pharmaceutical companies found a way to produce a safer—less reactive—shot (the acellular pertussis vaccine now used in the TDaP). In addition, the government created a special court designed to compensate families of children injured by vaccines, and the U.S. Centers for Disease Control and Prevention began ramping up its system for catching future reactions to shots. Despite these measures, people were spooked. Small whooping cough outbreaks began to occur as some parents opted to forgo the shot.

The next wave of reaction began with the publication of Wakefield's *Lancet* article in 1998, proposing a link between the MMR vaccine and autism. Then, in 1999, U.S. Food and Drug Administration scientists calculated that, in the first 6 months of life, the mercury children were getting from injections was higher than the EPA limit. The ultimate fear was that thimerosal might damage developing brains and cause the autism-like symptoms seen in some children exposed to high levels of methylmercury (scientists soon learned that the ethylmercury in vaccines was about four times less toxic than methylmercury). Oddly, the mercury hypothesis became entangled with Wakefield's MMR hypothesis, though the MMR vaccine never contained mercury of any kind.

By the time Thea and I began our research these scandals were old news and, with the benefit of hindsight, neither looked like an argument for abandoning vaccines. Children were certainly exposed to more mercury than they needed to be. Others may have even died unnecessarily for lack of an acellular pertussis vaccine.* But vaccination has always required the weighing of relative risk, and in the grand balance of total lives marred and saved, these cases barely made a blip.

As the years had passed, Wakefield's paper fell apart. In 2004, the investigative journalist Brian Deer showed that Wakefield had altered or fabricated his results. Deer also dug up documents proving that Wakefield was being paid by a law firm to produce evidence with which to sue vaccine makers, and that he had a financial stake in a competing vaccine.

What about Robert F. Kennedy Jr.'s slam-dunk evidence that thimerosal caused autism? It turned out to be almost entirely exaggeration. According to Kennedy, Verstraeten's numbers showed that thimerosal "appeared to be responsible for a dramatic increase in autism and a host of other neurological disorders among children," but actually Verstraeten's data just showed a slight trend that didn't even reach the level of statistical significance. Kennedy wrote that Verstraeten then cited "the staggering number of earlier studies that indicate a link between thimerosal . . . and autism." But the transcript of the meeting shows that he cited just a handful of studies—all on methylmercury, not thimerosal. There simply weren't any studies linking thimerosal to autism to cite—they didn't exist. Every credible study after that exonerated thimerosal. Most convincing of all was the fact that, after mercury was removed from childhood shots, autism rates continued to rise.

---

* The best examination of the old, whole cell pertussis vaccine—performed in the United Kingdom where socialized medicine does a better job of tracking injuries—estimated the risk for death or serious injury was 1 for every 310,000 shots. Children who got the disease rather than the vaccine were more likely to have seizures, and brain damage, and they were far more likely to die.

The most surprising thing I learned about the grass-roots struggle to force authorities to get thimerosal out of vaccines was that it was largely irrelevant. The authorities had acted before the movement had started: In 1999, when it was revealed that the combined load of mercury exceeded EPA guidelines, officials opted to err on the side of caution. They moved quickly. In just over a week after learning of the problem they asked vaccine makers to phase out thimerosal and advised pediatricians to delay some shots so as to minimize infant exposure. It looked like the authorities were actually doing a pretty good job. So why did people like Thea and me feel this innate suspicion?

There's a pattern that repeats itself throughout the history of inoculation: A flowering of vaccine fear needs first legitimate concerns based on real dangers; second, demagogues who use pseudoscience to magnify those dangers; and third, members of the medical establishment who defensively refuse to admit that any danger could possibly exist. The flat denials from drug makers and public health officials have frequently heightened fears rather than putting them to rest, observed Arthur Allen in *Vaccine,* his book on this history. In describing the efforts of smallpox vaccinators in the United States around the turn of the century, Allen wrote, "Medicine was not powerful enough to be self-critical, so it persisted in its blinkered unanimity: whatever the dangers and drawbacks of vaccinating, it had to be done, unquestioningly."

For those interested in avoiding the repetition of history it's worth noting that this approach didn't work so well. In fact, this lockstep mentality galvanized the nascent antivaccination movement. Medical officials who stopped up their ears against dissent were also deaf to legitimate warnings and found themselves in the unfortunate position of having to hide or explain true dangers. Public-health workers gave immunizations by force with the help of hired toughs (one unfortunate laborer was caught and vaccinated three times in as many months). And the mistakes began to pile up. In 1895 renowned doctor Walter Reed found pathogens contaminating syringes of the six largest pharmaceutical companies. In 1903 Edward Martin, head of Philadelphia's health bureau, performed trials of smallpox vaccines and found that only 1 in 10 worked. And in 1904 bacteriologist Joseph McFarland filed a report showing that one pharmaceutical company had rushed contaminated vaccines through production and in doing so, had given patients tetanus along with their shots.

These disclosures hurt the smallpox campaign, but they were also the first steps in proving that vaccinators were capable of honesty and self-criticism in the face of unfortunate facts. These qualities were personified by C.P. Wertenbaker, a federal public health official whose story was unearthed by historian Michael Willrich.

"As smallpox raged across the American South," Willrich wrote, "Wertenbaker journeyed to small communities and delivered speech after speech on vaccinations before swelling audiences of townsfolk, farmers and families. He listened and replied to people's fears. He told them about the horrors of smallpox. He candidly presented the latest scientific information about the benefits and risks of vaccination. And he urged his audiences to protect themselves and one another by taking the vaccine. By the time he was done, many of his listeners were already rolling up their sleeves."

Wertenbaker's principal tools were respect and humility. Instead of dismissing those who were suspicious of public health orthodoxy, he approached them as equals. He acknowledged the limits of medical knowledge and responded frankly to fears and criticism. And the public, when treated like intelligent adults, responded in kind.

The relationship between vaccinators and the public further improved as years passed, especially when soldiers began to come home from World War II. The GIs had witnessed the power of vaccines in their theaters of combat. In 1942, for instance, 60,000 Algerians died in a typhus outbreak, while not a single one of the half-million vaccinated U.S. soldiers in North Africa was felled by the disease.

Back in the United States it became clear that medicine had grown confident enough to admit its failures after two scandals involving the polio vaccine. First, sloppiness at the company Cutter Laboratories in 1955 led to the inclusion of virulent polio (rather than the inactivated viruses) in the vaccine, killing 10 and paralyzing 164 people. Then, in 1960, scientists found that a monkey virus was hitchhiking in some polio vaccines. In both cases, the whistleblowers were asked to pipe down by pharmaceutical representatives. But something fundamental had shifted in the scientific establishment, and these grumblers were overruled: Cutter was driven out of the vaccine business and the monkey viruses were quickly eliminated. Medicine had risen from its defensive crouch.

TRUST

When Thea gave birth to her son, Silas, she still hadn't entirely made up her mind about inoculations. She wanted an expert to thoroughly explain the rumors. Someone trustworthy who could say, for instance, "Okay, here's what you might have heard about formaldehyde in vaccines. Here's the real deal. Here's the evidence." She was reminded that the hepatitis B vaccine was recommended at birth only when a nurse asked permission to give it to her new baby. Things were pretty hazy for her at that moment, after 18 hours in labor. Someone reassured her that the vaccine was one of the safest out there, and that when babies caught the disease it was really, really bad. She still didn't understand how Silas might contract a sexually transmitted disease that she didn't have, but she was too exhausted to ask for an explanation.

In reality there is only a tiny risk that babies will contract hepatitis B unless someone in their family has the disease. From 1984 to 1992, infants were only immunized if their mothers tested positive for hepatitis. The rationale for universal immunization (which began in 1992) had to do with stigma: Few adults have the gumption to sign up for a shot that mainly protects those who engage in promiscuous sex or illegal-drug use. Giving every baby the vaccination solved this problem. But it also forced doctors explaining the shot into a tight spot. It was easier to gloss over the details—to deceive parents a tiny bit—than to make the argument for the larger common good. The introduction of two more vaccines—for chicken pox in 1995, and rotavirus (the common illness normally identified as stomach flu) in 1998—compounded this problem. Like hepatitis B, both these vaccines eventually* proved to be safe and effective, but their introduction made even some vaccine enthusiasts ask if they weren't using a sledgehammer to swat flies. All three immunizations raised complex public-health questions that were hard to sort out in a 15-minute doctor's appointment.

Of course, Thea had just experienced something far more profound than a hurried checkup. In a few hours, she'd gained the kind of trust for the medical professionals around her that would have taken years of office visits to develop.

"I was in awe of the nurses and doctors who had delivered Sy, and who were handling him with such confidence," she said. "It seemed impossible and, frankly, crazy to question them at that time. I was so grateful."

She was elated, and at the same time, terrified by the sudden realness of this strange, helpless creature, whose well-being now depended on her choices. When a nurse pressed again about the vaccine she just nodded.

When she parted company with those doctors and nurses, that trust disappeared. She hadn't found a pediatrician she liked, and when the time came for Silas's first set of shots 2 months later, Thea's lingering doubts and unanswered questions coalesced into implacable fear. The inoculation date came and went without a visit to the doctor.

---

* There were 112 cases of intussusception (a painful, sometimes fatal, condition in which the bowels bunch up on themselves) among the 1,200,000 children who got the RotaShield vaccine. This was slightly higher than the baseline rate at which infants are admitted to the hospital for intussusception, and the CDC pulled RotaShield out of use in 1999, less than a year after it was released. In 2006 a new vaccine, RotaTeq, was released. It has proved to be a safe immunization.

"I just had this gut horror at the thought of sticking up this tiny critter and pumping him full of crap," Thea said. "He just seemed way too vulnerable."

It wasn't until months later, after the family had moved to Eugene, Oregon, that Thea made another appointment. The office was in a prefabricated mobile unit surrounded by warehouses and lumberyards. Inside it was clean and bright. The doctor was good-looking: tall, thin blond hair, blue eyes, square jaw.

Thea nervously disclosed her reservations and mentioned a book on the subject that she'd liked by Bob Sears, a pediatrician from Southern California whose parents had written a series of popular books on attachment parenting. The doctor snorted. Sears was a quack, he told her. "The research in that book is seriously flawed," he said. "I don't even know if the studies he cites are valid."

It was a perplexing reaction. Thea was sure she hadn't been taken in by some self-styled guru peddling vaccine fear. Sears's *The Vaccine Book* had seemed balanced and practical.

There are some real problems with *The Vaccine Book*. Sears could have done a better job of drawing a distinction between the concerns backed by evidence, and those based on anecdote. He often elided correlation with causation (though he did briefly explain that many supposed side effects probably have nothing to do with vaccines). And sometimes he got his facts plainly wrong, warning—for example—that vaccines are not tested as thoroughly as drugs, when vaccines are tested far more rigorously. At times Sears came across as an enthusiastic cub reporter who hadn't bothered to interview all the experts, rather than one of those experts himself. Still, this informality was attractive. It provided a sense of the man behind the words, rather than some guarded, clinical stranger in a lab coat. Moreover, the book was genuinely helpful. It explained the dangers of the diseases, addressed each rumor, and described the rationale for taking each vaccine. It offered evidence instead of assurances.

Thea had been delighted to find in Sears a doctor who would address her concerns directly, and so she was baffled and upset by the effect of Sears's name. But her doctor may have read a well-circulated critique by rotavirus vaccine creator Paul Offit, which pointed out Sears's mistakes, and was convinced that the book was worthless.

Thea's doctor took a deep breath and drew himself together. "Look," he said, leaning in close. "I understand it's scary." He smiled. "But listen: Vaccines prevent diseases. They are necessary, and they are safe. You really, *really* don't have anything to worry about." He called for the nurse to prepare the shots.

"I wish I was the type of person who could have just gotten up and walked out," Thea said. Instead, she sat and watched Silas getting the injections, feeling about as benighted and helpless as the doctor seemed to think she was.

Thea hadn't gone looking for someone to pander to her, or to dignify false fears. She'd only hoped to find a pediatrician who would be a guide to help her come to an informed decision. Instead, two doctors (one in Oakland, one in Eugene) told her to take the lead, while two (both in Eugene) simply dismissed her doubts.

OUR SHIFTING VIRAL ECOLOGY

If she'd found a pediatrician willing to coach her, Thea might have asked about whether too many vaccines at once might overload the immune system. Indeed, autoimmunity can be triggered by a challenge to the immune system, and a few studies suggested that vaccinated kids were slightly more likely to develop a variety of autoimmune disorders, hinting that vaccines were part of the problem in the hygiene hypothesis. But as epidemiologists weeded out confounding factors in these studies, the association between immune problems and vaccines evaporated. Further, and more extensive, studies have since found no elevated risk among the vaccinated population. The originator of the theory that too many vaccines at once will overload the immune system, moreover, turned out to be none other than Andrew Wakefield. The science actually now seems to point in the opposite direction: One of the largest studies, of more than 850,000 Danish children, showed that those who got the measles, mumps, and rubella vaccine were actually a little *less* likely to get asthma than unvaccinated toddlers. Another suggested that immunizations were protective against allergies. The implication is that vaccines helped tune the immune response, rather than knocking it out of tune. And this actually fits more comfortably within the hygiene hypothesis: Unlike antibiotics, which remove immune-system stimulating germs, vaccines do just the opposite, introducing microbes and allergens at an early enough age to allow children to develop a normal response.

For most of human evolution, babies carried a far heavier load of viruses and bacteria. As the standard of living has improved in developed countries over the last century, it has upset the balance of power between human immunity, wild viruses, and other inhabitants of the human superorganism. But vaccination generally works to restore these old relationships. Polio, for instance, though it has afflicted humans for thousands of years, was so insignificant before the 19th century that nobody paid much attention to it. In those days everyone was infected with polio but very few developed symptoms: Babies were inoculated naturally, while still under the shield of maternal antibodies. It was only when polio became rare—when people began encountering the microbe for the first time at the age of 7 or 9—that it became dangerous. The first major outbreak ever reported in the United States occurred in 1894. The disease quickly became more serious, and in 1916 polio killed 6,000 Americans and left 27,000 paralyzed.

Polio became a cause célèbre, in part, because it struck those who lived in the newly sanitized world. It was a disease of patrician presidents, not sharecroppers. The epidemics floated into cities on a current of clean water: The public health officials whose sewage systems and food safety laws saved untold numbers from cholera and tuberculosis, probably were also responsible for the iron lungs and leg braces of polio. The polio contaminated water had worked like a vaccine, albeit a very dangerous vaccine. The Salk vaccines—which came 50 years later—restored the balance that had been lost in modernization, replacing the inoculation that babies had once received in their mother's milk.

Thea, though she hadn't investigated the state of microbial ecology or read the history of polio, came to the same conclusion. In the end Silas got all his shots, even though Thea herself hadn't been vaccinated. It had seemed entirely possible to her that most people were accepting vaccines without thought because that was the norm. She'd simply been looking for advice from someone who had considered objections to vaccines thoroughly, rather than dismissing them. It was enough for her to see the arguments and counterarguments laid out by Sears. He was her C.P. Wertenbaker.

NATURAL TECHNOLOGY

There are low levels of toxins and dangerous chemicals wherever you look. They are certainly in vaccines—an infinitesimal trace of formaldehyde here, a drop of aluminum gel there (the claim about antifreeze in vaccines, incidentally, is nonsense). They are in the vegetable staples of our diet, also in tiny amounts. There may never be proof that vaccines are safe, just as there may never be proof that vegetables are harmless. The trick, as Wendell Berry put it, is not to find certainty, but to act thoughtfully with partial knowledge. When my daughter was born, the choice was easy for me—though the experience was still nerve-wracking. She got her shots, on schedule.

I'd set out to reappraise my feelings about natural and technological toxins after considering these two cases side by side, and the results surprised me. I hadn't expected to catch myself redefining the terms of my thought experiment so that the technologies that won me over fell into the natural column.

Just as I had decided that cooking was more natural than eating raw, by the time I'd finished researching vaccination, I'd started to think of it as an ecological, rather than technological, intervention. The very word *vaccination* refers to the interconnected ecology of viruses, the human immune system, and animals. Vaccine comes from *vaca* (cow), a reference to cowpox and the folk knowledge that came from living with livestock. The shots we get today are simply an advanced form of the protection people used to get through their interactions with animals and microbes.

There are other ways that immunization predates Edward Jenner's cowpox shot: Before vaccination became an alien tool of the medical establishment it was an accepted product of cultural wisdom that rose out of Eastern medicine. There are written accounts of inoculation from 8th-century India. Tibetan monks carried the knowledge across the Himalayas, and there is evidence that a Buddhist nun popularized the practice in China. Only in the 1700s did inoculation reach the Occident.

"Unnatural," it seemed, was simply what I called things I didn't understand. The more I learned about something, the more natural it became. Instead of revealing a winner, this contest between nature and technology revealed the cultural deficiency that led me to make this arbitrary division in the first place: I'd resorted to separating the world into natural and unnatural only because my threadbare cultural inheritance provided me no better rules for making sense of the frightening mysteries around me. The real problem with vaccines was not their unnaturalness, but the reaction they created when combined with culture: They revealed tremendous failures in our system of sharing knowledge. Unlike the Yolngu, where the elder women are trusted to sort the poisonous seeds from the healthy, in the United States there were few bonds of trust connecting the public to the oracles of our accumulated cultural—and therefore medical—knowledge.

The irony is that the United States actually has set up highly sophisticated systems to separate—instead of seeds—the dangerous medicines from the useful. Before a vaccine is recommended, the federal Advisory Committee on Immune Practices wades through the science, often asking for further testing. Then the American Academy of Pediatrics and American Academy of Family Physicians also study the matter. Then each state decides how much money to spend on the vaccine and how forcefully to recommend immunization. At each step risks are weighed, doubts debated, and hypothetical dangers considered. But somehow, this system breaks down before the debate reaches the people it's designed to serve. (The responsibility for that last broken link falls not just on medicine, but also on my field, journalism.) For the average parent this discussion is stripped of its nuance and reduced to little more than a single directive: Get the shot.

If we wanted to emulate the success of the Yolngu, we'd forge a network of trusting relationships to absorb and disperse cultural knowledge. Such a solution would create a way to make sense of science, to convert facts into meaning. In societies where this kind of structure exists, it not only spreads information, but also supplies some comfort and support when the information available is utterly insufficient. But as globalization and technological innovation has created indispensable new networks, it's also made us more isolated—it's now difficult to have a comfortable conversation with the local doctor about vaccines, or to seek out the opinion of some resident running guru on the value of raw food. The Internet has substituted for some of the loss of real-world connections, but on the Internet it's all too easy to simply find an answer that affirms one's suspicions. It takes bonds of trust to change a mind.

The answer that's often proposed for this problem of grappling with the unknown is to attain scientific certainty. That, of course, does work: We no longer have to consider risks of either the smallpox virus nor its vaccination because we have eliminated that uncertainty. But such mastery takes a long time. For at least 1,000 years, between the development of inoculation in India and the discovery of the more benign cowpox vaccine in 1796, people not so different from Thea and me had to weigh the dangers of a nightmare disease against an immunization hundreds of times more dangerous than even the worst scenarios presented by antivaccinationists today. Humans have never had the luxury of waiting for complete knowledge. We cannot postpone eating until we fully understand the elements of our food. We cannot wait to have children until we come to understand the causes of autism. We cannot delay sickness until every vaccine is demonstrably harmless. Instead we must—with as much grace as possible—make choices from a position of ignorance. The provision of aid to those attempting that feat is best accomplished by culture—it both allows the transmission of available knowledge and provides assistance where that knowledge falls short.

Culture, in fact, might be defined as the collective capacity of people to create beautiful stopgaps for the problem of ignorance. Poetry, politics, and philosophy are all improvised measures that allow humanity to go on in the face of the unanswerable. This doesn't change the fact that culture looks weak next to certainty. Unlike technology, it can't ever promise a cure. But culture is more powerful than it appears: It takes culture to foster good science, and in the decade, the century, the millennia that it takes to find that cure, culture can make life rich. It's only a provisional, jury-rigged sort of happiness that culture can offer, but then—is there any other kind?

CHAPTER FIVE

SEEING THE FOREST

ENVIRONMENT

I n high school, once I'd ended my epoch of sprouts, I found a new preoccupation in an environmental club. Though I wasn't conscious of it at the time, it was a logical progression: After losing faith in nature to serve human health, I turned to the one field in which it still seemed self-evident that nature was in the right.

My discontent with environmentalism, however, had already been simmering. The entire endeavor seemed long on talk and short on action. A series of teachers had done their part, screening documentary horror films about the destruction of the planet. But evangelical movies weren't helpful for those of us who were already convinced. When teachers did suggest token measures, they were so obviously inadequate that, even to an idealistic teenager, they appeared condescending and ridiculous. I still find it fundamentally unfair for a teacher to show children images of the rainforest's cathedral groves burning or fishermen butchering a foundering population of whales, and then turn to the rows of stricken faces and instruct them to make dioramas about recycling. My generation was bequeathed ecological anxiety, but not the tools to change anything. Some of my friends grew prematurely jaded and started dropping their Twinkies wrappers on the field during recess.

All this was especially upsetting for me, because in my mind, my health and happiness were inextricably bound up with a misty conception of environmental purity. But the best thing I could do for nature, I was learning, was stay out of it. When human touch can only spread ugliness and decay, the role for a young environmentalist grows claustrophobically narrow. His only course of action is to restrain people, pick up their snack wrappers, and find ways to soften their casual destruction. He is reduced to a scold, forever battling humanity's sprawling exuberance.

By the time I joined the environmental club, I'd decided that the real problem was not people's penchant for casual pollution, but people themselves—humanity in its totality. The only solutions to that problem were desperate ones: We would have to be forced, en masse, out of the technological incubator that fed, clothed, and protected us; or, if not that, dramatically reduced in our number. I saw, in our little group of misfits, the beginnings of a campaign for the end of civilization.

The club was led by a tall and handsomely gaunt vegan with a Mohawk. The other members were either similarly decorated in piercings and safety pin–armored fatigues, or in beads and embroidered peasant blouses. We gathered after school on a patch of grass at the end of the English wing to deliberate over international treaties, the superiority of Marxism versus Buddhism, the carbon footprint of condoms, and the ethics of whale adoption.

I looked up to Mohawk—it was exciting to have a leader through whom I might channel my ecological anxiety. He handed out scraps of printed propaganda and suggested that we post copies around school, which I did dutifully. But a creeping sense of futility accompanied this labor as it dawned on me that, at best, I would only create more people like myself: angry but impotent. Finally, after months of meetings, Mohawk announced that we were going to do something to change the facts on the ground. Something that would transform us from passive consumers to righteous shapers of destiny. We were moving into action.

The demonstration would be in the desert at the southeastern edge of California, a 12-hour drive from Nevada City. I strained to hear the explanation of what we were protesting above Ani DiFranco's rage, which was being expressed at high decibels from the speakers of the sport-utility vehicle a club member had borrowed from her mom. We were headed for Ward Valley—a place sacred to Native Americans and home to the endangered desert tortoise, just 15 miles from the Colorado River—to stop the nuclear industry from dumping tons of radioactive waste in shallow, unlined trenches.

I don't know what I had been expecting to see when I arrived— flowering cacti perhaps, or graceful rock formations, or maybe a glimpse of a desert fox atop a boulder—whatever it was, it wasn't waiting for me in Ward Valley. Instead, we drove into a flat, unremittingly ugly landscape of low brush beneath high-tension power lines, a haze of dust, and a punishing sun. A man with a missing tooth and blond dreadlocks waved our SUV into a parking area and pointed out where we might lay our sleeping bags that night. The people milling around the encampment were dressed like us in the unofficial but immediately recognizable mufti of the millennial nomad. I was among my kind, I thought, the bright new lights of the next rebellion.

Two large military surplus tents were set up at the center of the encampment to serve as temporary meeting rooms. I would spend much of my daylight deployment in Ward Valley beneath these canvas roofs, thankful to be in the only shade for miles in any direction. The lectures given in those tents were designed to hone the activist's edge. But over-education can also blunt that edge, and the more I listened the more out of place I felt. For instance, the speakers sneered at the government's temerity in suggesting that a radioactive waste dump would actually help the desert tortoise. But then they went on to explain that biologists had come to this conclusion after accounting for mitigations funded by the dump: roadside fences (to prevent roadkill, the most common cause of tortoise demise), new underpasses to allow wildlife corridors beneath

the highway, and an area of high-quality tortoise habitat to be set aside
elsewhere. The more detail the educators gave, the more reasonable the
government naturalists actually seemed. Ditto for the plans to bury
nuclear waste so near the Colorado River. The waste, it turned out,
wouldn't be glow-in-the-dark goop, but more mundane materials: uni-
forms worn in the plants, irradiated wrenches, and concrete from old
reactors. Still, if water carrying radioactive isotopes from this garbage
began to pool, there were a number of underground faults through
which it might find its way down to the water table, and perhaps eventually to the river, though geologists said this was unlikely given the valley's lack of rainfall. I began to speculate about the geology beneath labs
and power plants scattered all across the United States, where the waste
was currently accumulating. There are fractures everywhere, and surely
few of these sites could be as hot and dry as the one where I was sitting.
By the end of the first day, the people perpetrating this presumptive evil,
which I had so blithely supposed I would fight, were looking more like
beleaguered public servants than demons.

After the sun's heat faded into an orangey miasma, I picked my way
out through the sage hoping I might find some tortoise tracks, some
flowers, or frankly anything redemptive about this place. When I
brought my eyes close to the ground to examine my surroundings in
detail, I could see that there were tracks everywhere, but not the type I
had hoped to find. I identified instead several species of tire tread. Many
of the sage bushes had been beaten down to nubs by their passing. There
were decaying plastic bags and a McDonald's cup tangled in the creosote
bushes, but I found no sign of animal life.

When I returned to the encampment, a man with a mass of hair
tucked into a pendulous crocheted Rasta hat handed me a plate and
glopped big spoonfuls of something brown on top. I said thanks, and he
winked at me. The food was filling and it was free. Sitting there, eating
with my fellow activists, I felt the tide of queasy uncertainty that had
risen in my stomach during the lectures begin to subside. When the girl

eating beside me struck up a conversation, I made a somewhat incoherent plea for help, hoping she might reel me back into the comfortable self-assurance I'd felt on the ride down.

"I don't know," I concluded lamely. "It just seems less clear than I'd thought."

She stared at me. "It seems pretty clear to me, man. Radioactive-waste dumps are bad. I don't have to think too hard about that one."

I winced. A woman sitting immediately to her right, however, offered an argument that I could understand: "There's not that much of nature left. If they really have to build this dump, they should do it in a strip mall."

This made perfect sense to me. If you are prepared to give nature some ethical standing (and I was), it is inarguably more just for the estate of civilization to swallow its own waste than to dump it on the estate of wilderness. But there seemed little chance that, aside from a small group of conscientious environmentalists, people were ready to make sacrifices in the name of justice. I laid out my sleeping bag that night envisioning a caper in which radicals surreptitiously piped spent uranium into a strip-mall Burger King. Maybe, I thought dismally, the best hope for the world would be for all our environmental efforts to fail spectacularly, and for my turtle-strangling, baby-seal-clubbing, clear-cutting, radioactive-waste producing species to collapse on its own trash heap.

In the end, no law-enforcement officials or nuclear energy executives would dignify our protest with their attention. I'd driven the length of the state to stand in this dusty scrap of desert and shout, "Stop!" but instead of saving the environment, I'd somehow ended up at a self-congratulatory rave. On the drive home I sat in the back, searching for a way past my sense of futility as my friends joked and flirted.

The government eventually decided against building the dump, though it was populist fears about radiation in the drinking water, rather than any noble effort to aid wilderness and tortoises, that tipped the balance. Self-serving desires would, it seemed, always outweigh justice. But after this experience I began to wonder if there was some way that the selfish aims of civilization could mesh with the aims of environmentalism.

I had assumed that civilization and nature were, by definition, in conflict, an assumption that had its roots in a tradition of environmentalist thought that goes back through John Muir to Henry David Thoreau and Ralph Waldo Emerson. The conflict is absolute. Civilization plunders nature. Nature withers where civilization plants its foot, though perhaps—as mushrooms buckle asphalt and jungles blanket fallen monuments—nature is destined to recover its territory. The point is that the two are like oil (spilling from a crippled tanker, perhaps) and water: Civilization and nature can't occupy the same place at the same time. The besieged grandeur we learned about in school was grand precisely because it was so remote, both uncorrupted by civilization and awesome in its strangeness. This vision of nature was so big, and so distant, that it strained the mind to imagine how we might help.

But what if this assumption of opposition is wrong? Instead of framing the problem as a desperate battle to rescue the last bits of nature from mankind, environmentalism could simply be defined as the effort to improve the neighborhood—to make the earth a better place for civilization. After all, though environmentalism sometimes presents itself as an ethic of self-denial, it's still anthropocentric: We don't protest for slime mold habitat and the rights of viruses—instead we protect the places and species that humans find meaningful, beautiful, or useful. Crucially, if the fundamental goal of environmentalism were to serve people—rather than to constrain, corral, and chide them—it would be much more likely to succeed.

I doubt that either Emerson or Thoreau would have approved of erasing the dividing line between nature and civilization. The qualities of nature that they loved—its purity, its quiet—depended on this division. The transcendentalists wanted people to go out into the woods and be moved by nature (as Emerson put it, "To the body and mind which have been cramped by noxious work or company, nature is medicinal and restores their tone.") but they didn't want people to stick around in nature and build houses. The transcendentalists gave wonderful advice for weekend mountaineers and off-hours stargazers, but were silent on how to be an environmentalist from 9 to 5, while sustaining oneself. Thoreau tried growing food at Walden Pond, but eventually decided his gardening was an unacceptable corruption. Instead, he carried his food in from town—the uncultivated wilderness he celebrated required the corruption he disdained elsewhere. And this approach was mirrored in environmental policy: Each park or wilderness implied more intensive use of land in its shadow.

The transcendentalists, the romantics, and just about every nature writer in the English language appreciated wilderness for its power to affect people. When they expressed any sentiment about the reverse—about people affecting nature—it was usually dismay. Perhaps this is why my youthful lessons about environmentalism were so freighted with dire warnings, and so light on practical advice. The only *doing* that the philosophical tradition allowed in nature was the *undoing* of another human action. The idea that humans acting on pristine nature might improve it was anathema.

The problem, as I found when I began thinking about my own environmentalism, is that people can't help but influence nature. It's vitally important that we develop some credo for acting on nature because, as the human population has grown, it's become inescapably clear that the wall between wilderness and civilization is illusory. Nature thrives within our cities, our homes, and our bodies. Every one of civilization's burps and sneezes troubles the remotest wilderness. Civilization and nature are not mutually exclusive; rather, they are inextricable.

All this philosophizing may look like splitting hairs. As I write I'm all too aware that what I'm doing here is uncomfortably similar to what my environmental club was doing behind the English wing. But there's a good reason for that: I think that in those embarrassingly unsophisticated bull sessions we were actually at the beginning—okay, the very beginning—of the right path. Thinking isn't as satisfying as action, but it's more important, since action without thoughtful direction tends to be expensive, counterproductive, and maddeningly frustrating. Our environmental failures, I suspect, are really philosophical failures. In the 1990s ecologist Daniel Botkin wrote that his fellow scientists—driven by an unexamined vision of nature as a fragile machine that must be protected—made one bad decision after another. He'd noticed this in the Tsavo National Park, in Kenya, where park managers had so successfully protected elephants from poachers that their population boomed. The elephants then devoured most of the park's trees and brush, until the landscape resembled a desert. When a serious drought hit in 1970, six thousand elephants died. Botkin wrote: "The potential for us to make progress with environmental issues is limited by the basic assumptions that we make about nature, the unspoken, often unrecognized perspective from which we view our environment." If there is any hope of dealing with our global environmental crisis, he observed, we must first "break free of old assumptions and old myths about nature and ourselves."

Our current state of ecological confusion has a lot to do with the lack of a philosophical tradition that shows us not just how to be *in* nature, but how to be a functional part of it. By the time I began this book I was ready to abandon my old environmental ideology in exchange for some other guiding credo—one that actually had a chance of making things better. And so I began my search for humanity's place in the world.

Option One: Natural Law—
Step Back and Let Nature Rule

It's possible, of course, that there is a place for civilization in nature only if we allow ourselves to submit to nature's laws. This is the idea most compatible with the traditional split between humanity and nature: We are allowed back in nature only when we somehow become natural ourselves.

There's a whole school of thought built around the idea that humanity took a turn down the wrong path when we first began controlling the environment through agriculture. The argument goes like this: First, farmers subverted nature's plan for a piece of land by placing it under technological control. Next, these ancient agronomists had to defend their crops—creating private property for the first time. As some accumulated more than others, property gave rise to hierarchy, which in turn led to the oppression of the weak. The higher population densities allowed by agriculture also provided breeding grounds for disease, and inevitable competition between swelling tribes led to conflict. In sum, agriculture (cum corruption of the natural order) was the cause of poverty, plague, war, and slavery. It's a Genesis-like creation story, in which human pursuit of technological control upsets Edenic harmony. But perhaps it's only Genesis-lite, because there's a road back to Eden: If humanity is able to surrender our and desire for control, we could become pristine.

Supposing we accepted this idea of giving up all technology, including agriculture, and went back to nature—would nature accept us? That is, if we gave up our sloppy attempts at control, would the environment revert to some nurturing Eden?

The forests of my youth offer a case study in the power of technology to upset the organic order, and the power of nature to restore it. Nevada City is the heart of California's Mother Lode, and in the mid-1800s the land swarmed with prospectors bent on skinning the earth and turning it inside out. The pictures of the town during the 19th-century California gold rush show a landscape denuded of forest except for a few scattered pines, looking skinny and knock-kneed. The lumber had gone to build cabins, rock-crushing machines, mineshaft stays, and mile upon mile of wooden aqueducts. These flumes still stand: Their crisscrossing timbers leap over gorges and snake along the contour lines. They, more than any other gold-rush technology, blighted the ecosystem because, besides gobbling up forests, they powered water cannons that could wash away mountains. The combination of hydraulic mining and erosion from clear-cut slopes filled the San Francisco Bay with sediment (to this day most of the bay is less than 10 feet deep at low tide). Sacramento was inundated with so much mud that workers gave up the excavation and rebuilt so that the old city blocks lie buried beneath the new ones. Entire hillsides were slumping down rivers.

It's hard to imagine a more thorough disruption of an environment; yet—once the gold was gone and the miners had disappeared—nature bounced back. When I got to Nevada City a century later, the population within city limits had fallen from its peak of 10,000 to 2,500, and the hills were thick with trees. I could see the stages of recovery in places touched more recently by humans: An area that had been cleared down to the orange subsoil would be covered in blackberry brambles and thousands of manzanita sprigs within a year. These stabilized the ground and blanketed the soil in a layer of leaf litter. Meanwhile, a crop of ponderosa pines would shoot up, outstripping the lower shrubs. Animals and insects took part in this terraforming as the pines rose: Birds and rodents carried in seeds, beetles and fungi worked leaf mulch into the soil, and predators (coyotes, hawks, spiders) arrived to regulate populations. Finally, shade-tolerant trees, like white fir and incense cedar, would rise beneath the ponderosas. Hardwoods—California bay laurel, perfuming the forest; silky-skinned madrone; and big leaf maple—would find their way into the margins and fill in the gaps as pines fell. Dogwood and buckeye would flower at eye level. One set of species subtly altered the soil chemistry, the rate of erosion, the moisture levels, until conditions were right for the next. As a boy, I learned that ultimately this process of succession led to—in ecology lingo—a climax community: a jouissance of biodiversity, each species playing its part, sustaining itself in perfect balance.

Today, the rivers that were choked with mud during the gold rush run blue over polished white granite. The forest that starts above the high-water scour line sponges up winter storms then seeps water into creeks throughout the dry season. People walk through this forest every day on a track just outside Nevada City, called Independence Trail, which runs along the canyon wall above the South Fork of the Yuba

River. The trail follows a hydraulic mining flume, an instrument of destruction repurposed as an instrument of appreciation. The air is cooler there in the summer, and in the fall newts plod onto the track and stare at passersby with a comically self-serious mien. It feels good: Step into this wood and you trade the messiness, the arguments, and the politicking of civilization for the order, the balance, the self-sustaining health of nature's law. The fact that nature could take a man-made wasteland and—through this intricate process—transform it into something beautiful seemed evidence enough of its wisdom. But that was before I started talking to the people who study this sort of thing.

NATURAL LAW IS INCONSISTENT

When I began chatting with academics and naturalists, they were able to speak in general about succession and climax communities, but none of them had expertise in the forests around Nevada City. Several suggested contacting Yuba Watershed Institute, which turned out to be organized (in part) by the parents of my friends from high school—artisans and writers from the Ridge. I spent a few pleasant evenings dialing once-memorized phone numbers and catching up. But these old friends passed the buck: The person I needed to talk to, they said, was Don Harkin. He knew more about the forest than anyone else; he had been trained at the Yale School of Forestry and spent nearly every day walking through the woods, taking measurements, and observing the changes from year to year. They also cautioned that Harkin was a difficult fellow. He was mostly deaf, lived in a cabin without electricity or refrigeration, and generally refused to answer questions directly.

I left messages for Harkin. He ignored them. Every three days or so I would call again. Eventually he realized I wasn't going to quit and called back, addressing me with gruff displeasure, as if I'd interrupted his hibernation. He'd stopped doing interviews with journalists, he said, because they never thought for themselves.

"I could tell you that the forest should be managed one way or another, but you'd have no way of assessing that information," he growled. "You'd have to make a faith-based decision to either trust me or not."

The only way I could learn about the forest, he said, was to spend a decade or two living in it. Harkin only softened when I explained that I *had* lived in it, that I had grown up in Nevada City, playing among the trees. Eventually, he agreed to at least entertain a few of my questions, but on some other occasion. It was getting late, he said, and he liked to be in bed by 9 p.m. And so began a series of conversations over the telephone. When next we spoke I started to ask Harkin to detail for me the stages of natural recovery around Nevada City, but he cut me off.

"You're talking about succession," he said. "So you will be familiar with Clements."

I admitted I was not.

"Frederic Clements, University of Nebraska. It's a very old idea, turn of the century. I suppose there is still some validity to it in certain limited areas." Then he reeled off a list of citations from ecology and forestry journals.

As we talked, I learned that I'd glossed over a lot of important details in constructing my story of forest succession. First, it turns out that there's not any one inevitable climax forest for any particular piece of land. Instead of succession proceeding inexorably toward a predetermined goal, it's more like a choose-your-own-adventure with many possible endings. Harkin reminded me of half a dozen examples of places where succession has stalled: creeks smothered in blackberries, hillsides dominated for decades by dense stands of manzanita, and land that had never recovered from the mining—like Malakoff Diggins on the Ridge, where the water cannons cut so deeply into the earth that it still looks as if an acre of southern Utah was dropped incongruously into the middle of the pine forest. For Harkin, as he walked through groves year after year, it became clear that there are so many variables affecting any given plot of land that the principles of succession were only a rough guide to predict the patterns of growth.

Also, succession doesn't always lead to what we'd think of as richer, more majestic landscapes, he said. Occasionally, the process can create a profusion of life, a moment of peak biomass, but then proceed on to something lesser. In Alaska, for example, you can walk through a century of succession by hiking from the base of certain glaciers into the land they once covered: You'd first encounter alders (quickly thickening into a near-impassible tangle), which add nitrogen to the soil and allow (a little farther on) spruce trees to grow. But as these conifers replaced the alders, they'd mine nitrogen from the ground. As you walked you'd soon notice you were stepping over many decaying spruce trunks and, eventually, you would find yourself squishing through a mossy sphagnum bog too acidic for trees. While succession is real, it's too unpredictable to serve as evidence that nature is purposeful.

FAILURE OF THE STEADY STATE

My second problem was that the very idea of a climax forest made Harkin uncomfortable. Forests don't ever stop changing, he told me. Fires sweep through, rainfall patterns shift, climates change, and new species muscle their way into the mix. My conception of nature in equipoise seemed to be flatly wrong. Even in a well-protected environment, populations spike and crash. Trees still compete for sunlight and water. If one species can gain an edge on its fellows, perhaps through some evolutionary innovation in seed design, it will gradually transform the forest.

Daniel Botkin likes to use the example of Hutcheson Memorial Forest, in New Jersey, to illustrate the same point: In 1954, when an oil company helped Rutgers University buy these 65 acres of old-growth forest, the company announced its charity in advertisements, bragging:

"[N]ature has been working thousands of years to perfect this 'climax' community in which trees, plants, animals, and all the creatures of the forest have reached a state of harmonious balance with their environment. Left undisturbed, this stabilized society will continue to perpetuate itself century after century."

But as scientists watched, sugar maples began to replace the dominant oaks and hickory, the once park-like woods grew crowded with shrubs, and exotic species like Norway maple and Japanese honeysuckle muscled their way into the mix. Life is forever moving. Edenic stasis is achieved only in death.

THE HUMAN FOREST

The third complication, and the coup de grace for my faith in natural dominion, was that humans contribute to nature's dynamism even when they are trying hard to keep things stable. Botkin attributes the changes in Hutcheson Forest largely to fire suppression. When counting tree rings, ecologists found charred evidence of fires about once a decade before Europeans settled the area in 1701. After that, the fires stopped. It took 300 more years, but as the big oaks and hickories fell, up sprang a generation of trees that are more susceptible to fire. "We're managing the forest," Harkin said, "even if all we are doing is trying not to manage it."

The forests of my youth were also being shaped by the human suppression of wildfires. Without periodic flames to clear them, needles and leaves will carpet the ground, thwarting ponderosa pine seeds. The sprouts dry up before they can reach the mineral soil. Incense cedar and white fir, on the other hand, can penetrate this duff layer. These trees form a darker, denser forest. Quieter too: Their groves tend to have more chickadees (which grow fat on cedar bark insects), but a lower overall diversity of songbirds. What I'd thought of as a climax forest was, in actuality, a human forest. Doubly so, because once established, this human forest held us hostage to the policy of fire suppression. Incense cedar is vulnerable to flames (it's the fire-starter of choice for wood stoves in Nevada County), and the resinous needles of white fir provide a ladder by which mild ground fires may climb into canopy-engulfing infernos. If there is any doubt that fire-sensitive trees have us in a full nelson, consider that for every dollar it received in timber sales in 2010 the U.S. Forest Service spent $8.60 on fire suppression.

We now know that humans have shaped the landscape by lighting fires as well as suppressing them. The environment that Europeans discovered as they settled the Americas had been sculpted by Indians. In *1491*—a colorful analysis of American history before Europeans—the writer Charles Mann showed that the land was not a sparsely populated wilderness. Most archeologists now agree that the Americas were densely peopled with civilizations that often used fire to shape the environment to their desires. "Rather than the thick, unbroken, monumental snarl of trees imagined by Thoreau, the great eastern forest was an ecological kaleidoscope of garden plots, blackberry rambles, pine barrens, and spacious groves of chestnut, hickory and oak," Mann wrote. "The first white settlers in Ohio found woodlands that resembled English parks—they could drive carriages through the trees." Much of the Great Plains in the middle of the continent were, in fact, man-made pasture created by seasonal burns. Prairie fires killed trees and encouraged the growth of grasses, which in turn encouraged the growth of bison.

By using fire to create habitat for the animals they hunted, the Indians controlled—or at least acted upon—their environment. There was also, contrary to the conventional wisdom, widespread agriculture throughout the Americas. When a wave of microbes, advancing ahead of white settlers, demolished these civilizations—or, to put it in ecological terms, when invasive species displaced the apex predator—the animal populations they had managed boomed. "Suddenly deregulated, ecosystems shook and sloshed like a cup of tea in an earthquake," Mann wrote. The passenger pigeons that blocked out the sun, the bison that shook the earth for hours on end, the profusion of shellfish in Cape Cod—all of which Europeans took as evidence of nature's virgin bounty, might instead have been symptoms of a radically destabilized environment.

In the United States, the debate over what is natural has high stakes because in 2003 the federal government made it policy (through the

Healthy Forest Restoration Act) to reduce "unnatural" conditions and re-create the forests that existed before the era of fire suppression. Logging companies like (and underwrite) science showing that the pre-Columbian forests were characterized by frequent, stand-replacing fires (much like clear-cuts). Environmentalists prefer to talk about the findings that show how much more old growth once existed.

To Harkin, the debates about how the forest looked a century ago seem about as pointless as the religious wars fought over the question of whether the Communion host is the literal or metaphoric flesh of Christ.

"If we return the forest to 1910 conditions is that natural?" he asked. "Why not 1210? Or 10 BC? What about after some happenstance ice-dam breakage sent a hundred million gallons of water flooding over everything, maybe that's what we should be aiming for."

Where is Eden to be found?

————

I abandoned the idea of natural dominion wistfully, I have to admit. The belief that nature is always driving toward paradise is comforting and, like the romantics, I was attracted to the notion that there is a higher power (be it the law of nature or God) that is inclined toward beauty and life. The idea had aligned with my childhood feeling that places like Yosemite, sheltered from humanity, were both wholesome and holy. It's an old idea: 18th-century Christian philosopher Thomas Derham was convinced that nature's order "is manifestly the work of a divine wisdom." Long before that, Aristotle argued that nature wastes nothing and that its perfection implies a designer. The problem with this line of reasoning is that its advocates must explain away the imperfections that inevitably crop up in nature (or else accept them as proof that there is no designer). As a result, the blame for every annoyance and flaw must be foisted upon human interference. We're the postlapsarian fall guys. After seeing enough examples of nature acting arbitrarily without the aid of humanity, I was prepared to consider an even older proposition: that humans must take dominion over the earth.

OPTION TWO: SCIENTIFIC DOMINION— STEP IN AND TAKE CONTROL

Harkin, by this point, had grudgingly accepted the inevitability of my phone calls, and he even seemed to take pleasure in making me his student. It became clear that he was extraordinarily well-read—keeping up to date on the academic literature—and keenly intelligent. But prying straight answers out of him was impossible. Whenever I posed some permutation of the question of how he thought we should be managing the forest, he would respond by asking, "Well, what do you want?" I came to hate this question, as he repeated it in nearly every conversation we had. I puzzled over several possible interpretations of this koan, one of which was simply the recognition that human desire tends to trump the facts on the ground. Perhaps there was nothing wrong with that, I reasoned. If nature can't be trusted to behave rationally, the obvious alternative is to control it. Rational environmentalism seeks to save the earth with both eyes open, subordinating sentiment to the practical fulfillment of human needs. Leaving the company of the romantics and transcendentalists, I found myself among the Enlightenment philosophers.

The romantics had thought that nature was fundamentally mysterious and only accessible, as Emerson put it, "by untaught sallies of the spirit." (Science, he maintained could explain less about the universe than could poetic reflection: "A dream may lead us deeper into the secrets of nature than a hundred concerted experiments.") The rationalist project of the Enlightenment, on the other hand, was to do away with all this haziness and uncover clear, unequivocal rules by which nature could be governed. Even more importantly, these rules would govern people: Hard facts would put an end to politics, posturing, and demagoguery.

There would be no need for endless debates, or war, once the nations were guided by science.

That has proved to be an elusive goal. In the centuries since Descartes, scientists have only found a few solid, argument-ending answers. And, in the complex morass of forest ecology, certainty is especially hard to come by. When I'd started talking to people at the Yuba Watershed Institute, I learned of one scientist who had attempted to bring this sort of clarity to the debate. In 2002, forestry professor William Libby had delivered a lecture in Nevada City that stood out as an example of how rationalism could cut through objections and ideologies. Talking about timber in my hometown is almost as perilous as talking about abortion politics. But Libby, undaunted and wielding the power of scientific certainty, set out to convince the environmentalists assembled before him to love clear-cutting.

California, Libby explained, imports 80 percent of its wood rather than growing its own, which spurs logging around the world, some of it illegally cut from the jungles of Southeast Asia, where the last orang-utans take shelter. After crunching the numbers he pronounced that, for every 1,000 acres of national forest in California taken out of lumber production, 10 species go extinct on the other side of the world. Then he asked everyone who wished to reduce logging in California to stand and take responsibility for these extinctions. "This is what America is about," Libby said. "We have freedom, we have responsibility, and if we're causing damage somewhere, we want to take responsibility for it." There were cries of disbelieving outrage, but Libby wasn't done.

"California has the most productive forestland in the world," he insisted. And if the environmentalists of California turned their public lands into scientifically managed tree plantations, they might double the timber harvested on each acre, relieving the pressure to log the rainforests. What's more, he explained, clear-cutting was good for the environment— it enhances biodiversity when large patches of forest in various stages of growth provide several different types of habitat, each with its own set of plants and animals. There are other frequently cited benefits to clear-cutting as well: The land yields more water since there are no trees to soak up rainfall and catch snow; destructive fires are rarer; and—of course—clear-cutting supports the local economy. Those were the facts, Libby told the angry crowd. They didn't have to like them, but they were still facts.

Though determined to accept reality, no matter how harsh, I didn't like those facts. I hated the idea of turning something I thought of as beautiful (a forest), into something I thought of as ugly (industrial farm-land), but I also knew that I might have to readjust my romantic aesthetics. When I saw what people from earlier times had to say about natural beauty, I was shocked to discover that they often turned my rubric of beauty upside down. Before they were beautiful, forests were feared refuges for bandits and wild animals. The vestigial association between trees and danger lingers in the word *savage,* which was derived from *silva* (a wood). Before the 18th century, nature was not magnificent, but grotesque and lacking in symmetry, becoming beautiful only once it was tamed. "[Man] cuts down the thistle and bramble, and he multiplies the vine and the rose," wrote George Leclerc, sometimes called the father of natural history, in the 18th century. "View those melancholy deserts where man has never resided. Over-run with briars, thorns, and trees which are deformed, broken and corrupted." When the *Mayflower* first dropped anchor at Cape Cod, William Bradford saw not a pristine garden, but "a hideous & desolate wilderness, full of wild beasts & wild men." I had assumed that an appreciation for natural splendor was time-less. But it made some sense that wilderness could not be beautiful unless it was controlled, at least in part: It's hard to appreciate the beauty of a wolf as it pursues you. Could it be that my preference for nature's beauty was not based on some universal truth, but simply a prejudice of my era?

While in Nevada City, I went looking for a clear-cut, to see if I could learn to find beauty in its rational order. When I spotted a likely-looking dirt road branching off the highway, I parked and walked into the woods. After passing through a strip of pines I reached the clearing. Here was a truly melancholy desert: Rows of weeping stumps extended across a ragged gap in the forest that sloped steeply into a ravine. Torn limbs tangled so thickly on the ground that I quickly abandoned my plan to walk across. It was like a battlefield—the carnage left by two armies of trees. I wasn't having much luck finding the beauty in this blasted landscape, but I could see its logic. Clear the land and it allows machines to move freely, simplifying the logistics of transporting logs. Plant a new crop of optimally spaced pines and they will grow quickly in the full sunlight, without competition. They will all be ready for harvest at the same time.

I suspect that even those 17th-century forest fearers would have found the clear-cut ugly. Aesthetics are intricately wedded to meaning: Danger is ugly, goodness is beautiful. And a field of stumps feels menacing. Individual trees, moreover, were always beloved—even when forests were not—because they gave shade, shelter, and fruit. To Alexander Pope, writing at a time when woods were dangerous, a tree was nonetheless nobler "than a prince in his coronation robes," and to Walter Blithe (in 1653) a tree was "a thing of delight." It's much easier to find beauty in something that's hospitable to humanity. In this sense the clear-cut was almost objectively ugly: It was a landscape utterly opposed to comfort and the sustenance of human life. Even foresters who see dollar signs in the stumps have said they find such remnants unappealing.

Perhaps clear-cuts are beautiful to the machines whose needs they are designed to serve, but the only humanly aesthetic argument I could muster in favor of clear-cutting was Libby's: By doing everything possible to maximize the timber production on this land, other land might be devoted entirely to pleasure and wildlife. I accepted this proposition reluctantly, aware that this reasoning could be extended to justify all sorts of ugliness: strip mining, factory farming, Soviet-style apartment blocks. It turns environmentalism into an echo of Union general William Tecumseh Sherman's total war (the idea that "War is Hell," as he put it, and the more hellish it is made, the more quickly it can be ended). Cities must be burned, beauty destroyed, cruelty doled out, to preserve the larger ecological union. If California wanted to supply all its own lumber, Libby had estimated that 20 percent of its land area (only 28 percent of which is forested) would have to become a tree plantation, and when he considered future population growth, he said, "I get a little grim." But accepting the clear-cut had the advantage of shielding me from Libby's charges of hypocrisy and myopia. As someone who lives in a wooden house and makes his living selling words printed on paper, I couldn't very well condemn this particular timber harvest unless I had another source of wood in mind. There are alternatives, like hemp or bamboo, but large-scale replacement would require similar plantations of these crops and chemically intensive processing. Analyses tend to show that timber is among the greenest of building materials. Better to accept this particular blight than to push other—fragile or pristine land—into production. At this terrible expense, I could enlist nature in the rational, ordered service of humankind. It might not be pretty, I figured, but at least it was real. Or real-ish. As soon as I began poking around the guts of this line of reasoning, I found that—like the idea of nature's law—there were wobbly assumptions hidden beneath its surface.

CERTAINTY IS POLITICAL

When I began researching Libby's facts, their initial persuasiveness slowly wore down until they began to look not like indisputable truths, but those soft romantic things we call values. Don Harkin told me, sure, clear-cutting can turn a forest into a patchwork of different habitats that could improve biodiversity. But it would also threaten those rarer species that had already been driven to the brink by habitat fragmentation, while encouraging those that thrive on human disturbance. And although it's true that land produces more water after a clear-cut, on steep terrain it's usually the worst sort of water: the kind that comes all at once when it's least wanted (and carries a lot of soil off with it).

As for forest fires, it seems that either an overgrown forest or a poorly managed plantation can set the stage for catastrophic infernos. The details quickly become complicated, but it isn't a simple fact that uniform forests of same-aged trees are safer.

Libby's explanation of extinction trade-offs drew some perplexed sighs from environmental-policy experts and foresters as well: California imports most of its lumber from the Pacific Northwest, not Southeast Asia. This demand creates competition for softwood building materials—a fairly different market from rainforest hardwoods. If we really wanted to preserve forest habitat, some said, it would make more sense to reduce consumption rather than spur production.

While most experts agreed that it made sense to grow timber in places where it was efficient, I was becoming less enthusiastic about turning the Sierra Nevada into an industrial timber plantation, once the shine of scientific certainty wore off. It's important to remember, a biologist reminded me, that scientists are just people, each subtly influenced by a set of assumptions and beliefs, each guided by a unique assortment of ambitions, passions, and incentives. Most science is plastic enough that it can be influenced, consciously or otherwise, by the desires of the experimenter. Several surveys of peer-reviewed articles have showed that those studies done with the support of an interested party were more likely to produce a result favorable to that party. The facts researchers produce are constructed in part from observation of reality and in part from the forces that constrain that observation.

SEEING THE FOREST FOR THE LUMBER

There are many facts, of course, that are bolstered, rather than eroded, by scrutiny. Most of the foresters I talked to agreed that if you simply want to maximize production, a plantation system is the best way to do it. When I asked Don Harkin about this, he responded with the kind of Jesuitical complication that I was learning to expect from him.

"Well," he drawled, "that depends what you mean by 'production.' Usually that refers to timber, but it could be game, for instance. Or, for national parks, it's production of public support—but that can be tricky because the public isn't one single entity. Some people want grizzly bears in their parks and some people don't want to get chewed on. Tricky."

Forests yield many resources, and the notion of optimizing production of just one element while ignoring all others is regarded among many silviculturists as hopelessly outdated. The water that drains into the Yuba River from the forests of Nevada County is annually worth a minimum of $66 million in hydropower generation alone, which is more than the value of the watershed's annual timber harvest has ever been. The ability of forests to soak up rainwater and release it slowly—thereby preventing floods, cleaning water, and recharging aquifers—is ignored by a perspective that focuses solely on wood. This calls into question the Sherman-esque proposition that some forests should be clear-cut so that others might remain pristine. Rather than optimizing land to yield either lumber or beauty, savvy public land managers now look for strategies to maximize a forest's net production of wood, water, oxygen, wildlife habitat, and human pleasure.

THE LURE OF SIMPLICITY

One reason that plantation forestry so efficiently produces timber is that we have 250 years of science showing how to do it. Humanity, in other words, has invested the bulk of its forestry research resources in the study of clear-cutting. This is curious, given that the first major experiments in plantations (in what is now Germany and Poland) were disasters.

In the 1760s Prussian bureaucrats devised a mathematical model to predict the amount of wood (and ultimately of money) that would be produced by a forest each year. This form of scientific forestry also provided a valuable service: It allowed a single authority to exercise management from afar. By reducing the woodland to a number, a ruler might see his entire forest at a glance and make informed decisions about how much to cut in any given year.

The ambitions of this Prussian project, however, went far beyond mere approximation. Early scientists thought that they could deduce universal rules through abstract reasoning, which would make tree counting, and direct observation of the forest, obsolete. As Heinrich Cotta, one of the founders of Prussian forestry, proudly explained, the principles of his science were "determined mathematically" by applying logic to postulates, and not from "direct real measurement." The on-the-ground reality, in other words, mattered less than the theory. Measurement was subordinated to abstraction.

Mathematician Johann Hossfeld wrote in the early 1800s that this approach to forestry was justified because nature "makes no leaps." In other words, forests were uniform. Anyone who has walked in the woods will recognize the absurdity of this assumption, but it became a self-fulfilling prophecy. Rather than constructing a theory to accurately represent reality, the foresters shaped reality until it fit the theory. After years of management, the Prussian forests turned into pure stands of even-aged Norway spruce arranged in a checkerboard.

The results were initially good. Production jumped in the first generation. In the second generation, however, timber yields dropped 20 to 30 percent, and great swaths of trees withered. A new compound word consisting of two concepts that had not had been previously associated— forest and death (*Wald* and *sterben*)—appeared in the German language. The causes of *Waldsterben* are still debated, but at least two forces were at work. First, the "cleaning" of forests in the name of regimented order—though it allowed the spruce trees access to nutrients without competition from other plants—also removed the system for replenishing those nutrients. Second, the cutting of grand old trees destroyed the network of water drainage conduits provided by their deep roots, and trees in low-lying areas drowned.

There was no place in the mathematical models for root systems, water drainage, or symbiotic nutrient exchange among trees, shrubs, and fungi. But that was precisely the point. The goal of silviculture was to rise above the laborious trial-and-error forestry of peasants and join the Enlightenment sciences based on elegant formulae. After the 100 years that it took to grow the first successful crop of intensively managed spruce, and then to witness the sickly growth of the second generation, the technology was already locked in. It had spread to France, where Gifford Pinchot (father of the U.S. Forest Service) learned its methods and brought them to the Yale School of Forestry. German forestry science had become dominant around the world. Despite the *Waldsterben,* scientists opted to further alter the facts on the ground, employing empiricism to refine the model and better force forests to its order, rather than throwing out the model and seeking one that better fit the forests. They did this in part because they lacked a sophisticated alternative, and in part because the Enlightenment dream—that science could provide unchallengeable guidance on how to proceed—still lingered.

Simplifying the complexity of an ecosystem is attractive. Once you scrape the ground to bare soil, apply herbicide, plant in legible rows, fertilize, and spray for moths, you can expect a reasonably foreseeable outcome. Three centuries of silviculture research on this model has led to plantations that are far more productive than any natural forest. The way to make nature predictable is to strip it of variables, confounding factors, and contingency—all of which, unfortunately, are synonyms for life and (at least in the eyes of this beholder) beauty.

———

Even the most rigorous of plantation systems, Harkin reminded me, rely to some degree on the earth's mysterious bounty. And yet there are still those who believe we are ready to cast free of nature's patronage.

The most complete test of what happens when humans fully take over occurred in the early 1990s, in Oracle, Arizona. You may remember hearing about the Biosphere 2 experiment, in which eight people entered an airtight greenhouse to live for 2 years in an entirely man-made ecosystem. The idea was to provide a way to sustain life on a ruined planet, or in space. Futurists imagined similar greenhouses at the center of space stations: capsules of green converting starlight into oxygen as they slowly tumbled through the vacuum.

The result, however, was an ecological nightmare. The water turned acid and the atmosphere became so toxic that the team had to pump in oxygen from outside. Seventy-five percent of the vertebrate species inside went extinct, along with all of the pollinating insects. Morning glories formed tangled mats against the glass, ants swarmed, and—as always—cockroaches thrived. Throughout, the biospherians worked ferociously to eke calories from failing crops. They lost, on average, 18 percent of their bodyweight and turned orange from an imbalance of nutrients. They woke up choking from lack of oxygen and some may have suffered nerve damage from high levels of nitrous oxide. Their experience is captured in a chapter title of *The Human Experiment,* by biospherian Jane Poynter: "Starving, Suffocating, and Going Quite Mad."

All this discomfort despite $150 million invested in technology to control 3 acres, along with an energy bill of $1 million each year: (This was a contradiction never adequately explained: The project required its own gas-power plant.) Extrapolating from the Biosphere 2 experiment, ecological engineer William Mitsch estimated that the cost of replacing nature with technology would be $10 billion per square kilometer each year. Ecologists reflecting on the project in the journal *Science* wrote: "The major retrospective conclusion that can be drawn is simple. At present there is no demonstrated alternative to maintaining the viability of Earth. No one yet knows how to engineer systems that provide humans with the life-supporting services that ecosystems produce for free. . . . Despite its mysteries and hazards, Earth remains the only known home that can support life."

It's awfully tempting to call on the power of science to trump debate, as Bill Libby had done when trying to get Nevada City environmentalists to embrace plantations. But, rather than cutting off debate, this only intensifies the vitriol as each side assembles its own raft of experts insisting that they have the Truth. The assertion of science as Truth compresses the nuances of evidence and counterevidence down to competing dogmas—it becomes a matter of faith that you can either accept or reject. Things get very black and white. The people who think that science can provide incontrovertible certainty are the same ones likely to say that science is worthless because it provides less than that.

In point of fact, scientific certainty is an oxymoron. Science derives its great power from humility. It encourages challenge—no question is off-limits, and no finding is too sacred for falsification. The expectation that science will establish indisputable truths is, in the end, antiscientific.

My experience with vaccine science had shown me that certainty isn't essential: It's possible to act on the basis of partial knowledge. But without absolute certainty you can't force people to agree with you. Good science is useless without good culture and good politics. Moreover, convincing people is only half the battle. I was convinced, for example, by the evidence of the greenhouse effect, yet I still contributed to the burning of jet fuel by buying airplane tickets. My love of forests didn't stop me from buying books. If I were a zealot I would have moved next door to a library and refused to travel. But I wasn't a zealot. I was just a guy who hated watching others nullify years of my sacrifices with a single excursion in their private jet. In other words, I couldn't stand being a sucker. Despite the clear economic incentive for humanity as a whole to sustain its home, there was no economic incentive for me, as an individual, to do the right thing: This misalignment of what's good for an individual and what's good for the commonwealth was precisely the problem Adam Smith had set out to solve with his *invisible hand*. Perhaps with a tune-up and a few replacement parts, that hand could be induced to shoo humanity away from the irrational destruction of its patrimony.

OPTION THREE: GREEN GREED— TRUST THE INVISIBLE HAND

The business suit of free-market economics chafes in a dozen places when worn by a child of countercultural nature lovers, even one who finds himself rebelling against the rebels. I'm more interested in natural beauty and biodiversity than in the bottom line. The free-market fundamentalist's claim that we can pollute without remorse—and trust the market to create a solution—struck me as blindly credulous. But I'd also read an essay that succinctly addressed these concerns and, at the same time, convinced me that, if I wanted to preserve the wild places I loved, I'd have to accept the sovereignty of either the market or of authoritarian government.

This essay is a classic: Garrett Hardin's "The Tragedy of the Commons," published by *Science* in 1968. Hardin made his case with an imaginary scenario—a village commons for cattle. If the grass were overgrazed, the field would become a mud patch, and everyone would lose what had been a free resource. For any individual cowherd, however, it made sense to use the pasture as much as possible—to get the grass before anyone else. The benefits to the cowherd increased linearly as he brought in more cows, while the costs for overgrazing were shared by all. The upshot: Whenever there is competition for a shared resource, legitimate self-interest will destroy the commonwealth.

"Therein is the tragedy," Hardin wrote. "Each man is locked into a system that compels him to increase his herd without limit—in a world that is limited. Ruin is the destination toward which all men rush, each pursuing his own best interest in a society that believes in the freedom of the commons. Freedom in a commons brings ruin to all."

The commons, of course, is a metaphor for clean air, fresh water, fish stocks, and all the shared resources we refer to as nature. Saving the commons with appeals to conscience inevitably fails, Hardin argued, because scolding ("If you don't do as we ask, we will openly condemn you for not acting like a responsible citizen") is always accompanied by a contradictory economic message ("If you do behave as we ask, we will secretly condemn you for a simpleton who can be shamed into standing aside while the rest of us exploit the commons"). This perfectly captures the impasse I experience whenever I waver between buying an organic head of lettuce or a conventional one for half the price; whenever I hesitate over the option to buy carbon offsets to cancel out the pollution of a flight.

Hardin's essay cut through my moralizing with the clarity of a geometric proof. Rational decisions made by individuals in their own interest cause society to act irrationally, *quod erat demonstrandum.* We have, therefore, only two choices: Do away with the commons, or do away with freedom. Hardin preferred the latter—the kind of coercive government control that Thomas Hobbes describes in *Leviathan.* The former, the idea of selling off the air, water, and right to reproduce, Hardin wrote, was "too horrifying to contemplate." I wasn't sure if I agreed. Much had changed between the time Hardin wrote that paper and when I read it. Most prominently, several big experiments in totalitarianism had broken down, or opened up, and revealed how catastrophically centralized control of nature can fail. Under Soviet control millions starved in Ukraine, and in China centralized land management during the Great Leap Forward led to the largest famine in history. (Hardin also proposed population control, whether through forced sterilization or some variation of China's one-child rule. This seems slightly more humane.)

When I called my forester-philosopher, Don Harkin, to ask about this choice between the free market and Leviathan, he reminded me that during the gold rush the government had set up a textbook demonstration of the tragedy of the commons. Back then, the country's frontier resources were divvied up according to a national policy of, as Harkin put it, "It's yours if you can grab it." The resulting mud floods in downstream agricultural towns provoked an outcry for government regulation and prompted some of the first environmental laws. After allowing unrestricted access to the commons, the state had opted to restrict freedom, but in doing so it generated a set of problems that have dogged land administrators ever since. People interested in exploiting resources on a large scale set out to manipulate the rules and the regulators, while those who could profit by small-scale exploitation simply continued illicitly.

The law of "It's yours if you can grab it" always applies to some extent, no matter the form of governance, and those who consider grabbing make calculated decisions about how much opposition they are likely to meet. Doing away with the commons—that is, turning the land into private property—can solve some of these problems. Harkin, who had grown up amid similar frontier lawlessness on a ranch near the Clark Fork River in Montana, had regularly participated in vigilante sorties to establish the cost of appropriating his property.

"The old man would tell one brother to get the Krag," Harkin said. "And he'd say, 'Don, you better take the Winchester. And Doug, I guess you're going to have to take the shotgun.' And we'd take a little ride to find out what really happened to those calves that had gone missing."

When owners live on their land they are in a position to both police it and to see how different management techniques work in relation to its various idiosyncrasies. And after learning what central-ized authority in Prussia had done to forests, I began to lean toward privatization of the commons, rather than Leviathan. How could Washington make good decisions about managing land around Nevada City, where every acre demanded a unique strategy? Whatever the faults of the market, at least it allowed individuals who understood the complex facts on the ground to exercise local knowledge. So, I asked: If Garrett Hardin had not been too horrified to contemplate market solutions, what would he have found?

The quarrel I (and many environmentalists) have with free markets is their failure to assign value to beauty and health. These qualities are outside of the market—externalities. But these external commons could be brought in from the cold if we began paying for those $10 billion worth of services that William Mitsch calculated are provided by each square kilometer of land. This notion of bringing ecosystem services into the market is popular around Nevada City: Landowners know that, once it reaches the cities, the water that comes from their forests sells for as much as $500 per acre-foot (the amount of water needed to cover

1 acre to the depth of 1 foot), but they don't see a cent for maintaining a landscape that soaks up rain during the spring flood season and releases the water in the summer when it's needed.

My father spends considerable time maintaining the steep strip of land where he lives, and as a result his woods work year-round, slowing rainfall so that it can seep into the ground, pulling carbon dioxide out of the air, creating oxygen, holding the topsoil in place, and providing habitat to creatures like the black bear that plundered birdseed from his garage in 2009. Dad thinks it would only be fair if he were reimbursed for his stewardship. Imagine for a moment a world in which this actually happened, a world in which we all paid people like my father for the air, water, and erosion control they provide. Instead of simply weighing the value of his standing timber against his own romantic feelings of duty to the land, Dad could maximize the common good by maximizing his profits. After looking over the going rates, he might see that he should allow his water production to fall a little bit while taking advantage of the increased value of wood by logging— some of this wood would be sold cheaply for burning, while some would receive an atmospheric-services premium for locking up carbon in two-by-fours. Downstream, I would see the ripple effect in my increased water bill. To compensate, I might work with my landlord to build rain catchments on the roof, which would provide me with free water. Afterward, the city would pay my landlord for absorbing rain when storms threatened to overwhelm the water-treatment plant and flush raw sewage into the ocean. Fishermen, in turn, would pay the city for the right to cast their nets in the newly pollution-free habitat along the coastline. And all of these decisions would be made purely out of self-interest. Privatize the commons and greed becomes not only good, but green. The invisible hand would rescue the environment in order to rescue the goods and services nature provides.

Of course there are problems. It's very tricky to measure how much oxygen and water Dad's land is producing at any given moment, and just as tricky to calculate how much I am consuming. Making these estimates would require an army of auditors, each of whom would have to operate under assumptions that would make the Prussian bureaucrats blush. The dilemmas would pile up to absurd heights: Who should be billed for the value a tree brings for providing dappled shade, for slowing rain-drops, for offering twigs and branches suitable for nesting? Exactly how many dollars and cents for the song of a ruby-crowned kinglet?

Ecosystem economics is afflicted by that ultimate cause of market failure: lack of information. There are so many natural services that we don't fully understand—not to mention those we have not discovered—that it would be impossible to provide the market with the information it would need to operate efficiently. When a fisherman hauls a tuna out of the water, how does he determine whose habitat it came from? Would every minnow have to be equipped with a LoJack? And the fish food—the plankton, diatoms, and other microscopic wigglers—those would require tracking devices as well. The more we struggle to maintain the construct of private property, the more easily nature makes a mockery of it.

There are ethical problems on top of the logistical ones: Presumably, these auditors would be backed up by a police force to hunt down illegal polluters and those caught stealing. What would happen when the enforcers collared people too poor to legally breathe? Leviathan lurks in the alleys of free-market utopia.

During one conversation with Harkin, I asked him to explain how he would estimate the value of a tree near his house. He gamely walked me through the techniques, but then added: "So we could check this tree and find out it's worth $6,500, right? Okay, next we might also want to measure the age and dimensions of your three female cousins and find their value, if I sold them on the white slaver's market, what I could get for that." He let the point sink in. "Why is the baby Jesus any more important than a Douglas fir tree?"

I'd hoped to find not only economic half measures for improving the environment, but economic certainty—the kind of muscular philosophy that would sweep away objections and force change. But Harkin was right; it did seem like a problem that in my free-market utopia there would be no difference between Jesus and a tree. I could hope that the market would correctly assess the value of each, but history suggests that Jesus's relative value as Messiah, versus a sort of decorative overlay to complement the joining of two timbers, is utterly subjective.

———

A fog of depression set in once I'd decided that neither the market, nor submission to nature, nor mastery over it, could be counted upon to protect the landscapes I loved. Around this time I came across a similarly gloomy paper by the famous English ecologist Robert May, who presented three arguments for the preservation of biodiversity that roughly correlated with the three categories I've sketched out here. May said species might be shielded from extinction by the technological rationalist because they could provide medicines and materials, by the capitalist because they provide ecosystem services, and by the Romantic because it's ethically the right thing to do. The problem, May wrote, is that, "no one of these three arguments is necessarily compelling":

> First, it seems likely to me that tomorrow's Biotechnological Revolution will design its new medicines, new materials, and other new products from the molecules up, based on our increasing understanding of the molecular machinery of life. Second, I fear that we may be clever enough to create a world that is grievously biologically impoverished, but nevertheless sustainable—the hateful world of the cult movie *Bladerunner*. And although I find the third, ethical argument totally compelling, I wonder what force it would have if I were dirt poor, struggling to feed my children. These are uncomfortable admissions.

At first, the ideologies of the rationalist, the romantic, and the free marketeer had seemed irreconcilably opposed, but as I worked through them I saw that I was attracted to each for its similarities. All were employed as a means to bypass the messiness of debate. All exalted transcendent laws beyond human reproach. Each had its supernatural force—Mother Nature, Scientific Certainty, The Invisible Hand—which supposedly would put the world aright if allowed the freedom to operate. Each spawned fundamentalists, convinced of the rectitude of their own path.

For me, the best argument against this trinity of faiths was their failure to slow environmental degradation. The attempts to make certainty—whether divined from nature, Cartesian logic, or the market—put an end to partisan bickering had, instead, only intensified the debate. Still, I was afraid that without a bulwark of inarguable certainty, people would simply pave nature. Would it be possible to address problems like climate change without invoking higher laws?

There is one other credo beyond the three that I (and May) found lacking—one that has to do with relationships, humility, and compromise. This approach would incorporate economics, science, and a passion for nature, without invoking their capitalized deities to circumvent politics. But this alternative for defining humanity's place in nature is so vague in its dimensions, and so dependent on context, that at first I found it intellectually unsatisfying and impossible to defend as a single world-changing philosophy. This fourth strategy abandons any pretense at certainty and, instead, relies on the political process in all its messy, exasperating disorder. I only began to take this idea seriously after I decided to take Harkin's initial advice and spend some more time in the woods. I requested an audience with Harkin and, somewhat to my surprise, he agreed to meet me.

HUMAN SOLUTIONS

It was a gentle spring morning when I arrived at our rendezvous point: the whitewashed Columbia Schoolhouse on the San Juan Ridge. An orchestra of birds was tuning in the sunshine, and chickens quarreled on the farm across the road. Harkin rumbled up in a gray Mazda van, and we shook hands. Over the weeks when we'd spoken by telephone, I'd gained a wry affection for the man. He was startlingly smart, sly, erudite, and uniquely well-informed about the local ecology. In the mental picture I'd developed of Harkin he was a professorial hermit surrounded by books, bent and slightly unkempt, perhaps in a worn corduroy jacket. The man before me, however, looked less like a scholar than a hobo. The hand that gripped mine was hard as rawhide and dark with geologic layers of dirt and calluses. His eyes were a watery blue and his cheeks were clouded by a week's worth of white bristles. An old Band-Aid clung to the ridge of his ear like the abandoned shell of some metamorphosed insect. He wore a red flannel shirt and blue jeans—though grime was worked so thoroughly into the fabric over his thighs that they had turned from blue to brown. Later that day, when a piece of hard candy slipped from his mouth onto the dirt road, he absently wiped it on those jeans before returning it to his lips. The aroma that accompanied Harkin's person was, improbably, the clean Christmas-tree scent of sawdust.

"Pleasure to meet you in person," he said. "You can relax completely. Whatever you want to know, we can talk about it." When I began to respond, he interrupted. "One of the things you've got to know about old Don is that he did not use ear protection when working with a chainsaw. So you have to speak loud, and close."

There was a jumble of dusty tools in the van, and a dog, which Harkin introduced as Meryl. He produced a battered plastic bag containing cookies, a chipped bowl, and half a grapefruit, then motioned for me to follow him to a picnic table nearby. What I wanted to know, I said (then repeated myself much more loudly), was whether he had a model for managing the land, since he'd convinced me of the inadequacy of all the ideas I'd brought to him.

He mashed a spoon into the grapefruit and slurped up the dangling pulp. Meryl observed, keen-eyed. A model, he said, is a difficult thing. It can provide a framework to organize findings, a scaffolding that allows knowledge to build up rather than simply spread out, but it can also become a trap. "If you don't have a model, you are just like milk oozing across the table, but if you get stuck on it you'll become dogmatic, like it's a religion or something." The forest is complex enough, he said, that firm models for how things work tend to have a short lifespan. In the end, he said, returning to his infuriating riddle, "It all depends on what you want."

Harkin told me to follow him in my car, and we drove off into the woods. Occasionally, he'd stop to comment on geography (Spring Creek, Holden Creek, Bald Mountain), botany (bleeding heart, kitkitdizze, hazelnut), and geology (serpentine, decomposed granite, Franciscan mélange—at this last name he groaned, as if it brought physical pain to permit something so highfalutin through his lips). I asked my questions with effort, approaching intimate proximity, then shouting into Harkin's Band-Aid encrusted ear.

Our route took us through various governance systems: private property, state park land, and federal areas. To my eyes at least, there was no obvious winner. In some places the trees had been allowed to grow willy-nilly into impassable thickets ("that there would burn like gasoline"); others had been thinned, or the underbrush had been cleared by a masticator (a massive crushing and chipping machine). The most pleasant spot—shaded by maples, the leaves forming a glowing-green scrim between the sun and a brook—was a private mining claim on public land.

It was noon by the time we reached our destination. Harkin suggested we lunch before we started work, and offered me a worn glass bottle of what looked like motor oil.

"Taste it first," he said. "I make it myself, so naturally it's a little weird."

This homebrew, he explained, was made by mixing a malt liquor called Pitbull with molasses, cayenne, and other spices, and then allowing it to ferment further. "During the summer you can't let a bottle roll around under the seat of your car too long, or it'll explode," he said.

It was surprisingly pleasant, like a sweet version of Guinness, with a yeasty alcoholic kicker. We sat in the dappled shade and ate. The trees around us were conifers, 80 to 100 feet tall, and a waist-high regiment of madrone saplings rose throughout the grove. Madrone has shiny, magnolia-like leaves, and silky red bark that peels off in papery curls. I'd never before seen so many young madrones growing in such close proximity. This land had last been logged sometime in the 1880s, Harkin speculated, creating the even-aged stand of conifers. A few years earlier the Bureau of Land Management (BLM) had conducted a controlled burn here, removing brush and small trees. The madrone had come up after that. Harkin's plan for the day was to lay out a transect, a random swath of land which he would study in detail, to see if he could learn something about how the area responded to fire. With a compass and measuring tape we plotted the dimensions of the transect, pounding in metal stakes to mark the corners. He kept up a running commentary as we worked.

"One big question is, why are all these madrone coming up here? Now madrone is a stump-sprouting tree, which means it has a head start after a fire, but this is clearly more than a stump. It's possible we are looking at an underground network of roots shooting up, but I don't know that anyone has shown that in this species. It's more what you'd expect to see with aspen."

Clearly there were more questions than answers to be found in this forest. And the questions of consequence, such as how a plot of land might be kept from turning into a brush choked firetrap, were the most difficult of all. You could clear by hand, Harkin said, or bring in a masticator, but both methods became prohibitively expensive over any large area. Controlled burns were even more costly. Herbicide spraying was cheaper, but often upsetting to people who live (and gather food) in the forest. Ideally, an ecologist would manipulate the species mix and density so as to cajole the growth toward an idyllic, open, park-like, fire-safe, and productive forest. But when I inquired (*fortissimo voce*) if Harkin knew of a way to achieve this, he shrugged: "That all depends on what you want."

There are so many variables at play in any cubic foot of dirt that the development of vegetation there can seem almost random. Harkin ticked off a few: slope, water table, light and heat, geologic substrate, orientation toward the sun and prevailing winds, proximity of other species, depth of leaf litter, and the nutrients available in the soil. This last, alone, is infinitely variable: The matrix of dirt—roots, minerals, mycelium (the mushroom filaments throughout the earth), insects, decaying needles, and bacteria—is so elaborate, so rococo in its internal economy of mineral goods and chemical services, that most compounds synthesized there are utterly novel. One soil scientist has been quoted as saying, "It is possible that no two humus molecules are or ever have been alike."

If each molecule of humus is new, never before seen on the face of the earth, how can we possibly presume to predict its behavior? Ideologies driven by faith in unchanging, universal truth are not suited to such rampant creativity. The forester who wants to work with nature's disordered abundance must be an eternal student, listening carefully, tinkering, allowing the forest to lead, experimenting, ready to take advantage of the genius of the mistake. Of course Harkin didn't say any of this to me—not in so many words. He was happy to point out where I had gone wrong, to discuss esoteric pieces of forestry science, to ruminate on philosophy, to gossip about national politics and local history, or wander tangentially from one subject to another, but he would never concede a direct answer. His deafness aided in these evasions even when I took care to enunciate loudly, and I started to suspect that he was deliberately mishearing the questions he did not want to answer. Throughout the day I probed with increasingly elliptical queries, hoping he would let something useful slip in his denials (his answers always seemed to start with "not exactly"). I came closest when I asked if it was simply impossible to manage a forest for wildlife, lumber, and people all at the same time.

"Impossible? No, that's too pessimistic." The forestry itself wasn't a problem, he said, that management could be done. The problem was managing the people. Politics was the crux, not science. When I pushed him to explain further, Harkin grew irritable. "I'm not involved in the political leadership around here," he snapped. "You're pretty tight with the people running the Yuba Watershed Institute, right?"

I nodded.

"Well if you want to talk about politics, you should be talking to them."

"But I don't want to talk about politics," I protested. "I'm here because I want to learn about the ecology. I mean, how would the forestry work if politics were no object?"

Harkin nodded sagely. "In that case . . ." He started speculatively—and I saw at once that I'd fallen into his favorite rhetorical trap, despite all my calculated bank-shot questions; he had managed to bring the conversation back, yet again, to the place we had started—"I guess I'd say that it all depends on what you want."

My growing frustration with this answer stemmed not just from its repetition, but from the fact that it skipped lightly over my main concern. I'd set out in search of a fitting place for humankind in this landscape—for a way to mesh profitability, scientific forestry, and natural beauty. Harkin would tantalize me by suggesting that this was technically possible, but then refused to tell me how.

At the end of my day with Harkin, after we had finished laying out the transect, I asked him if we could take a core from one of the conifers to see how fast they were growing. He grumbled that this was an inaccurate technique, but he was happy to teach me how to use an increment borer. He pulled two slender rods from his backpack and affixed them to form a T. The bottom of the T was hollow, with screw threads spiraling up around the outside of the tube. We selected a tree, a big sugar pine, and took turns turning the top of the T. The screw bit into the wood, pulling the borer inward and cutting free a cylinder of tree flesh. The dowel that emerged was light and fragrant, its surface glistening with moisture. Harkin put a gnarled finger at the end and counted the rings backward from 2011, occasionally noting an expected congruence: "1977 is a small ring, that was a drought year." We'd only taken half a foot, and Harkin slid it into a slit drinking straw for safekeeping; then, with a wad of pitch, he plugged the hole we'd made. Before we said our good-byes he handed this little rod to me.

"It's not worth a damn until it's dried and sanded," he said, before hustling Meryl into his van and driving off.

After we had parted company, I flipped through my notes ruefully. They were mostly fragments—sometimes just a single word jotted down for later research—all as hopelessly jumbled as Harkin's conversational peregrinations: warblers, sooty mold, 1872 mining law, ponderosa pine over grass in Arizona, "Native Americans didn't have chainsaws and they didn't have D8 cats," Montpellier's phytosociology, western gall rust, Bitterlick's basal area, axins, Soviets say root grafting proves the solidarity of the working class, and, revealingly: "I think there is no answer; the only answer is to bring up the most I can and let people make of it what they will."

It was only after struggling for weeks with this mess that I began to see I was being as obstinate as Harkin had been obscure: I wanted to erase the line between humanity and nature, and yet I insisted on maintaining a strict distinction between ecological feasibility and political feasibility. I'd wanted to subordinate politics to physical possibility, while Harkin had essentially responded: It's all politics.

Could this possibly be true? There are certainly problems that politics can't solve. A group of people working to build a perpetual motion machine will never succeed, no matter how robust their system of governance. Then again, our goals usually aren't so specific. The proposed perpetual motion machine (or an environmental plan) is merely a means to an end—a means that can be scrapped or revised when it fails. Politics, done well, is the process of finding goals people can agree on, and then identifying the right ways to get there.

This definition of politics has in it the hopeful echo of Garrett Hardin's despondent cry. In "The Tragedy of the Commons," Hardin saw politics as a coercive force, a police state's manacles needed to restrain humanity from exceeding nature's limits. But as I learned about the politics governing the forests on the Ridge, it became clear that this grim picture could be upended: Good politics can expand nature's bounty. When people find a common goal and focus their cumulative creativity on achieving it, they often find that nature is, as if in response, miraculously abundant. The solution to the political problem can be the solution to the ecological problem.

THE 'INIMIM FOREST

In 2009 Elinor Ostrom won the Nobel Prize for economics (the first woman to do so) for showing how to defuse the tragedy of the commons. Ostrom had found a crack in Hardin's seemingly airtight logic. While he, in his abstract reasoning, had assumed that people would behave like rational actors, she observed that people behaved instead like people: creatures capable of making deals, earning trust, and holding one another accountable. Hardin had argued that the only alternatives to environmental destruction were privatization or coercion. Ostrom added a third option: cooperative management of the commons.

People all over the world manage common resources without summoning Leviathan. Dairy farmers in the Swiss Alps share high-meadow pastures, and these meadows are not overgrazed because the farmers also engage a shepherd who will report anyone trying to add more than his share of animals on the sly. In Japan there is a long tradition of collectively managed forests, by which villagers take turns being the regulatory "detective" to police the commons. In the Philippines, workers often give 2 months of hard labor each year to maintain commonly owned dams and canals—an obligation taken so seriously that a farmer's land may be confiscated by the community if he misses too many work days. Cooperative management, however, isn't something that only happens in faraway lands where people rely on archaic traditions. You can find well-managed commons anywhere equals work together: Law partners and doctors often share pools of secretaries, or assistants. Municipal water departments share aquifers. And under my nose, 2,000 acres of cooperatively managed forest had developed on the Ridge.

In 1989, Don Harkin had spotted a legal notice in the newspaper announcing a land swap, which would turn over public land on the Ridge to Sierra Pacific Industries in exchange for parcels elsewhere. Sierra Pacific is a timber corporation that rotates clear-cuts across its holdings. When Harkin informed his neighbors of these plans, they were alarmed. Whether they were artists who had moved to the Ridge for its beauty, or marijuana farmers who appreciated its isolation, just about everyone had a reason to fight the land swap.

It's likely nothing would have come of these complaints if the man responsible for the land swap had not already had one run-in with the community on the Ridge. That man, Deane Swickard, field manager for the Bureau of Land Management, was no bookish bureaucrat, but a former Marine pilot who had returned from combat in Vietnam and then set records for the swiftness with which he rose in government service. A year earlier, he'd drawn the ire of Ridge residents with his plan to build a radio tower for the transmission of calls for backup when rangers confronted squatters or drug growers. The people on the Ridge had sent the BLM a wave of letters complaining, as Swickard remembered, "because the Buddhists chanted and the Indians sang there."

"Well, I gotta say," Swickard chuckled, "that kind of put me off. Chant and sing somewhere else because I've got a law enforcement problem here. To some extent they were a bunch of sandal-wearing, granola-chewing hippies. And my background is the Marine Corps. So you've got a little gap there."

When Swickard had taken the job, however, he had pledged to himself that, rather than run things from his office, he would touch the land he governed and look the people he was dealing with in the eyes.

"So I chug on up to the San Juan Ridge," Swickard said. "We meet up on Bald Mountain, and I've got this posse of people peppering me with questions. I expected some hostility, and it was a little hostile—it is not a trusting group of people up there, at least when it comes to the government. But they were also willing to listen."

Swickard was impressed by the tenor of the conversation—these were not simply narrowly focused environmentalists. He didn't know then that one of those people was Gary Snyder, an internationally recognized poet, often thought of as one of the elder deans of environmental thinking. Snyder's presence had drawn many of the other residents to the Ridge—eccentric, scientifically minded, freethinking people.

"These people were genuine," Swickard said. "They were interesting, bright people that I could learn from."

The residents were concerned, it became clear, about how the tower would look. He offered a compromise: The BLM would check to see if there were any other feasible locations, and set up a model so that people could see exactly how intrusive it would be. The Ridge residents agreed. And after they saw the model they gave the plan their approval.

"There was a little spark of communication and trust there," Swickard said. "I thought: 'This might be an interesting place to try out some bigger ideas.'"

He got his chance when residents assembled against his land swap. Swickard told them that if they wanted to contribute to land management decisions they had to organize and offer solutions rather then simply try to stop everything he wanted to do. He promised that if the locals could come up with a cooperative management plan he would enforce it, and cancel the land swap. Len Brackett, who lived down a fire road from Harkin, knew enough about bureaucracies to see that Swickard was sticking his neck out.

"Isn't this a little risky for you?" he asked.

"I'm not afraid of trying anything that makes sense," Swickard said. "As long as it's consistent with law and policy, I'll do it. C'mon, there are no bullets flying here, we're just talking. Where's the risk?"

And so a motley group of Ridge-dwellers assembled in Snyder's barn and drew up an initial document outlining their mission. It read, in part: "The guiding principle of the partnership is that of a cooperative stewardship of the land to ensure that existing resource values are not lost or reduced, but sustained and enhanced for the long-term benefit of not only local residents, but the American people as a whole."

Figuring out how to do that was maddeningly difficult. One resident objected to plans for thinning the forest on the grounds that it might make his illicit crops more visible to agents of the Drug Enforcement Administration. Others were simply suspicious of any government representative and any change. "There were people who pretty much hated our guts," said Bob Erickson, a furniture maker who found himself devoting more and more time to this enterprise. Representatives of every ideology chimed in. There were those who believed the forest should not be touched; those who wanted to manage it according to strict scientific principles; those who wanted to utilize the power of commerce; and those who recoiled at the mention of money. The hours spent reconciling these differences were frustrating for Swickard, who had no budget to pursue the project and had to squeeze in meetings around the gaps in his schedule.

"I remember at one point this woman was in tears," Swickard said. "She was shaking, and literally crying, begging me not to kill the manzanita. 'Well lady, we're going to clear brush so that this whole place doesn't burn. So yeah, some things are going to die.'"

Despite the raw emotions, the meetings made progress. People found that it was impossible to cleave to their abstract convictions when they were talking about something so tangible, so readily observable in their backyards. They could all see what worked and what failed, and this provided a check on ideologically driven debates. As they talked, the rednecks and hippies got to know each other and became less guarded. Compromise became conceivable. Curiosity replaced militant certainty.

When public land administrators produce a management plan they usually conduct thorough environmental assessments but, because there was no money, Swickard suggested that the residents begin surveying the land themselves. The community ably took up the task.

"One of the things this has taught me is to trust the intellectual power of communities," Swickard said. "I had 30 absolutely great employees, but they all went to land-grant colleges and read the same textbooks and had pretty much the same ideas. But in a community a couple of hundred people will come out with totally different points of view. One guy was a dentist, but he'd spent 30 years watching how things worked in his backyard. On the Ridge we got this top-flight birder, a guy from the Yale School of Forestry [Harkin], and Erickson who has ideas from working with wood. We used Gary Snyder as our scribe to take notes. And all of a sudden you've got a hundred minds working with you, rather than being cynical and suspicious. You get fresh ideas."

One of the most audacious of these fresh ideas came from Len Brackett, a builder of traditional Japanese houses, who suggested that instead of managing the forest like a plantation—to quickly produce cheap lumber—they manage the land to produce the high-value wood that timber-framers like him need. These woodworkers look for timbers that are fine grained, free of knots, and large enough to form the center beam of a barn. That kind of wood only comes from old trees. This idea fit with something Swickard had been pondering for years. Industrial clear-cuts may make sense in some situations, he said, "but it doesn't make so much sense when you are doing it in someone's backyard. It's a pretty violent assault on the landscape. It doesn't look good, and it doesn't feel good."

If Brackett's idea was implemented with care, it might be possible to reap profits from timber while maintaining the aesthetics and the wildlife habitat of the land. In 1996, six long years after the first discussions began, the community finished its management plan. It was crafted to achieve four goals: more big trees, fewer big fires, diversity of wildlife, and soil conservation. This meant they'd do some selective logging for fire protection, while allowing most trees the decades they needed to get big. Eventually, they'd start selling this high-value timber at a sustainable rate. As Swickard had promised, the BLM adopted the plan.

This could have been an opportunity for the locals to appropriate resources that belong to the country as a whole. But, instead of pillaging the woods, these residents adopted them. They named the land the 'Inimim Forest, after the native term for ponderosa pine, and began cataloging wildlife sightings, noting the trees that housed pileated woodpeckers, and conducting formal frog counts and bird-banding projects. They also began policing themselves. Once, while I was talking with Erickson, we heard the coughing roar of a chainsaw starting up. He swore under his breath and dashed off into the BLM forest near his house. Moments later, the chainsaw hiccupped and died. Locals had been illegally cutting wood from the public land for years—now it's hard to get away with it. Once the community began managing the forest, they also began to take pride in it, and enforce the rules they'd set.

Formerly murderous tensions—between factions, and toward the administrators caught in the middle—eased. "The BLM could have a lot of trouble up here," Don Harkin told me. "Instead, they have no trouble at all." This peaceful accord was remarkable, given that—in the "Timber Wars" of the 1990s—loggers and environmentalists were trying (sometimes successfully) to kill each other with tree spikes and car bombs.

In the years after the residents began managing the land, more creatures seemed to show up in the woods. At a time when biologists were warning that the number of yellow-legged frogs had fallen to dangerously low levels, this species was increasing around the 'Inimim. Members of the Yuba Watershed Institute sighted mountain lions. Spotted owls established nests on adjoining parcels. It's too early, however, to tell whether the forest can be profitable as well as beautiful. By definition, old-growth forestry takes a long time. The BLM has sold more than $90,000 worth of timber from the land, but this logging consisted only of small thinning projects, and the receipts came nowhere close to covering the costs of management.

There are older forests, however, that provide proof of concept. Arcata, a coastal California town near the Oregon border, owns and manages 2,000 acres of redwood forest, which provides a view for many east-facing windows, and trails for hiking and mountain biking. When I suggested to Arcata Environmental Services manager, Mark Andre, that the only real way to make money in forestry is through intensive plantations, he scoffed. For years, the Arcata Community Forest has stoked the city's treasury with profits. "The bigger the trees, the less expensive it is to get them out of the forest," he said (it's cheaper to build one road to one big tree than to build 10 roads to a lot of little trees). "So we have bigger margins. And when you are thinking about the long term, you have more options as the market goes up or down—as opposed to an even-aged plantation forest where you pretty much have to cut everything at once." Though truckloads of redwood come out of the forest every year, the city manages the land so that the total board feet standing in the trees has always increased.

Len Brackett, the Japanese-style builder, was hopeful that the 'Inimim could achieve something similar. He'd taken cores from some of the big sugar pines near his house and found that the trees are adding about 2 inches in diameter every 5 years. A younger tree grows faster (and this provides the usual argument for cutting at 60 to 80 years), but because these old trees were easily 8 feet around and 200 feet tall, each inch added to the radius constituted a tremendous volume of wood. Brackett performed some rough calculations and estimated that each tree was growing 300 board feet of wood a year. More importantly, because the trees were tall with few branches for the first 100 feet, the lumber would be what carpenters call "clear" wood: gentle, even-grained, unlikely to warp or crack—the kind of golden wood that sells for over $5 a board foot.

"Three-hundred board-feet of clear sugar pine timber," he told me, marveling. "That's the equivalent to $1,500 a year, just from one tree."

Being in possession of a sugar-pine core myself, I decided to drive out to Len Brackett's house. It's an elegant structure with a slate roof and sliding rice-paper walls, held together by joinery rather than nails. The air indoors is perfumed by cedar oils. Brackett, who had finished his day's work, asked if I'd have a drink with him. He juiced a lemon and made a pair of whiskey sours. We sat on his deck, looking over the creek, and sipped.

My measurement of the sugar pine core put its growth at 1.8 inches in diameter every 5 years—just a little less than his trees had been growing. But I wondered if it was reasonable to expect more people to buy wood at $5 a board foot. Brackett nodded. Most builders would blanch at that price when cheap lumber sells for less than 30 cents a board foot. But, he'd, it wasn't always logical to build with cheap materials. He'd been convinced of the value of high-quality wood during his apprenticeship in Japan. One of the buildings he'd worked on was part of the Daitoku-ji, a famous temple in Kyoto that had been built in the 13th century.

"We were replacing the roof, and the wooden roof-structure underneath—all made of local pine—was in perfect condition. It had been built around the time they were starting up the Crusades. I'm sure it was expensive, but if you look at the cost over however many generations that is, it makes some sense."

"When it comes to forest sustainability," Brackett said, "one thing I would suggest is that you build houses that last a long time and that are so beautiful that no one would ever want to tear them down."

During the last half of the 20th century, the United States took the opposite tack. After World War II it became federal policy to provide cheap lumber as part of the effort to put veterans in their own homes. When the U.S. Forest Service began to manage its lands more intensively, it didn't bring in much money (most—often all—of the profits were sucked up to pay for foresters, bureaucracy, and fire control) but that wasn't the point. The point was cheap timber for cheap houses. By flooding the markets for lumber and housing, the government drove down prices and spurred a new kind of sprawling growth. Levittowns sprang up around the country.

This history, which I considered while sipping a second potent cocktail, cast the imperative for ultra-efficient logging in a different light. It's true that, if we want wood, we need to cut down trees. But the number of trees required to serve the market, and the land-management strategies demanded by those numbers, all depend—as Harkin says—on what we want. Suburban sprawl and ticky-tacky McMansions require quickly growing trees, and the small-diameter mills that generate two-by-fours and chipboard. They demand, in other words, a style of forest management that efficiently produces low-cost, low-quality lumber. The wood does not need to be perfectly straight or free of knots, it just needs to hold up a roof. The ugliness and uniformity of an even-aged plantation is mirrored in unlovely cookie-cutter developments. Ugliness begets ugliness.

When I said goodbye to Brackett he asked if I was sober enough to drive, and I insisted I was. But I caught myself swaying on the path back to the car, and I decided it would be wise to pause for a moment to think before descending the twisting dirt road back to Nevada City. I was feeling physically clumsy, but mentally lucid. There, in Brackett's driveway, I was filled with an unfamiliar sense of optimism. What lifted me (with a little assistance from Jack Daniels) was the notion that beauty begets beauty: Beautiful homes could yield beautiful forests, not just the other way around. Instead of a zero-sum game in which any additions to civilization's side of the ledger must be subtracted from nature's account, here was a glimpse of land that was growing healthier and more beautiful under the influence of civilization. The 'Inimim Forest was small, but its significance—at least to me—was huge. It was the first concrete example I had seen in which the landscape I'd come to love as a child was both thriving and supporting people. I'd grown up in a world of environmental absolutes: Yosemite Valley and the Central Valley, old growth and clear-cuts, nature trails and strip malls.

Under the old system of environmental thought, land was either virgin and therefore sacred, or corrupted and therefore fit for exploitation. As Michael Pollan once put it, "This old idea may have taught us how to worship nature, but it didn't tell us how to live with her. It told us more than we needed to know about virginity and rape, and almost nothing about marriage."

On the Ridge I'd witnessed a richer form of relations—this was not just détente between civilization and wilderness, but something that looked a lot like matrimony. For someone who had seen nothing but the ecological equivalents of prostitution and unrequited love, the possibility of loving family relations struck like a thunderbolt.

As a metaphor for the human relationship to the land, marriage acknowledges the failure of tyrannical dominion by either partner: There is no single solution for a marriage, but a million tiny solutions that must be improvised and refined. As a result there are always mistakes: the misplaced word that causes an argument, the controlled burn that licks up into the canopy. Such missteps can be revelatory, and ultimately can improve the relationship, but only if there is someone not blinded by theory who is paying attention. A marriage creates a community of two, while a marriage of people and the land creates something larger: This, wrote Gary Snyder, scribe of the 'Inimim Forest, is the real definition of a commons. Both land and culture depend upon this union of human and nonhuman:

> There will be no "tragedy of the commons" greater than this: if we do not recover the commons—regain personal, local, community, and peoples' involvement in sharing (in *being*) the web of the wild world—that world will keep slipping away . . . And, it is clear, the loss of a local commons heralds the end of self-sufficiency and signals the doom of the vernacular culture of the region.

When the question is not how to manage something far away, but how to shape the neighborhood, it's easier for people to put aside their abstract ideas about what is natural. It's easier for people to give up absolute allegiance to Mother Nature, or Scientific Certainty, or The Invisible Hand. And when people let go of these abstractions, it can free them up to combine their love of nature with good science and pragmatic economic incentives to devise a system that works with the realities on the ground.

I'd resisted this idea because, to be blunt, I didn't trust people. We seemed too venal, too cruel, and ultimately too stupid to solve such large problems. But abandoning the search for some universal straitjacket to make people behave, and instead giving them the keys to the asylum, has advantages. Sure, humans turn mean when they think they might be cheated, and cold when faced with a problem beyond their ken, but more frequently they are generous, hospitable beyond all reason. Humans, at their best, are noble, patient, and humble. My teenage-activist self would have objected by asserting that, even at its best, humanity would eventually collapse under its own weight: No matter how clever the forestry scheme, it would be overwhelmed as population rose, would it not? I had to admit that the situation seemed desperate: If it took 6 years for a small group of neighbors to solve a local problem, how long would it take the earth's billions to ever find solutions for quandaries that are global in scope? But the 'Inimim had kindled a small flame of hope that could not be stifled.

I took this hope back with me to San Francisco. There was a forest around me that I'd never acknowledged, and I resolved to get to know the trees as I knew them in Nevada City. I found there were carob trees a block from my house. I registered the change of brilliant yellow flowers to purple seed pods in the Bailey's acacia. I noted when the plums blossomed and when the gingkos turned yellow. I noticed for the first time how afflicted with thrips the myoporum trees were, their malformed leaves swelling into clubs around the infections. I began to perceive a new layer of activity around me. And I began to see where I might fit in.

In cities, it's the streets, rather than the woods, that are the commons, and I began to take an interest in how they were managed. The discussions weren't so different from the land-management talks in Nevada City—rather than arguing about trees people argued about cars and bikes. I did my best to steer clear of the endless policy discussions and the vitriolic online debates, but eventually I broke down and started going to planning meetings, and occasionally volunteering. I began to find dozens of little 'Inimim Forests—places where small groups of patient people had improved the land by working together, like the timed lights that allow bicyclists to coast through one green after another on Valencia Street. These efforts were designed to make San Francisco more hospitable, but they have also improved the larger commons. As a result, the city has reduced its carbon dioxide emissions by 14.5 percent below 1990 levels. The work is slow and frustrating. But that's the nature of tinkering. It can take decades (if not centuries) of attention to work out a political accord that allows civilization to fit comfortably within nature. When more people pitch in, however, it speeds things up.

Before the word *politics* implied holy war between immovable certainties, it had a meaning associated with the relations of neighbors. The word originally comes, not from notions of scheming and domination, but from the Greek terms for *citizen* and *city:* It concerns the tangible question of how best to live together. The 'Inimim Forest was a humble experiment, one that has not yet even fully proven itself. Still, it's enough to provide hope of a *polis* that includes the wild, and a wilderness that includes humanity. It's modest enough that it just might work.

CHAPTER SIX

MASTURBACON

AGRICULTURE

I took the first job I was offered out of college and began working as a general-assignment reporter at a newspaper in Burley, Idaho. I liked the idea of being a journalist because, in my mind, journalism represented the polar opposite of flaky health-food-store credulity: It meant getting to the bottom of things. It meant *just the facts.* But I had absolutely no newspaper experience, which is how I ended up in Burley. You can find Burley on a map by following the Utah–Nevada border north until it encounters Idaho's southern limit, and then continuing on 40 miles northeast. From above it's a blotch of green pivot circles spreading along the canals that web out from the Snake River.

When I arrived I found—to my frequent mortification—that I had entered a world where the laws of social physics as I knew them no longer applied. I learned to say that I'd gone to a small university in California rather than confessing I'd attended a *liberal* arts college. Likewise, you could hardly find fewer sympathizers for an all-natural ethic than in Idaho's Magic Valley, whose name celebrated the technological conquest of nature and the engineers who had transformed the parched sagebrush flats into farmland.

For the first 6 months in the Magic Valley, I struggled miserably. It was fraying to hear the derision of the principles that I had previously taken to be self-evident. But those jeers also put me in the fortunate position of having to either abandon my beliefs, or dig into them and discover what precepts at their core I found truly worthy of defense. Before Idaho, I had known it was possible for a conservative to be either intelligent or selfless but was unconvinced that those qualities could occur in the same person. In Burley, I found countless living examples of kindness and wisdom to remind me of my prejudice.

I grew to love the wrinkled cowboys, the hard-dealing sheep ranchers, and the enterprising dairymen who appeared at the local meetings I covered. Their speech was grammatically creative in a way that transcended error and became a sort of poetry. After one land-use meeting, a rancher approached a lanky white-haired man who unfolded himself from his chair to shake hands.

"You still breaking horses out there?"

"We is."

The rancher whistled "That's a hard way to serve the Lord."

One way or the other, however, these cowboys seemed destined for history's manure heap. Either the consolidated beef packers would squeeze them into penury (a project well under way), or the ranching families would give up raising cattle on rangeland in favor of feedlots: Modernize, or dry up like the tumbleweed.

As I scribbled my way through Cassia County commissioner's meetings I began to see that what I was covering was, in sum, a second transformation as big as the one that had created the Magic Valley in the first place. The hearings I attended were ostensibly about setbacks and variances, zoning and budgets, but in reality the agenda was always the same: How could the region serve the world market without selling its soul?

Burley and the other surrounding towns were gap-toothed with decaying storefronts. It was clear from the police blotter I typed up each day that there was pervasive drug addiction beneath the surface of this pious Mormon region. I could see the ravages through my own windows. I lived in an apartment complex—a set of three-story units of pinkish-orange brick and aqua-blue trim, clustered around a blighted weed patch—which called itself the Norman Manor. No matter how thoroughly I scrubbed, I could never entirely exorcise the humid nicotine ghost of my apartment's previous occupant. When I boiled pasta, condensation rolled down the walls in sticky yellow rivulets. From my front window I had a view of an auto mechanic's shed, a set of Simplot grain towers, and a school bus parking lot. Beyond was sagebrush and wind—always wind. Locals sometimes joked that Burley was accidentally founded when a wagon train of pioneers, driven to distraction by the wind, had vowed to halt and take shelter until it stopped blowing. In the winter, storms whooped round my apartment and harried the windows with the desperation of a starving animal. And as I got to know the residents in my complex I began to fancy that the wind, eddying into the corner formed by the apartment buildings, had piled up everyone too rootless or poor to buy a house, like so many leaves.

All of us were merely pausing, hoping for something better. There was a woman raising her grandchildren while her daughter was in jail, a couple whose fights filtered through my walls, a hollow-eyed neighbor who smoked ceaselessly at the base of my stairs and stared through me when I said hello. My downstairs neighbor was a withered alcoholic who would join me at my kitchen table on the Sundays when he was sober enough to help me do the crossword puzzle. I played chess with the apartment manager who told me how the police had raided an apartment where a resident had been cooking methamphetamine. He had torn up the carpets and periodically applied another layer of paint, but no one knew if there was any way to make a home safe again once those toxins had leached into the walls. The rise of meth only made sense, he opined one evening as I puzzled over the chessboard. As farms got bigger and more industrial they'd brought in the chemicals needed to make the drug. They'd also brought monotonous, low-paying jobs—feces pumpers, graveyard-shift milkers, slaughter-house cutters—precisely the sort of thing that begged for a drug that turned users into fanatically driven, untiring dynamos. The changing economy provided both the supply and the demand.

These changes clouded the clear libertarian vision with which the land had been governed for years. One old-timer, protesting the use of grant monies to rehabilitate drug addicts, informed the county commissioners that there was a better way. "In my father's time we'd ride them to the county line," he said. "And tell them not to come back unless they was so fond of the Cassia County soil they wanted to spend a lot of time in it."

A commissioner inclined his head to one side and chuckled. "Well now," he said. "It's not so simple anymore."

For many respectable residents the aesthetic changes they noticed in conjunction with the Magic Valley's second transformation were just as disturbing as the rise of poverty and the crime that went with it. The new form of farming that promised to heal the region's ailing finances depended on the concentration of thousands of animals. These confined animal feeding operations, or CAFOs, created economies of scale. They allowed milking machines to run 24 hours a day, and trucks to pick up an entire load of animals in one stop. But they also made the landscape less pleasant. The aroma of feces was inescapable, and the wind freighted dirt around by the spade-full. In those rare windless moments, black hailstorms of flies fell from the sky. The simple tenets of rangeland justice offered little guidance in regulating these plagues. When I drove out to a prairie home to ask the 79-year old Wendell Pierce why he'd quit the planning and zoning board, he lifted his palms skyward. "I joined up because I thought it would be a good place to protect property rights. But then, whose rights do you protect?"

I knew what he meant. Both the CAFO operator, and the homeowner who complained of diminished quality of life, could legitimately claim his defense. And while the CAFOs might rescue the region from insolvency, they might not leave anything worth rescuing.

Residents, complaining of mysterious illnesses, showed me how chemists had detected pesticides and nitrates in their wells. Hydrologists, furthermore, confirmed the existence of excremental plumes seeping into the water table. Locals began to triangulate the addresses recently visited by cancer and they demanded that I expose the causes, Erin Brokovitch style. I was seized by the clean symmetry of the notion: the ugliness and stink above ground spreading through dark passages, to metastasize into a mirror-image corruption inside bodies. But my story fizzled when scientists told me that, unless the chemical readings were 10 times as high, they would not suspect that pollution had been the cause of these tumors.

There was an element of truth to the idea that human health and the health of Cassia County were linked, but as always, it was not a simple matter of mechanical cause and effect. The connections were complex, too complex for an easily distracted newspaper reporter with daily deadlines. I would never have dug deeper had prurient fascination not led me back into the details. And this fascination would never have been kindled if my friend Becky had not been so frustrated with her job the night we met for a beer, shortly before I left Burley.

Becky worked at a big hog farm outside of town. Each day she faced an unending line of sows filing into the room where she worked. Occasionally one of the 200-pound pigs broke ranks, knocking Becky down.

"Sometimes they get nervous when you stimulate them," she said.

I set down my beer. "Stimulate?"

"Yeah, for artificial insemination. Usually if you bring a boar around they'll get in the mood. But if not you just have to get in there and start rubbing away."

At my urging, Becky obligingly laid out the intricacies of coaxing sows to conceive, along with equally piquant methods of harvesting boar semen. This seemed, at first blush, like an awful lot of effort to expend on something creatures normally do without encouragement.

It began to make more sense, of course, as I gathered the facts. The science of pork production has made tremendous strides, and one wouldn't expect to find pigs doing anything the old-fashioned way at state-of-the-art hog facilities. But artificial insemination ("AI," in the industry) is more than a byproduct of modernization. It has served as the enabling technology for a process that has transformed pigs from affable, pot-bellied forest dwellers to panicky, torpedo-shaped clones that cannot survive outdoors, but can produce monstrous, lean hams.

Though I'd been reporting on the tide of CAFOs flooding Cassia County for 2 years, I'd never learned exactly what went on inside their walls. Previously, any concerns I might have had about hog farming always vanished right about lunchtime. But when I discovered the ubiquity of this breeding technique I became curious: If swine masturbation was required to produce my bacon, what else was involved in bringing pork to the table? Traveling down this rabbit hole (or pig hole, if you like), allowed me to trace the proximate causes of AI back to their final perfect logic. It was this logic that was driving CAFOs into being.

THE MODERN FAMILY HOG FARM

I'd asked Becky if I could come witness the modern fertility ritual she had described, but she didn't have enough clout to bring me into the bio-secure inner sanctum. Over the course of the next year, I called anyone I could think of who might better help me understand this practice and the industry that had come to depend on it. This reporting carried me, one frosty December morning, to the Sleezer Fertility Clinic in Aurelia, Iowa.

The Sleezer family keeps two red metal barns full of pigs, spaced 3 miles apart, off a county road. I passed the first barn and, following Derrick Sleezer's instructions, drove on between barren winter fields of plowed earth. Then I turned down a dirt road and drove toward the second barn and the little cluster of buildings behind it. These hog houses are long, low affairs, built in a simple barracks style, designed to house as many porcine bodies as possible while conserving materials.

But as I drove closer I could see the barn design had evolved beyond a devotion to simplicity. White fans dotted one wall like jet engines, making the barns look like a cross between a barracks and a power plant. I parked under a copse of trees between a little prefab office and the farmhouse where Derrick's parents still live.

Derrick Sleezer welcomed me with an earnest handshake. He showed me into the office's brand-new conference room and offered me a soda. He sat down and, looking at me through wire-rimmed glasses, told me his primary goal was to maintain the family's reputation for integrity. I knew I could trust him immediately. Then he sat back and asked how he could help me. He'd be happy to tell me anything I wanted to know about the farm.

"So, the Sleezer Fertility Center," I asked, "what is it?"

"We're a boar stud," Sleezer said matter-of-factly.

"Oh, right." I scribbled "boar stud" in my notebook, then paused a beat as I reread the words.

"Um, what exactly do you do?"

"We keep the boars here and make fresh semen deliveries."

In the early 1990s, Derrick said, farmers started asking his father, Butch Sleezer, to artificially inseminate their young sows. Then they asked him to hold on to their boars. That was when big streamlined hog farms were moving into the Midwest and pork producers were converting from generalists who kept a few pigs on the side, to swine specialists. Tending to the boars, which had once been a single task in a busy day, became a business of its own.

In 1990 artificial insemination accounted for only 7 percent of America's swine breeding. At that time large confinement operations were just emerging as industry leaders. These big operations aimed to maximize their efficiency by producing standardized pigs, which grew at predictable rates and produced predictably uniform meat. To make a standardized pig, these companies needed standardized genetics, which they could most easily distribute in the form of semen. By 2000, more than 90 percent of large hog farms depended on artificial insemination. And with the rise of AI, boar-stud operations, the Sleezers' among them, began to sprout up across the country.

The Sleezers' boars live in the first barn I had passed on the way in. It's 3 miles from the other barn, which contains only sows, in order to reduce the risk of the wind blowing pathogens between the two herds. A chain-link fence, topped with razor wire, keeps away people and animals, which are also potential disease vectors. Nothing meant for human consumption comes out of the building; it produces only semen, delivered to a nearby lab via an underground pneumatic tube. The tube carries the fluid in containers that look very much like those at drive-through bank-teller windows.

In the old days, a prize boar would provide natural service to sows on the local farms. Today, this would be economic suicide for large producers and a literal death sentence for the pigs. The modern pig is so susceptible to disease that producers must take extreme measures to transform their barns into pathogen-free bubbles. The pigs are vulnerable because they live in close quarters, and because they are genetically uniform—a bug that breaches one pig's immune system can hop to the next. A bacterium stowing away between a traveling boar's toes could wipe out half a herd. Producers expose their hogs to fewer germs when they bring only the semen from outside rather than the whole hog.

Sleezer's protective measures are not limited to fencing and pneumatic tubes: He keeps new boars in quarantine for 60 days and tests their blood three times before moving them in with the rest of the herd. The Sleezers run the farm as a family, but to avoid transporting germs, only Derrick ever enters the boar barn. When I visited, the swine were also getting a small amount of antibiotics in their feed, which helped them fend off sickness. It's a controversial practice because bacteria eventually develop resistance to the antibiotics—and antibiotic-resistant bacteria kills more than 14,000 Americans each year (though it's hard to tell which bacteria evolved on farms and which in hospitals). At the time, almost all hog farms used low-level antibiotics in feed because, besides improving health, antibiotics boost animal growth rates. Antibiotic use for growth promotion was outlawed in 2012, but there are no penalties for those who ignore the rule, and the drugs are still allowed for preemptive disease prevention.

Other operations often maintain even more stringent measures than the Sleezers. One company required a father and son who worked in different barns to eat their dinners apart in order to avoid exchanging germs. The most high-tech facilities start their herds with piglets fresh from the womb, delivered by Caesarean section, scrubbed clean and nursed by a mechanical sow.

Before I even had a chance to ask, Sleezer told me there was no way I was getting in the boar barn. I was glad for a reprieve from my rendezvous with boar spunk, but also disappointed after traveling so far. I could see I wasn't going to change Derrick's mind, so I asked if I could look inside the other barn, where they keep some 800 sows. That would be up to his father, Derrick said. Butch Sleezer, a tall, square-jawed man, agreed, on one condition:

He fixed me with a look of deadly gravity and asked, "Now, you've got to be honest with me here. You haven't been around any other pigs recently, have you?"

Since I had not, Butch took me to the house to dress. He gave me a blue jumpsuit, an orange hooded sweatshirt, and a pair of plastic booties. We paused just outside the barn while I, feeling awkward in my makeshift biohazard suit, pulled the thick plastic slippers over my shoes. This, I thought, is what it must have been like to call on the aging Howard Hughes. As Butch explained, the coverings would protect both the pigs from germs on my clothes and my clothes from the ammonia fumes in the barn.

"I'd pull that hood up if you don't want it to get in your hair," he said, before we entered the barn. We stepped into a narrow hallway, well lit, with white plastic walls. Machinery hummed softly. The concrete floor was spotless. It might have been a hospital. Around a corner stood a row of doors, each with a control panel. Butch opened one and I put my head inside. The atmosphere was as I imagine it would be on Venus: thick, warm, and caustic. Butch was pleased.

"We spend more money on propane for heating so we can keep the ventilation going," he said. "You go into some of these places, you can't hardly breathe."

There were about 25 sows inside, each confined by a metal crate to an area about two and a half by seven feet. The sows filled their cages. They had a foot or two in which to move forward or back, and enough room to lie down but not enough to turn around. Each had a litter of suckling pigs. The Sleezers sell the piglets to other farmers, who raise them for meat.

Butch pointed to a panel on the hallway wall.

"Everything is controlled right here," he said.

The machinery sets the angle of the louvers that draw fresh air from outside; it monitors the ventilation fans, adjusts the heat, and turns on the lights. Should the room fall 6°F below the optimum temperature, the control panel calls all the Sleezers' telephones. I grinned at Butch. There was something delightful in the thought of this ever vigilant mechanical farmer making minute adjustments in the atmospheric composition and heat.

Keeping pigs at just the right temperature allows them to devote every ounce of energy to one purpose: growth. Well, growth and survival. The modern pig is bred too lean to survive Iowa's winters. The blanket of fat that insulates pigs against the cold does not fetch the price of muscle—that is to say, meat. But producing a layer of back fat takes energy, and energy means feed, which in turn means money. So geneticists have bred most of the lard out of the hog in the last 50 years. Now many of these pigs cannot survive outside the womb of the thrumming, computerized barn.

Butch led me down the hall, and we peered into two other rooms.

"Look at the uniformity of these litters," he said with pride, counting. "Two, four, six—ten in that one."

The piglets scampering around their enclosures looked as if they had all been cast in the same mold, and they almost certainly did have the same father. Meatpackers want identical pigs, the better to give customers identical hams. Artificial insemination makes this possible, because breeders can distribute semen from a single exemplary boar all across the country.

This cookie-cutter perfection, of course, becomes a liability when a pig gets sick. But the demand for uniformity outweighs this risk. The more similar the swine, the more easily they fit into the mechanized system, increasing efficiency. As swine carcasses move down the conveyor belt in packing plants, for instance, they hit a curved knife, which slices the cylindrical loin from the inside of the body cavity. If the animals don't have just the right proportions, the knife will hit the wrong spot, wasting meat or cutting into bone. The meatpacking plant is the model for the efficiencies we associate with factories. After paying a visit to a disassembly line at a slaughterhouse, Henry Ford went back to his Highland Park auto plant and designed something he called an "assembly line."

Before leaving the barn, Butch Sleezer showed me the gestation room, a much larger space, which houses about 700 clean, white sows. The hogs stood in tight formation, row upon row stretching off to the end of the building under dusty, yellowish lights. Crates held the pigs in line with their noses next to a water trough and their tails over a slatted floor. The pigs had scattered the remains of their seed-meal breakfast across the floor. The animals eat where they stand and deposit their dung at the other end of the crate. Their own feet, or a shot with a hose, sends the waste through cracks in the floor.

Producers sometimes keep sows in group pens, which allow them to walk around. But in confinement, pigs can go a little crazy. They often attack one another, even killing and eating their pen mates. Group pens do not provide enough room for a bullied sow to escape her tormentors.

As we walked down the narrow path between two rows of pigs, the barn filled with the crash of metal and unholy screaming. The sows bellowed, squealed, and recoiled. Others lunged against the bars as we passed.

"They can tell when a stranger comes in," Butch said.

Partway down the aisle, Butch stopped and pointed to the ceiling.

"Feel the air? It comes down from there and hits there—right across the shoulders." He made a slicing motion down the line of pigs. "That way every one of them has fresh air."

Fresh air is especially important in a room suspended above an open sewer. The feces fall through the slatted floors into a pit and gases from the decomposing slurry rise back into the barn. (I've since received notices, via my subscription to an industry newsletter, urging me to "Prevent manure pit explosions" by allowing enough ventilation so that methane doesn't accumulate.)

We stepped outside and came into view of the lagoon, where the contents of this cellar are periodically flushed. Beyond, a more modern sewage unit was under construction: a concrete swimming pool, bristling with rebar. At the far end, a backhoe muscled loads of mud out of a drainage trench.

A soil study had shown that the earthen lagoon might leak, Sleezer said, hence the concrete tank. A grant from the U.S. Department of Agriculture had paid for almost half of the $150,000 tank, but not for the unforeseen cost of the backhoe after a rainstorm clogged the drainage pipes with mud.

The Sleezers also grow crops, so they can apply manure to the fields as a fertilizer in the spring. But when pork producers reach a certain size, this tidy cycle—manure to corn to pig to manure—breaks down. Bigger producers must use other methods to dispose of waste, because there is not enough nearby land to absorb it. One of the biggest producers, Circle Four Farms in Utah (owned by a Smithfield subsidiary), uses the simple miracle of evaporation to spirit away the equivalent of almost 200 Olympic-sized swimming pools of liquefied manure annually. The fecal matter dries and vanishes on the wind.

There was nothing pleasant about the smell that pooled in the car as I drove away, or the feeling of dull shock I felt at the memory of the sows hurling themselves against their bars, but the logic of the system was irrefutable. The Sleezers had taken on the cost of this barn with the hope that they could use it to make a little more money. Every square foot of barn space added to the debt. Every square foot not occupied by a pig decreased their ability to pay it off. And when the competition is using such methods to produce more pigs for less money, how can they not?

By combining crops, hogs, and semen, the Sleezers have retooled the family farm to survive in this era of giant pork producers. But the future of even such modern operations is in doubt. A 1997 paper published by the Federal Reserve Bank of Chicago coolly observed, "The standards set by the largest hog producers now suggest that some 50 producers could account for all the hogs needed in the U.S." Such efficiency has driven down the cost of food and decimated Midwestern farms. As I drove away from the Sleezers', along back roads, I passed one empty house after another—relics of the old rural economy. Outside of the town of Manson I slowed to peer at a small, hand-painted sign. WE APPRECIATE YOUR BUSINESS, it read, in faded script. The ineffectual plea for salvation struck a tender spot within me. I could imagine the local economic-development meeting where the sign had been dreamed up. I'd attended ribbon cuttings for similar initiatives in Idaho.

Before I left the Sleezer farm, I'd asked Butch if taking on the debt to build his high-tech barns made him nervous. He nodded grimly. The technology evolves so quickly it's impossible to keep up, he said. Yet it's also impossible not to try. "That's the thing about being in the hog business and building these buildings," he said. "They're tombstones."

A Date with the Inseminator

Rain was falling hard on the walnut groves that surround WD Swine Farm in Modesto, California, when I arrived. I had come because Ryan Watje had agreed to let me observe the way the pork chop begins. I knew I was in the right place when I saw the Ford F250 with a vanity plate reading WDSF and a license-plate frame proclaiming, "I smell $ Money $."

Money, on a hog farm at least, smells of ammonia and boiled eggs, and it burns a bit as it slides past the palate. But the scent was not over-powering, and after a few minutes it faded into the background. The fact that the stench intrudes on consciousness only for a brief period of familiarization is testament to the size of Ryan Watje's farm; with just 200 hogs, it's tiny by modern standards.

I found Watje behind his barn; his curly brown hair was wet and his jeans were spattered with mud. Watje, who was 35 at the time, but seemed younger, breeds hogs that routinely win top honors in his state, and recently his pigs placed as grand champion and reserve champion at the National Barrow Show.

"I'm the guy everybody's after," Watje said, ending the sentence with a short, sardonic laugh, embarrassed to have said something so prideful.

Watje manages to make a living selling his prize pigs and semen from the boars that sired them. Although he is good at what he does, Watje is a small-timer. He sends most of his semen to people raising show pigs for 4-H or county fairs. He gets his business by word of mouth, whereas big genetics companies, like Lean Value Sires, issue catalogues full of boars. These catalogues display the top studs—each shaved, oiled, and photographed to display bulging muscles and swollen scrotums. The captions beside the pictures bristle with martial language: "With a head and neck made to cause panic and a butt that exceeds all the limits of man and nature," reads the blurb next to a pig named Hung Jury, "he's a cold blooded killer out to eliminate the competition."

Sometimes Watje will buy semen from these boars to bring in "extreme traits." But mostly he uses semen from his own boars to breed "a good functional, all-around pig." His hogs live in open-air, steel-barred pens with an awning to keep the rain off. Because the pigs live outside, they need immune systems strong enough to block the occasional disease. For this reason, Watje uses vaccines and anti-biotics only in emergencies. He prefers to let diseases pass through the herd, allowing the animals to develop immunities and weeding out the weakest pigs.

Show-pig breeders, who select for attributes like disease resistance and aesthetic appeal, maintain a small but crucial well of genetic diversity. John Mabry, director of the Iowa Pork Industry Center, says that since big farms started taking over, the number of independent breeders has plummeted, and people like Watje now play an important role as stewards of rare genes. Whereas industry geneticists strive for uniformity and move in roughly the same direction, chasing the market, show-pig breeders make decisions based on their personal judgment, intuition, and whimsy. In the past, when large companies found they had overbred their swine, they have dipped into this well of genetic diversity to revitalize their herds.

"The impact of the independents has been invaluable," Mabry said. "We would never have gotten to where we are without them."

Without genetics from these independents, the industry could not have developed such highly efficient, lean pigs. Unlike plant seeds, animal genetics cannot simply be put in the freezer—it's too iffy to freeze and revive eggs and embryos. The only sure way to maintain diversity in pigs is to maintain diversity in farmers.

On the day I visited WD Swine Farm, Watje had decided to mate a Yorkshire sow with one of his newest boars—an experimental and somewhat random pairing, he said.

The boars were as big and as furry as bears. Each had its own pen—but in the last stall, in place of a pig, was what looked like a blue plastic saddle standing a few feet off the ground. Watje opened this gate and led a white boar into the corral.

"I've been training this one," Watje said. "We'll see how he does."

The boar walked straight to the dummy and mounted without hesitation. Now, to be fair, this is a position few mammals are able to maintain with grace. But this boar, no doubt due to his lack of experience, made the pose look particularly awkward. One foreleg bent under his body. His back arched and his head lolled on the saddle.

Watje reached under the pig's belly with one latex-gloved hand and squeezed a stream of clear liquid onto the ground.

"You want to get all the urine out of there," he said. "Then you just hold on to the penis, which can be difficult because it's slimy."

He saw the look on my face and laughed. "Sometimes it's so slippery I have to take the glove off to hold on."

The tip of a boar's penis is shaped like a corkscrew, which gives the farmer something to grip. The hog doesn't need friction, just pressure.

The boar, meanwhile, was shifting, working his way around the dummy. Perhaps he had realized that things were not quite going according to plan and had hit on the idea that he had picked the wrong side. Watje rolled his eyes and hung on. When the moment came, he signaled me and I handed him the cup—an insulated coffee mug lined with a plastic bag and covered in cheesecloth. Watje pulled the penis— two feet long and pencil-thin—to the cup's mouth and held it for three long minutes as the boar ejaculated. Then Watje took the cup inside. It held about half a pint.

"Usually I'd dilute it, but I'm out of distilled water," he said, breaking what had become an uncomfortable silence.

"Do you ever stop in the middle of that and think, 'I'm holding a boar's penis'?" I blurted.

Watje laughed. "Sometimes my friends give me a hard time about it. But no, I've been doing this since I was a kid."

He poured some of the liquid into a squeeze bottle and affixed the bottle to a long straw with a sponge on the end. The remaining semen went in a refrigerator—he sends it overnight to buyers at $50 a dose. Depending on the boar, each ejaculate contains enough sperm to fertilize between 10 and 40 sows.

The sow was easy. Housed close to the boars, she needed no foreplay, none of the haunch and belly rubbing that Becky had described. Watje just sat on her back, facing her tail (this for verisimilitude: "Be the boar" advises the Pig Improvement Company), and slid the semen straw inside. The sow leaned her heavy head against my shin while he slowly squeezed the bottle empty. Then it was over.

The Chickenification of the American Pig

American hog farmers have experimented with artificial insemination (AI) since the 1930s, but it became standard practice only after vertically integrated megafarms began to dominate the business. Although the pork industry can claim the honor of showing Henry Ford the way to mechanization, it has only recently embraced the principle of vertical integration, which when combined with the assembly line brought Ford and other automobile manufacturers such splendid success. It wasn't until 1991 that anyone in the pig world succeeded in expanding Ford's principles beyond the slaughterhouse, back down the food chain, to hog farms. The innovator was Joseph Luter III, who took over Smithfield Foods in 1975. He saw that poultry companies were already turning big profits by building massive chicken farms and controlling every stage of production. If vertical integration could work for chickens, Luter reasoned, it could work for pigs.

Luter wanted to give customers something not often found in nature: predictability. He wanted shoppers to know exactly what a ham with the Smithfield label would taste like before they bought it.

"And the only way to do that," Luter told a newspaper reporter in 2000, "is to control the process from the farm to the packing plant."

With AI, Luter could distribute a single line of genetics across a thousand farms. Smithfield provided every farmer with the same pigs, the same feed, and the same detailed instructions. Producers only had to build up-to-spec barns and follow orders. This system lifted the burden, and the benefits, of innovation from the producer's shoulders. Some farmers resented being forced into the role of de-facto assembly-line workers, but they did not have much choice. They could not compete with the efficiencies of vertical integration. Megafarms sprouted up around Smithfield's packing plant in North Carolina, and in the mid-nineties other vertical integrators began moving into the Midwest, the traditional American hog belt. Now Smithfield turns some 27 million hogs into billions of pounds of pork every year, making it the world's largest pork producer.

Farmers who wanted to stay in business converted. Many quit. The most stubborn went bankrupt. Between 1979 and 2004, as pork production increased by 6 billion pounds, the number of hog farms in America decreased by 89 percent. It just took fewer hands to raise a pig. The motto of the more efficient, inseminating, vertically inte-grated megafarmer could be: More handjobs on the farm, fewer farm-hands on the job.

"Farmers with know-how and pride got eliminated," one pork pro-ducer who had chosen conversion told me. "This kind of farming doesn't take any talent. The company gives you a plan, a consultant, the feed, and the pigs. All you have to do is follow the plan. People who had no talent thought it was great."

Luter's system also required farmers to subtly shift the way they looked at their animals. The good farmer had to know his animals. The successful Smithfield producer has to know his inputs, death rates, and his feed conversion ratios. Trade magazines are full of advertisements for the tools needed to optimize such abstractions:

"Tylan helps minimize attrition losses and maximize economic returns," read one ad for an antibiotic growth promoter. "On average, 30–35% of pigs born never reach full-value market weight because they die, are culled or are lightweights at marketing."

Instead of paying attention to individual pigs, producers focused on herd efficiency. As one Midwestern veterinarian put it, his role has changed from something akin to a family doctor to a technician—supplying vaccinations en masse. "The days when I would get called in to see one sick pig are long gone," he said. Instead, workers dispatch sick hogs with a bolt gun, or simply swing the runts by their hind legs against the concrete floor. Healing is inefficient.

As the way producers looked at pigs changed, so did the animal itself. Luter needed a brave new pig for his new system, and in 1990, Smithfield purchased exclusive U.S. rights to the genetic lines of extraordinarily lean pigs from the National Pig Development Company. These hogs excelled at efficiently converting feed into salable protein, because they wasted little energy on fat production. As an added benefit, the lean meat they produced appealed to lard-fearing Americans. At that time, health-conscious consumers shied away from fatty meats but considered chicken lean and virtuous. In 1986 the National Pork Board had begun an advertising campaign that would recast the pig as a second type of chicken. Pork, advertisers asserted, is "the other white meat." Smithfield made this claim a reality.

As other pork corporations turned to the Smithfield model, breeding companies designed pigs to accommodate the desire for leaner, more efficient swine. Today geneticists have developed tools to reshape pigs almost as ably as Ford's engineers reshape radiators.

WE HAVE GONE TOO FAR

In 2004 I attended the National Swine Improvement Federation Conference in Ames, Iowa, to find out what the leading lights of the hog industry thought of the animal they had created. Surprisingly, meatpackers, academics, and private-sector scientists all gave me the same answer: We have gone too far.

Geneticists have made great gains. Between 1995 and 2010, the portion of the hog that people can actually eat (as opposed to the skin, bones, and fat) has increased by 1.49 percent—more than an extra pork chop per pig. Scientists have shaved 20 days off the time it takes the animal to reach market weight and increased the area of the loin eye (used as an indicator for general muscle size) by 3.6 centimeters. Sows give birth to an average of 2.62 more piglets per litter (making litters of about 13). Today's pigs are impressively uniform and grow large, lean muscles quickly. But the pork has become so lean that packers often have to inject saline marinades directly into the meat—and chefs must drown it in heavy sauces—to make it palatable. What's more, a combination of overbreeding and stressful living conditions makes a percentage of our pork more acidic and less tasty than it used to be.

Standing in an Iowa State University lecture hall, flanked by dual PowerPoint screens, food scientist Ken Prusa told the swine improvers that the future of the industry lay in providing customers a "positive taste experience." And providing a positive taste experience means providing less acidic pork, Prusa said.

In pork, acids break down muscle tissue, turning it to mush, bleaching it of color, and giving it a slightly sour taste. The industry calls this condition "pale soft exudative" or PSE. Prusa held up a plastic-wrapped loin to the audience. The pale meat slumped around his hand.

"What's all this reddish liquid sloshing around?" he asked.

"Exudate," someone called out. "Purge," said another. "Water."

"Right," Prusa said. To be exact, the fluid is mostly water with some iron, proteins, and trace minerals mixed in. He clicked to a slide showing a microscope photograph of healthy muscle, honeycombed with cell walls. Then he clicked to a picture of pale, soft, exudative meat. The slide showed only a mass of gray.

"When the cell structure breaks down like this, the meat loses ability to retain water," Prusa said.

When cooked, this acidic pork (with a pH below about 5.5) grows rubbery and dry. But as the pH rises—growing less acidic—the pork becomes "a taste experience we can only imagine," Prusa said.

"At pH 6.2 and above—I don't know if anyone's ever eaten one of those, but you would not forget it," he said.

For years, the Japanese have been buying all the best meat from American slaughterhouses. They need meat that won't melt to mush in shipping, and they are also more willing to pay for quality food. So far, meatpackers have simply picked the best meat off the disassembly line— from one hog here and another there—to satisfy this demand. The Japanese choose the meat by color: Darker pork signifies less acid. Americans get the leftovers: the other white meat. But this is changing, Prusa said. If people want more perfect pork, geneticists may have to breed a different animal.

"What's your definition of perfect pork?" asked an audience member.

"An excellent eating experience," Prusa said.

"But commodity consumers aren't interested in that."

Prusa disagreed. Instead of settling for "commodity pork"—that is, the cheapest thing on the shelf—American shoppers seem increasingly willing to pay more for a brand they can trust or for some information about their meat's past. And although cheap, unbranded pork may remain on supermarket shelves, in the future it will probably come from countries like Brazil and Mexico—countries with cheaper labor and fewer laws preventing farmers from dumping their waste.

At the cocktail party after the lecture, I asked Dan Hamilton, a geneticist for the breeding company Geneti-porc, if scientists would be able to reengineer the pig to produce less acidic meat. It's a difficult problem, he said, because many factors govern acidity. It depends, for instance, on how quickly packers cool the meat after slaughter and how people treat the animal beforehand. But geneticists can contribute by breeding more docile animals—pigs that can endure trying conditions without becoming stressed.

When pale, soft, exudative meat first emerged as a major problem, scientists linked it definitively to stress. In breeding the Smithfield— type super swine, geneticists had inadvertently selected for a gene that made hogs prone to panic. Pigs exhibiting this trait might tremble all their lives and die of shock when a barn door banged shut too loudly. Hogs under stress (and humans as well) use an energy-production short-cut, rapidly burning glycogen in their muscles and creating lactic acid as a byproduct. Genetically stressed-out pigs live with their muscles immersed in lactic acid and, unless they die in unusual placidity, their meat goes quickly bad.

Iowa State University professor Lauren Christian is credited with discovering "the stress gene"—a segment of DNA that produced heavily muscled, ultra-lean, but also exceptionally high-strung pigs. In 1995 he called on the industry to eliminate the gene, and the breeders responded. Today most genetics corporations have purged it from their breeding pools. All the same, the problems associated with the stress still exist. Farmers still complain of pigs that drop dead when they drive their tractors too close to the barn, and the pork industry still loses money on pale, soft, exudative flesh. The American Meat Science Association found that the amount of PSE pork had increased from 10.2 percent in 1992 to 15.5 percent in 2002, when the problem cost the industry $90 million. Either the genetic causes of stress are more complicated than Christian thought or something else is making the pigs crazy.

If genes are no longer responsible for all this watery, floppy meat, animal living conditions may be the problem. Scientists have found that the modern pig's monotonous life in cramped quarters puts it on edge. Temple Grandin, a professor of animal science at Colorado State University, has shown that when workers petted pigs for 5 minutes a day, let them out of their crates for a brief walk, or gave them a piece of rubber hose to play with, the animals calmed down. Pigs are, after all, highly intelligent animals—probably more intelligent than dogs and, like dogs, they grow restless without anything to do. When swine cannot so much as turn around in their crates, they often develop repetitive movements, biting at the air and swinging their heads from side to side—movements that some students of animal behavior say signal frustration or neurosis.

As breeders have pushed for efficiency, they have also relaxed the standards for physical traits that allow pigs to stand on concrete their whole lives without going lame. Hogs can live up to twenty years in the wild, but large pork producers usually cull sows after less than four years. Sows can produce more than ten litters, and older sows birth larger, healthier pigs. In confinement a sow's health won't hold up much past three litters. Swine producers recognize the problem, and a faction at the conference argued that it was time to make a change.

In an effort to help breeders choose pigs that are less likely to go lame, Dale Miller, editor of *National Hog Farmer,* was distributing posters at the National Swine Improvement Federation Conference. The posters illustrated the good, the bad, and the ugly in hog body types. As I studied the pictures of pigeon-toed pigs, Miller chatted with Peggy Hawkins, a scientist from Monsanto, who had just ordered a set of posters. Monsanto, the agricultural biotech firm most famous for making the herbicide Roundup and Roundup-resistant crops, also sells sows under the registered trademark "Genepacker."

"This lack of soundness has become a real problem," said Miller, "I can't believe the producers have stood for it as long as they have."

"Well, if you buy a sow from Monsanto and it dies, we replace it for free," Hawkins said. "So it doesn't affect the producers one way or the other. We figure they're better off having the top genetics."

"It affects them when they have to drag dead sows out of the crates every day," Miller retorted.

It would be unfair to leave this bit of casual conversation out of context, since, to judge from its marketing, Monsanto recognizes that farmers need durable sows to maximize production, and it specifically positions the Genepacker as a pig with the fortitude to withstand the rigors of confinement. The solution to this problem of soundness, as far as Monsanto or those at the conference are concerned, is to breed "better" pigs—pigs that can stand on a 2-foot by 7-foot rectangle of concrete all their lives without going lame or insane with boredom. And if genetic modification doesn't work, technology often can provide a mechanical solution. Swine Robotics, for instance, has developed a device that removes dead animals from crates—a contraption that looks like a hand truck with a power winch. This "Boar Buzzard" helps eliminate the problems of poor employee morale and back injuries. And scientists have found they can reduce the amount of pale, soft, exudative meat by taking pigs off their feed 18 hours before slaughter. The hungry pigs burn off their glycogen reserves, and without glycogen they do not produce lactic acid, no matter how stressed they are.

As practical as they may be, there is something troubling about these technical work-arounds. Bit by bit, scientific breakthroughs have emancipated the hog industry from the demands of nature, but each freedom comes at a price. Each new liberty for pork producers depends on further control, further domination of the pig. No one at the conference suggested what seemed the obvious answer: doing away with the causes of stress and lameness. But then, swine geneticists are innovators, not policymakers.

In just a little more than a decade, the modern hog industry has produced a tower of efficiency-maximizing products, one stacked atop the next, each innovation fixing the problem the last fix created. It is a monumental if somewhat haphazard structure, composed of slatted floors and aluminum crates, automatic sorting scales and mechanized wet-dry feeders. It is constructed of Genepacker sows, Tylan antibiotic feed, Agro-Clean liquid detergent, Argus salmonella vaccine, Goldenpig foam-tipped disposable AI catheters, CL Sow Replacer milk substitute, and Matrix estrus synchronizer. The scientists who add their discoveries to this edifice do not see themselves as its architects. As they see it, their job is not to shift the foundations of the hog industry but to build atop its tower of technology, masking what structural flaws they can with new construction, reaching ever upward.

That night, at the National Swine Improvement Federation Conference dinner, I found myself face to face with three slabs of white pork smothered in gravy. One of the conferees held up the meal long enough to give an invocation.

"Dear Lord," he said, "thank you for giving us the gift of technology and showing us how to use that gift to help the industry we serve, the pork industry . . ." He went on for several minutes, giving me time to consider my meat, in light of all I had learned in the past months. ". . . and serve humanity without someone looking over our shoulder, amen."

The pork was tender and juicy, but I was having a hard time swallowing it. For the first time since I had had my illuminating conversation with Becky in that bar in Idaho, I knew exactly what I was eating.

There are plenty of good arguments stacked in favor of the system that had delivered the pork to my plate. Or if not good arguments, at least powerful ones. There is tremendous pressure to produce cheap food—and, adjusting for inflation, the price of pork has fallen more than a dollar a pound since the 1990s. The pressure to sell cheap lean pork leads to the building of uniform pigs—which leads to the need for biosecure confinement facilities. These factors, in turn, make artificial insemination, for all its absurdity, not only reasonable but necessary. And as I chewed my pork loin, I could not avoid the conclusion: All these powerful arguments for the transformation of hogs into predictable production machines imply the existence of an equally predictable consumption machine, someone like me who expected to find identical cuts of inexpensive pork every time he entered the supermarket.

I had gone in search of artificial insemination's original cause and now I had found it: It swallowed and gingerly took another gravy-laden mouthful. I had never thought of my bacon-eating self as part of the pig industrial complex. Corporations like Smithfield and Pig Improvement Company bear the responsibility for engineering the modern pig, but, as they will point out, they made it to the specifications of their master: the vast collective American maw.

Humanity was not always a blind and ravenous consumer: In reality, shoppers can see perfectly well. But by the time pork reaches the supermarket it has shed all markers that might allow consumers to evaluate their purchase save one, its price. It's no wonder that, when given this solitary criterion for judgment, shoppers choose the cheapest possible meat.

The industry has responded admirably to the demand for consistent, copious, and cheap pork. But in satisfying those desires, it has done away with the other qualities that once distinguished pork, like flavor and variety. In following the limited signals transmitted between farmer and eater via the market's crude semaphore, we have reduced pork choices to the extent that shoppers know few options. They can select only from what the industry decides to give them. If I wanted to replicate my revelatory meal, I could find identical pork in any American supermarket. In fact, I'd have a hard time finding any other type of pork.

CAFO County

On the other side of the Rockies, Cassia County was still in the growth phase, investing money in CAFOs. The region has proved more amenable to dairies than hog farms—in part because Idaho residents had time to watch what happened with the first wave of intensive pig farming elsewhere. Cows were next in line for chickenification. In the years after I left Cassia County it had permitted 20 new dairies with the equivalent of 89,700 full-grown Holsteins. Local leaders had managed to build a dairy processing plant and establish a milk-trucking business in Burley. This surge of investment had improved the economy, but Iowa's history made me wonder if it was a Pyrrhic victory. The same forces that depopulated Iowa would eventually squeeze jobs out of southern Idaho. In theory this is just as it should be—as technology improves fewer people are required to do the work, which frees others up to innovate. There will always be the next big thing, the next conquest in the series of transformations: desert to farmland, farmland to CAFO, and what next? Perhaps factories to construct as-yet unknown materials out of milk proteins? I worry that there's not much magic left in the Magic Valley. The close-knit families are already finding it hard to convince their children to settle in town. If Cassia County hopes to retain its best minds and foster high-tech innovation it would have to begin prioritizing beauty, pleasure, and health—rather than simply optimizing the efficient conversion of corn to milk and excrement.

On the other hand, milk and excrement is the only sane choice for now. If I were an economic consultant I would have advised the Cassia County to become a CAFO county—with some light caveats—exactly as it has done. It was a good bet in hard times—a proven way to make money. It's all very well for high-profile companies with high profit margins to sacrifice some efficiency for the sake of prettiness or justice, but farmers rarely have this sort of wiggle room. The farmers of Cassia County must serve a market which they did not design and which cares nothing for their aesthetics—only for their resources. The market is blind. If allowed to extract value from the region, it will do so eagerly until it has created one massive cesspool.

Sooner or later, after economic pressure has driven standards below the point of outrage, laws will be passed: If history is any guide they will be superficially reasoned laws that punish farmers for successfully following the market signals that allowed them to stay (sporadically) in the black. The destructive cycle of legislation and agricultural economics goes something like this: Consumers demand lower prices; farms respond by becoming fewer, larger, less pleasant, and farther from the people they serve; consumers are periodically horrified when they learn what happens on the now distant farms; laws are passed prohibiting these horrors and, their foe vanquished, consumers go back to consuming and signaling their interest in low prices; and (again) farms become fewer, larger, less pleasant, and farther from the people they serve. When Sweden, for example, passed strict animal-welfare laws for hog farms, they exported porcine suffering rather than ending it. The Swedes simply began buying their cheap pork from Denmark. Such legislation generally restrains the proximate cause of misery on CAFOs, but it leaves unchanged the incentives that called that misery into being in the first place. Of course, if consumers wanted to break this cycle they could simply pass laws regulating the ultimate cause. If Americans were willing to legislate on their own consumption (banning or taxing the consumption of food that creates ugliness), farmers in places like Cassia County would find a way to serve the market, as they have always done. Such laws would make food more expensive, but it would also allow small agricultural towns to hold on to a little dignity. The thing is, once a town accepts CAFOs, it's impossible to confine their ugliness. Flies can't be caged. Neither can odors. Cruelty also tends to spread. Once farmers become hardened to animal pain, it's a smaller step to also seeing their workers as unfeeling machines. Researchers have found that in 85 percent of households where animals are subjected to violence, there are also incidents of domestic abuse. Violence radiates out through society. As does poverty: These days middle class family farmers must make ever riskier bets to stay afloat, and their farms demand menial laborers—often undocumented and always poor— who claw at the slippery foot of the American dream, sometimes driven to drugs and crime by the hopelessness of the endeavor.

After 2 years in Burley, I decided I'd had enough. The town was growing smellier, more businesses had closed, and no young college grads were moving in. I had wonderful friends in Burley, but most were 20 years my senior. I quit my job at the newspaper and packed my worldly belongings into my car. Moving is always hard work, and by the time I made my last trip up the three-story stairs I was a frayed bundle of sparking nerves, cursing myself, and Burley, and the wind, and the layer of topsoil that was accumulating in my hair. I did a final walk from front to back of the empty apartment and pocketed a few odds and ends that hadn't made it into any of the boxes. Then I went to the front window to take in the view one last time. The sun was setting behind the seed towers, and I felt a sudden stab of jubilation at the thought that I'd successfully slipped every one of my obligations to this place. I was free.

There was a light knock at the door. I froze, considered making a run for it out the back, then lowered myself to a crouch and determined to wait until my visitor disappeared. The knock came again, accompanied by my name, called querulously.

I rose ruefully, and opened the door. My downstairs neighbor, looking even more booze-battered than usual, offered a greeting. After an exchange of pleasantries he explained that he badly needed my help. I didn't respond.

He gazed off into the middle distance, "Look," he said, "I'm bleeding from a place where I'm not supposed to be bleeding." Then turned his dolorous basset-hound eyes on me. I met them with steely displeasure. "Look," he started again, "there was blood in the toilet and—"

"All right, all right, I get it." I said, cracking. "Sorry, I just—I'm taking you to the hospital."

Later, when I had managed to extricate myself, and was nudging the speedometer up to 70, it occurred to me that I could not have dreamed up someone better than my neighbor as a symbol for the town: someone unexpectedly kind and intelligent, yet fundamentally self-destructive, with breath like refried death. The CAFOs hadn't made my neighbor an alcoholic any more than they had caused the cancer cluster that residents had asked me to investigate. But it was clear to me that the system had created a cancer in the body politic. It was a system that, in pursuing one kind of efficiency, had embraced other inefficiencies: Pollution, and all forms of waste, is by definition inefficient. Suffering is inefficient. As I sped away into the night I wondered: Was it possible to fashion an economy that saw the efficiency in keeping families together, the efficiency of healthy people, and perhaps even (dare I ask it?) the efficiency of beauty and pleasure?

POSTINDUSTRIAL PIGS

A few months after that swine conference I'd attended, the magazine *Pork* ran an editorial forecasting consumer demands. Quality meat, organics, and animal-welfare assurance, the editor predicted, would be trends in coming years. And though this is true, not all that much changed down on the industrial farm. Gestation crates are being phased out in many places, as big fast-food chains demand bacon from pigs with enough room to turn around. A few "natural" pork brands cost extra because they raise their pigs on organic feed and may even give them a little extra room to roam, but they still squeeze the pig to fit the same mechanized, indoor system.

The biggest change has occurred in marketing, which has begun to advertise natural pork and welfare assurance. This change is coming about because the pork industry has taken note of the success of a few pork producers who treat their pigs as sentient animals rather than pro-tein units. These farms account for less than 1 percent of the pork in the United States, but they have sent shockwaves through the industry because their profitability violates a fundamental axiom of efficiency-based agriculture: They have proven that consumers are capable of see-ing more than the price tag.

Probably the most successful of these farmers is Paul Willis, who runs the Niman Ranch Pork Company out of the brick house in Iowa where he was born. When I arrived, early in the morning, it felt the way I once imagined a farm should feel. Pigeons cooed in a cote and some-where a rooster proclaimed its wakefulness. It smelled earthy, not septic. But although Willis's place looks like an old-fashioned farm it is also a scientifically sophisticated operation based on a revolutionary idea: "We are trying to adapt to who the pig is," Willis said.

Instead of pushing the pig to the limit of what it can stand so that it will better fit into an efficient system, Willis has created a farm that works in cooperation with the animal. Give the pig what it wants, the theory goes, and in return the pig will thrive and someday make a tooth-some meal.

When pigs have their druthers (and though this seems obvious, it has been experimentally verified), they spend time grazing in pastures and rooting in the earth. Willis used these studies to refine traditional methods and created a system that would allow hogs to indulge all their grazing, foraging, socializing, and nest-building instincts. This system allows Willis to dispense with the great heap of gadgets and drugs that confined-animal feeding operations must buy, and when pigs have room to spread out, their manure enriches rather than pollutes the soil.

But it's the little things that count. For instance, Willis spends enough time with his sows so that they get to know him. They didn't protest when I entered the barn: Porcine heads simply swiveled to regard me quizzically. He firmly believes that a pig that lives a life of placid ease is more likely to become the best-tasting meat in the world—and it's his mission to create that meat. Willis isn't interested in maintaining strict genetic uniformity, and his hogs can survive the chance encounter with a germ or two, so artificial insemination is not of much use to him. And since his pigs spend most of their time running around outside, catching them for insemination would be a full-time job.

"A boar," Willis said, "is a cheap hired man."

There's no arguing with the price tag, however. A Niman Ranch pork chop costs significantly more than one from Smithfield. Nonetheless, the pork has been a hit. In 1997 the company was producing 120 pigs a week. Now, to keep up with demand, it sends more than 3,000 hogs to slaughter each week. Niman Ranch has 500 farmers growing swine according to its protocols, and Willis is recruiting more.

Willis is particularly proud to be giving these small farmers a way to make a decent living, though he knows Niman Ranch alone can't repopulate the dying towns of the Midwest. We drove together through the town of Thornton, Iowa, and Willis pulled up at his old high school. He had been a Thornton Thunderbolt—a dying breed. As large farms replaced small ones, the population of Thornton became too small to warrant its own high school. Now his high school serves as a middle school for both Thornton and three other towns.

Willis pulled away from his alma mater, and we drove in silence. But his mood brightened a moment later. He stopped the truck and pointed out a group of his pigs in a cornfield. The pigs frolicked. Yes,

anthropomorphism be damned, they frolicked amid the dried corn-
stalks. They dashed off in one direction, only to dash back again. They
rolled on the ground. They ran in little circles of porcine glee. They
drove their noses into the earth, burying themselves up to their ears.

"There it is," Willis said. "Porktopia."

CHAPTER SEVEN

WHEN MEDICINE ISN'T THE BEST MEDICINE

HEALTHCARE

My parents never entirely trusted Western medicine. "They're just treating the symptoms," Mom would say. By the family rationale, it was counterproductive to take painkillers to mute symptoms because, in doing so, you turned down the volume on urgent messages from body to brain. And true healing depended on listening to the body. Throughout my youth, I was inclined to agree. It was only near the end of my time in Idaho that I learned to love conventional medicine.

I'd come home from a road trip and was cleaning weekend detritus from the car when I found the pizza. It was really good pizza, from Boise, with the kind of delightfully prissy ingredients that were impossible to get in Burley: fennel sausage, heirloom tomatoes, sheep cheese. Lingering over all this were the subtle aromatics that can only be gained by slow baking for 8 hours in the back of a vehicle. I pondered this smell as I carried the box up to my apartment. At the kitchen table I dissected a piece of sausage and peered at its innards like a Greek seer searching for portents. It actually seemed okay, and I was hungry.

Around midnight I woke up with something sharp slowly, but inexorably, driving through my abdomen. It seemed plausible that my spleen was growing a horn, or that my duodenum had sprouted a disastrously pointy erection. The pizza, I surmised, had been a mistake.

I crawled to the bathroom and tried to throw up, without success. Then I took some aspirin, went back to bed, and visualized waves of electric blue pulsing around my intestinal tract. Dad had taught me this trick when I was 7. The idea was to cure the ailment by irradiating the area in healing light.

At that moment, however, what I wanted more than almost anything else was for someone—as Mom put it—to just treat the symptoms. The pain had grown from a piercing point to a generalized agony of stretching and compression, as if a pair of brawny belly dwarves were competing in an enthusiastic tug-of-war with my intestines, having first tied them into a complicated knot. I poured myself a tall glass of Wesson Oil and drank it, hoping to purge. The results were disappointing. Four in the morning found me drenched in sweat on the kitchen linoleum, which for some reason seemed like the most comfortable place in the apartment.

By dawn, the pain had resolved into a single rapier, planted resolutely in the lower right quadrant of my abdomen, an indication—I happened to know—not of food poisoning, but of appendicitis. I drove myself to the emergency room. There were a few hours of doubled-over waiting, a blood test, then more waiting. An attendant confided that they were taking bets on my diagnosis. Appendicitis was the five-to-one favorite. A few minutes later, the same attendant showed me to a gurney and wheeled me deeper into the hospital. Then an anesthesiologist was shaking my hand, and shortly thereafter time folded in on itself. I was hazily aware of being alone in a dark room with a new pain below my abdomen, in utterly the wrong spot. Had there been some terrible, unforeseen complication? My groping seemed to confirm my direst fears until a nurse explained that it was customary to insert a catheter during operations.

I drove myself home 12 hours later. My stomach was full of staples, but my appendix was gone, along with the rapier. I resumed work after a week, and sit-ups after a month—about the time it would have taken me to die if I hadn't had access to Western medicine. What did visualization have on that?

Dad suffered appendicitis about a year later, and afterward there was a change in the tone of our conversations about medicine. The nice thing about the allopathic tradition, we agreed, was that its effects were universally consistent. It didn't matter if the patient believed in the treatment, or what he thought about his sickness. It didn't matter if the surgeon was compassionate. All that mattered was that a competent technician carried out the correct procedure.

In a follow-up appointment I asked my surgeon what had caused my appendix to turn traitor. I wondered if I'd been wrong to blame the sausage. His response was vague: Perhaps an infection, he said. When I asked why infection had struck at that particular moment, he just shrugged. Mom's point about doctors caring more about symptoms than underlying causes seemed correct in this case. But my grateful post-operative self was disposed to put it a bit more charitably: Conventional medicine is concerned with helping pragmatically, using the information available to accomplish what it can. It focuses on the visible, pressing problems. You don't have to know why a fire started to put it out.

This philosophy has made Western medicine awesomely powerful. So powerful that I could see why its partisans feel justified in sneering at alternatives. The force of visualization, or of homeopathy or acupuncture, looks wan and anemic when placed alongside the muscular lifesaving effectiveness of antibiotics, organ transplantation, or surgery. Which made me wonder, for the first time, what was it that made alternative medicine so attractive?

MEDICINE'S DOUBLE EDGE

Of my immediate family, Mom was the most frequent adventurer in unorthodox treatments. She'd started exploring alternative medicine because Western medicine often failed to make her feel healthier; in fact, sometimes it made her feel worse.

In 2002, after some routine tests, her doctor told her she had osteopenia and hepatitis C. He explained that osteopenia was a thinning of the bones, and that the hepatitis C could destroy her liver. Fortunately, both conditions were treatable. He recommended a drug called Fosamax for the former and a regimen of antiviral therapy for the latter.

When she left the doctor's office Mom was upset. She hardly ever got sick, and—though her hair was more salt than pepper, and she had smile-wrinkles at her eyes—she looked a decade younger than her age. She'd felt vibrantly healthy until her doctor told her she was ill and decrepit. She wasn't sure she could trust him as she had trusted our previous family physician, Dr. Johnston, who had taken care of us for years. Mom had respected Dr. Johnston enough to keep asking questions until she felt completely confident in his directives—or until they had agreed on some alternate course. She knew he wouldn't think she was an anti-scientific crazy person if she explained her doubts. With this new doctor Mom didn't bring up her concerns, which all really amounted to one big question: Were his prescriptions tailored to serve her, in all her physical and psychic complexity—or were they tailored to serve her lab results? She assumed the latter.

"He basically said, 'You have X, so you need to take Y,'" Mom said.

Poking around on the Internet, she learned that a second hepatitis C test was usually performed to see if the disease required treatment. She also stumbled across people writing about how they thought Fosamax had made otherwise-robust bones weaker. She arranged to take the hepatitis test and ordered two books on osteoporosis.

As it turned out, Mom's hunch about her new doctor's guidance turned out to be precisely correct. The second hepatitis test came back negative, and the specialist who read the results said there was no need for antiviral therapy. The lifestyle changes she made after reading the books on osteoporosis also proved successful: She was eating more calcium-rich foods, spending more time in the garden to soak up vitamin D, and running more frequently. Her next bone-density reading showed that she was no longer in the danger zone.

Thanks to her skepticism, Mom saved some money that she would have spent on drugs—savings both for herself and society at large. When I started reading about the costs of healthcare I was shocked to learn that the people who study health policy generally agree that between a fifth and a third of all medical care delivered in the United States is unnecessary. One study pegged the minimum cost of this waste at $500 billion a year.

As boggling as the dollar amounts are, the physical consequences of overtreatment are worse. Every medical procedure—unnecessary or not—carries some risk. Fosamax may, in rare circumstances, *cause* femur fractures, and the antiviral hepatitis drugs often cause depression, fatigue, and fever. The small risks add up because inappropriate tests and surgeries are performed with alarming regularity. Elliott Fisher, a public health scientist at Dartmouth Medical School, has estimated that unnecessary treatment kills over 30,000 Americans each year (a minimum number, counting only those covered by Medicare), more than the estimated 26,000 Americans who die annually because they can't get medical care.*

At the root of Mom's suspicions was her fear that Western medicine is designed to create healthy profits rather than healthy people. It's undeniable that the desire to make money provides powerful incentives for pharmaceutical companies to advertise drugs of dubious efficacy, for doctors to choose lucrative surgeries rather than unprofitable therapy, and for hospitals to invest in flashy new technologies instead of searching for ways to keep people healthy. But, to understand the market, one must also understand culture. Market incentives are shaped by our desires and fears. We patients wouldn't be susceptible to pitches from medical advertisers if we did not believe them on some level. It's the patients who bear the costs

---

* Fisher's number is extremely conservative. We know, for instance that some 100,000 patients are killed each year by adverse drug reactions while in the hospital.

of medical sprawl, measured both in dollars and lives, and it's the patients who campaign most fiercely for its intensification. When researchers assemble evidence that some test or intervention is doing more harm than good, it's the patients who protest the reforms. Americans believe, at a fundamental level, in the power of medical technology.

THE FLINCH

The evidence that conventional medicine is dangerously overused doesn't make alternative medicine more valid. But as soon as I'd started looking at why people were attracted to alternative medicine, I'd found myself confronted with an equal and opposite quandary: What could explain the attraction to unnecessary conventional medicine? The solution to both mysteries, I suspected, was one and the same. When in distress, some people flinch toward nature, some toward technology. But both reactions are triggered by the desire to do *something*. The efficacy of the fix is less important than its availability. Doing nothing is intolerable.

Mom, for all the skeptical acuity she directed toward conventional medicine, became willingly credulous when offered untested New Age therapies. When I called to plumb her memories of the Fosamax incident, she prefaced her story by recommending a new practice she had discovered, called "Earthing." The idea was that, because our feet are generally insulated from the ground by rubber and foam, people build up an unhealthy electric charge in their bodies. Mom had bought a bed sheet woven with silvery carbon-fiber wires, and when she slept on this sheet, the filaments were supposed to conduct ions out of her body and into the grounding plug of an electrical outlet (a wire ran from sheet to wall socket). The results, Mom said, were obvious.

"It might just be psychosomatic," she said, "but the first night that I slept on it I went out so deeply that I was groggy the next day."

I read a couple of the studies supporting Earthing, and was not impressed. They were printed in the *Journal of Alternative and Comple-*

mentary Medicine, and the methods were sloppy: no controls, no blinding, no demonstrations of statistical significance. It looked like hokum.*

On the other hand, this treatment made sense on a metaphoric level. The lack of connection between humanity and the earth was, after all, a legitimate problem in my eyes. I couldn't remember the last time I'd set my bare feet on the ground. I wanted the kind of life that would allow me to dig my toes into the dirt every once and a while. There was a conceptual logic to this product that remedied the lack of contact between the human sole and the skin of the earth—it was just that the mechanism for this reunion didn't make sense. Inserting a silver-shot, plug-in bed sheet into our disconnected lives (even supposing it did provide some physical benefit) wouldn't address the deeper problem. It seemed like a classic case of just treating the symptoms. Nonetheless, this bit of ceremony, this gesture toward reconnection, seemed to be improving Mom's life. She felt less driven, she said, less scattered, better able to enjoy the moment. She was being healed, I think, by a metaphor.

METAPHOR AS MEDICINE

The place where metaphor meets medicine is difficult to study. If all Western knowledge were laid out on a parchment map, these particular seas would be represented by a vague cloudy mass, marked by depictions of strange creatures and the words HERE LIES THE PLACEBO EFFECT. Eastern medical traditions, which do not draw a hard line between mind and body, have devoted considerably more attention to sketching in these shoals and shorelines. But I worried I wouldn't do justice to ayurveda or Qigong if I examined them with Western expectations. I wanted information that had been credentialed by the scientific system I understood. And so I set course for the waters where placebo is known to reside.

---

* When I looked at more of the studies, during fact checking, I found some did use controls and presented results more uniformly positive than I had ever seen in a clinical trial. In other words, it seemed too good to be true. They were conducted by people with financial ties to the company selling the Earthing equipment.

Placebo was not originally a medical term. It simply means, in Latin, "I shall please." In the Middle Ages, however, it took on a connotation of obsequiousness: A placebo was a yes-man, a courtier who would say whatever his king wanted to hear. By the 1800s, the term was being used by doctors to describe fake pills given to please demanding patients. Then in the 20th century, placebo took on a slippery third meaning: a treatment that shouldn't work according to the rules of biochemistry, but does all the same. At first this was just an annoyance—evidence that a clinical trial was flawed or poorly designed. It's only recently that scientists have begun to see the placebo as a phenomenon to be investigated in its own right, rather than an inconvenient static to be weeded out of otherwise solid research.* Those who study placebo no longer see it as self-delusion or fakery, but as a little piece of something large and strange: a process by which information, symbolism, and cultural meaning modulate the body's normally subconscious functions. The placebo effect is like the reflective glint of eyes in the darkness, a small part of some massive beast whose shape our lights are as yet too weak to illuminate.

One especially intrepid placebo hunter, the contemporary Italian scientist Fabrizio Benedetti, has performed a series of experiments to show how something as intangible as belief can have physical consequences. In one experiment, Benedetti hooked up his subjects to an intravenous line with a saline drip so they could not tell if they were being given medication. He then instructed them to squeeze a hand exerciser while a partial tourniquet around their arms restricted blood flow. I've tried this. It hurts. The oxygen-starved muscles send out panicky pain signals as the lactic acid builds up. When Benedetti's subjects (perhaps the word is victims) rated their pain level at a 7 out of 10, he told some that he was providing a strong analgesic and that they should

---

* These aren't treatments that magically mend broken bones or perform any other mechanical sort of repair, but treatments that change the way the patient feels—reducing pain or dispelling nausea. Asbjørn Hróbjartsson, a researcher at the Nordic Cochrane Centre, has shown in meta-analyses that the placebo does not seem to have "clinically important effects" though it does have a clear impact on pain (which, I'd argue, is clinically important) and several other conditions.

relax as it took effect over the next few minutes—and it worked, even when Benedetti added nothing to the saline drip.

Benedetti's hypothesis was that the imagined analgesic had created a real one. When he had suggested to his experimental subjects that they were about to feel the effects of opiates, they had started producing them on their own. Our native opiates are called endorphins, and several other studies have shown that the belief that a palliative is coming is enough to trigger a release of these painkillers.

The real trick came 15 minutes later, when Benedetti secretly added Naloxone to the intravenous lines. Naloxone is an opiate blocker—it inhibits painkillers. And even though the subjects didn't know what was happening, those who got the Naloxone felt their pain rapidly increase. Benedetti had demonstrated that a physical chemical could block the effects of an imaginary painkiller.

Though this is incredible, it also makes intuitive sense. Anyone who has ever gone to the movies is familiar with the power of a story to produce measurable physical effects. Narrative and meaning can cause hearts to race, stomachs to clench, palms to sweat, and tears to flow. We tend to think of these effects as minor, and therefore unrelated to physical health, but in some cases emotion can cause lasting changes in physiology. Harvard neurologist Martin Samuels has documented scores of cases in which heart attacks seem to be triggered by fear or grief: the mother who learns her son has died, then goes into cardiac arrest. Samuels published a hypothesis (in the journal *Circulation*) to explain how a cascade of chemical reactions starting in the brain could stop the heart, providing a plausible mechanism whereby metaphorical heartbreak could lead to physiological heart failure.

The closer you look at placebos, the weirder they get. Large sugar pills work better than small ones, capsules work better than tablets, and pink pills perk people up, while blue ones slow them down. All of these disparities seem to be caused by the stories patients weave from whatever information they have: Big tends to be associated with more oomph than little; capsules (especially those cool dual-toned capsules containing tiny round balls) are associated with more high-tech power than tablets; and warm colors tend to be associated with energy, while blue is mellow (although Viagra is rapidly re-branding blue as an emblem of vigor). It's the meaning patients give these pills that charges their power. That's why anthropologist Daniel Moerman has suggested that we rename the placebo effect the placebo effect *the meaning effect*. The powerful-looking pill is a synecdoche, a part of Western medicine that represents its authoritative whole. Even when it contains no active ingredients, the pill is full of meaning. And meaning is the key that unlocks the pharmacies of the mind.

Of all the symbols of medicine's transformative power, the greatest is the surgeon's blade. Sham surgeries provide a stronger "meaning effect" than pills or even injections. For instance, a test of a controversial surgery for treating heart disease (bilateral internal mammary artery ligation) showed that most of the patients experienced substantial improvement. One Kansas City man said, "Practically immediately I felt better. I felt I could take a deep breath. . . . I figure I'm about 95 percent better." The number of nitroglycerin tablets he was taking fell from five per day to two per week. But this man had been part of the placebo group: He had been taken into the operating room, where a surgeon had made two incisions in his chest, and then stitched them back up. Of the patients receiving sham surgery, 87 percent experienced improvement, compared to 67 percent of patients who got the real thing.

Why do people ascribe such power to surgeries? Moerman (whose excellent book *Meaning, Medicine and the "Placebo Effect"* has been propped open by my keyboard as I write this) thinks it has to do with the mechanistic goggles through which we see the world. We understand our bodies by borrowing metaphors from machines: The brain is a computer, the heart is a pump, and the arteries are pipes, which sometimes get clogged. Surgeons speak at this level of metaphor. They reroute plumbing, patch leaks, and remove obstructions. Anyone who can change the spark plugs in an engine can understand the logic of surgery: It provides meaning that Americans can accept. And patients must not only accept, but *commit* to this meaning, allowing their chests to be cracked open and their hearts to be stopped on the faith that the coronary artery bypass, for example, will work.

People yearn for metaphor, and today the metaphor for healing generally comes packaged in technological medicine. The unnecessary surgeries and fruitless testing regimens that regularly occur in the United States are often requested by patients seeking to fill a vacuum of meaning. One physician, blogging under the handle Dr. Panda Bear, described what it was like to face the ever-growing demand for treatment:

"I have received a few patient complaints and many of them essentially boil down to, 'That doctor didn't do nothing,' after I sent them home with no testing and no strong medicine. I have also on a few occasions, in the course of a thorough history and physical exam, been interrupted by angry family [members] demanding that I shut up, stop wasting time, and order some tests. It's magic that they want; wonderful, deeply satisfying, mystical American Medical Magic. Blinking lights! Blood tests! X-rays!"

American Medical Magic is an expensive and dangerous way of generating ritual meaning. And yet, I could feel no scorn for this doctor's patients. They needed something done, even if it was only a ritual.

The Eclipse of the Patient

Clinical medicine was a latecomer to the Enlightenment, and two centuries after Newton, very little of what doctors did was backed by science. A review (by physician Paul Beeson) of treatments recommended in the 1927 edition of *Cecil Textbook of Medicine* found that 60 percent of the remedies therein were harmful, ineffective, or merely anodyne, while only 3 percent provided useful treatment. A scientific revolution occurred in medicine in the following years, so that by 2001 the Institute of Medicine (an arm of the National Academies) judged that 50 percent of all treatments were backed by evidence. This improvement was made, in part, by the avant-garde of science, and in part by a rear guard, which policed doctors whose techniques ran counter to the norm.

This rear guard's founding document was Abraham Flexner's 1910 report on North American medical schools. At the request of the Carnegie Foundation, Flexner toured institutions throughout the United States and Canada. Many medical schools lacked laboratories, up-to-date medical texts, or a means of providing clinical experience to students. Others taught techniques according to the experience of professors, rather than according to the objectively verifiable evidence. Some perpetuated long-debunked methods. In the years following the Flexner report, the number of medical schools fell by half. Those that remained embraced science.

To make science objective you have to strip away the imponderable, the confounding, and the messy—which effectively eliminates humanity from the picture. A scientific scope of focus excels in examining quantifiable lab results, but struggles to contain that mix of vague concerns and contradictions known as a patient. Flexner drove many dangerous quacks out of medicine, but he also drove out healers who were able to improve their patients' lives more by listening carefully to them than through physical repair. Medicine has, by and large, disavowed responsibility for the patient's overall happiness, instead defining itself narrowly as a contest between technology and disease. The medical system focuses so tightly on what must be done to fight disease that it sometimes cannot see what is best for the patient. As the physician Leo Galland wrote, "The eclipse of the patient is the most profound, lasting, and unfortunate effect of the Flexner report."

By the time I was born this eclipse was set in stone literally. As the doctor Esther Sternberg pointed out in her book, *Healing Spaces,* you can see it in the architecture of hospitals:

Often the hospital's physical space seemed meant to optimize care of the equipment rather than care of the patients. In the early 1970s, one could still find hospitals where the only department that was air conditioned was the Radiology Department, because the delicate equipment could not tolerate the summer heat. As reliance on and awe of medical technology increased in the mid-twentieth century, the comfort of patients was somehow pushed aside and their surroundings were often ignored. Hospital planners assumed that patients could adapt to the needs of technology rather than the other way around.

Some of the very same mainstream doctors who'd effectively rooted out snake-oil were also the ones who noticed problems with the revolution they'd brought about. Among these reformers was Leon Eisenberg, one of the first to rigorously apply the scientific method to clinical psychiatry. Eisenberg had always been something of an outsider—he was openly rejected, first from medical schools, then from residencies, because he was a Jew. He was skinny, and his cheeks were scarred by severe adolescent acne. He was also brilliant—he graduated first in his class. And he was easy to like—he had a joke (often a Jewish joke) for every circumstance. He eventually gained a place of respect in the Ivy League institutions that had rejected him, but he never lost the contrarian eye of an outsider.

In the early 1960s Eisenberg assembled enough evidence to show that Freudian psychoanalysis—then ascendant—was doing little to help children. He performed the first randomized clinical drug trials in child psychology. These trials laid the groundwork for the treatment of attention deficit disorder with drugs like Ritalin. He was aghast, however, at the way these medications were reflexively employed to treat an ever-wider range of problems. It became clear to Eisenberg that doctors were not thinking critically, but were instead simply trading one belief system for another.

More and more, Flexnerian medicine asserted a strict Cartesian divide between body and mind. The discovery of chemical treatments for the brain helped bolster the belief that all illness, even mental illness, was simply a matter of chemistry. It helped bring medicine closer to a state of Newtonian perfection, in which every action might be traced to caroming particles, in which disease, along with personality, love, and hope, might be controlled by a skillful shot in the great molecular billiard match. Eisenberg had helped turn the tide, moving away from a Freudian fascination with the individual and toward the study of chemistry and genetics; but in his last reminiscences before his death, he said that this change had constituted an "intellectual tsunami," a rush from one extreme to another that haphazardly knocked down whatever inconvenient evidence impeded its progress.

The evidence clearly showed that, as Eisenberg wrote, "A sizeable proportion (one-third to one-half) of the cases in general medical practice have a significant emotional or behavioral component. Some emotional problems are obvious anxiety states or neuroses; many more appear in the form of bodily complaints that have no ascertainable organic basis and reflect response to psycho-social stresses; an important minority (one or two percent) present themselves as severe psychiatric illness." Nonetheless, Eisenberg wrote, most physicians were either skeptical of the evidence that disease could have a nonphysical antecedent, or "downright arrogant in their dismissal of it."

Some physicians recoiled from this evidence because it was not their area of expertise. The skill of genuinely caring about patients seems foreign to the deductive skill of matching symptoms to disease, and disease to treatment. In fact, in the collective imagination these talents are so incompatible as to be mutually exclusive: The softhearted physician stands at the opposite pole from the hardheaded one. The medical ideal has become an emotionally stunted savant who, with cool Holmesian logic, puts together the solution while others are dithering with feelings—television's Dr. House. But only in television's projections of our cultural dreams can science so readily provide fixes. Often the doctor must help the patient create his own solution, a feat that can be infinitely more complex than matching illness with cure.

HEALING THE INCURABLE

If you want to see conventional medicine struggle, watch what it does when there is nothing more, physically, that can be done. Death, because it's a problem with no solution, can bring out the worst in our fix-focused culture. Nowhere is the temptation to fill the vacuum of meaning with medical technology more expensive or more painful than in the confrontation with death.

My parents suggested I look up an old family friend, a former doctor I'll call Francis, who, they said, had been thinking deeply about how he could help people who were beyond help. I called him, and he invited me to his house. Francis's hair and beard are white, and neatly cropped. He wears rimless glasses that magnify his eyes, giving him a vaguely owlish look. We spoke in his living room over cups of herbal tea. As we talked, the sun dropped behind the hill until we were sitting in darkness.

Francis said his interest in the end of life began during a short conversation with a postmaster. It was in a small town on California's coast, and the post office she ran was a trailer on the side of the road, lined with fake wood paneling and a few rows of brass boxes. She kept an electric heater by her desk. Every day she would wheel her oxygen tank out to her Oldsmobile, lower herself into the seat, and drive to work. It was only a few hundred yards, but she was too short of breath to walk even that distance.

Francis was aware of all this when he stopped in to check his mail. They were all neighbors in that town, and it was hard not to know each other's business. He waved hello, took the letters from his box, and asked if she had anything else for him.

"Actually," he remembered her saying in her smoker's voice, "There is something." She was suffering, she explained. Her emphysema was getting worse, and chemotherapy hadn't slowed her lung cancer. The doctors had told her there was nothing else they could do for her. She asked Francis to get her enough barbiturates for an overdose.

"I thought her request was reasonable," he said. "She was saying, 'Hey I can't take it now, and it's going to get worse. Let me get out of here.' And it—it just seemed intellectually reasonable. And, I think, emotionally reasonable."

If you follow Western medicine to its logical conclusion, when there are no more surgeries that can be done, or pharmaceuticals that can be taken, it only makes sense to find a final solution: one last fix. (Francis provided that fix, which is why he asked me to use a pseudonym. Decades had passed, but he worried that the story might invite harassment.)

Though it was utterly logical, there was something about this exchange that bothered Francis. Perhaps it had been the impersonal nature of the encounter, the frictionless sangfroid with which they had negotiated. He raised one eyebrow and said to me, "Funny that that conversation would happen in a post office, right?"

Post-office transactions are constrained to trivial exchanges. A few cents for a stamp. A few words about the weather. The color of the curb outside limits the length of conversations. Yet there they were, making arrangements to determine the question of existence for this woman.

Although Francis was discreet, word got around. People driven to extreme measures—prison inmates, rebel fighters, the terminally ill—become proficient in the transmission of illicit information. Before long, others approached Francis, and he gave them the pills they wanted. The way things were going, he could have become an undercover Jack Kevorkian—helping people die without the media spectacle. But Francis bristled when I compared him to this doctor. "He's a pervert," Francis protested. "He's insane. No, I was just interested in helping this woman end her suffering. If I could have found another way to end it without . . ." He paused, then settled on the bluntest way of putting it, "Without killing her, I would have."

Which is why it came as a shock to Francis when he learned from a mutual friend that instead of taking the pills, she'd let her illness take its course. Intrigued, he inquired after the other people to whom he'd prescribed barbiturates. Not a single one had hastened their death. What had made these people choose the long decline they had so desperately wanted to avoid? In the end, despite the fact that there was no cure for these people's illnesses, each of them had found a cure for their desire to die. It was a disturbing mystery. After all, Francis had been willing to help them die, ignorant of the further recourse that had made their lives worth living. Another doctor might have puzzled over this a while, then shrugged it off. But for Francis, it shook his already unsteady faith in his career.

"I was running an ER at the time so I could see these people—people who drank, people who smoked a lot, people who ate too much, people who were accident prone, people who had trouble with relationships. I started seeing that their sicknesses or injuries didn't come out of a vacuum."

Francis would treat the symptoms of domestic violence or alcoholism (set the broken arm, stitch the laceration), but a week later the same patients would return with similar wounds.

"We put Band-Aids on them and sent them back to the same crap. I began to see that I was mainly trained as a mechanic. Really what I was operating was a high-tech turnstile."

Perhaps it's obvious, Francis said, but at the time it was a revelation to discover that a person's culture, the way they conducted their relationships, their values and priorities in life, their fears and aspirations—that all these airy intangibles could result in real, visible, bodily harm. Francis had gone to medical school with the desire to help people, and patching up the same patients each week didn't satisfy this desire. Working in an emergency room is a noble vocation, he said, but he didn't feel as if he were really making lives better. After months of troubled consideration, he told his supervisor that he would be leaving the hospital, and leaving medicine. This was only partly true. Although he gave up the formal work of a medical doctor, it was a desire to be a better healer that drew him away. If the immaterial ephemera of emotions could make people sick, Francis reasoned, the reverse could also be true: Perhaps a patient's mind could salve physical infirmities.

LEARNING FROM CANCER

Francis started by reading everything he could find on holistic medicine. He taught a class on the subject at a community college. And he started practicing yoga. These days, you can find yoga offered between kickboxing and cardio pole dancing, but back then it had not yet been stripped down to a purely physical workout. Francis learned how to pay close attention to the way his body reacted, or failed to react. He learned to tease apart the physical reality of pain from its psychological attendants—the fear that the pain would grow worse, or that it would continue forever. He discovered what every Buddhist novice discovers: When you study pain existing in the present moment with genial curiosity, it often becomes bearable, even insignificant.

A few years later, a group of cancer patients asked him to attend one of their meetings and share some of these tricks for coping with pain. He stuck around afterward to listen. It was about what you'd expect. People rehashed what doctors had told them, chatted about the way they felt, made dark jokes about their common situation, and solicited advice. There was something in this that interested Francis. So much so that he asked permission to come to their next meeting. He kept attending for the next 5 years.

In these meetings Francis observed the cancer patients slowly unravel the snarled threads of their fear and sadness. Often these strands led to the least expected places. The true source of suffering was often only tangentially related to the indignities of disease. Once people understood what was eating at them, their pain often became manageable. These people, he realized, were knitting meaning from what had seemed a meaningless tangle of misery.

As he listened, Francis thought back to the postmaster and asked himself what meaning those barbiturates had held for her. There was no way of knowing for sure, but he suspected that the pills had represented control. He had diagnosed life as the postmaster's problem, and he had provided the appropriate prescription. But maybe he'd made a misdiagnosis. Perhaps the greatest cause of her suffering hadn't been physical pain, but the steady erosion of her agency: She was losing control of her body, her daily schedule, and her power of movement.

For those few people Francis had furnished with barbiturates, the drugs must have provided an off-label dose of metaphor. "Those pills—having that parachute in hand—gave them a sense of control," he said. "And that sense of control—maybe it was just the illusion of control—but it was enough to evaporate that particular kind of suffering. The result is that people wanted to be around longer."

These days Francis facilitates cancer support groups and he begins by asking people what bothers them about having cancer.

"Of course I don't say it that way. You can't ask straight on or people get pissed. You're supposed to understand that having cancer really bothers people. Okay, cool, but *what* about it bothers you? And after they talk about it a while they usually say, 'What bothers me about it is I'm worried I'm gonna die.' All right, next question: What bothers you about dying?"

Figuring this out can take weeks. "It's not the kind of conversation you can have in a post office," Francis said. The answers people come up with are often revelatory.

"Eventually, you might come back and say, 'I've thought about it for a while and what bothers me is I have unfinished business with my son.' Well, *vaya con Dios,* dude! Go do it."

The solutions aren't always so tidy, but when I went to one of the cancer support groups, patients told me these sorts of conversations sometimes felt more lifesaving than anything else the doctors were doing. For people with a poor prognosis, it can seem as if there are only two options available: Choke down more treatment, or accept that the time has come to die. Francis offers a third option. He works to separate the unanswerable fear of the unknown from those fears that spring from soluble problems: the fear of hurting a family member, the fear of pain. On its own, death doesn't always seem so bad. And when people confront their fears they often find themselves more vitally engaged in the substance of life than they have been in years. One support-group member told me, "If it doesn't kill me, cancer will be the best thing that has ever happened to me." She considered, then said, "And if it does kill me, I think that will still be true."

Francis is humble enough to know that his tools won't work for everyone. Sometimes, people would literally rather die than walk down the dark corridors of their souls to face their fears. Even the patient doesn't want to do this work, he insists that it's imperative for the doctor to give painstaking attention to the unique circumstances of each case before acting. It's the failure to listen to patients that makes medicine inhumane, he said. When I asked him for an example of what he meant, Francis recalled a meeting in which oncologists were discussing a patient's breast cancer. The patient had said she didn't want surgery for any reason, yet as the doctors took in her information and began to reason out the possible treatments, that bit of data failed to penetrate.

"And they all said, 'The only thing we can see here is surgery,'" said Francis. "They were thinking about how to fix the problem, not about what is good for the patient. And these are truly wonderful people. They care about their patients. They are personally warm. But the nature of our medical system is such that doctors must immediately come up with a solution, then move on. And that allows for our amazing technical expertise. But if you only see the problem, that obscures the real person."

Physicians and family members who decide how long to stave off death sometimes find themselves trapped between natural and technological ideals. We often default to the worst of both worlds, romantically insisting that life is sacred, while employing only coldly rational treatment to keep the motor running.

It's more important than ever for the medical system to combine technical excellence and empathetic wisdom because the bulk of ills afflicting Americans are not sicknesses that can be cured, but chronic problems. Obesity, heart disease, and depression are incurable by technology alone—these modern epidemics require practitioners who have the skills to address physical symptoms and the emotional intelligence to teach patients how to fundamentally change their lives. Perhaps this is asking too much of medicine, but there's nowhere else to turn. The doctor's examination room has become, Francis said, "the closest thing we have to confessionals in secular society. The problem is, doctors don't have priestly training." And the physicians best situated to provide this sort of pastoral care, the primary care doctors, have year after year been afforded less money and less respect.

THE DECLINE AND FALL OF PRIMARY CARE

Johns Hopkins doctor Kerr White was one of the first medical leaders in the United States to notice the gap between what medicine could provide and what patients needed. White was the lead author of a 1961 paper in the *New England Journal of Medicine*, entitled "The Ecology of Medical Care," which demonstrated that of any 750 people who become sick, 250 would see a doctor, nine would go on to be hospitalized, and only one would require the services of a high-end university medical center. This meant that primary care medicine (a term popularized by this paper) was doing most of the heavy lifting. But the country was investing its best resources in serving that single patient who filtered through to the research hospital.

This paper became a frequently cited classic, but the tide was flowing in the other direction, toward the laboratory and away from anything resembling priestly care. In the same period that public health leaders accepted the importance of primary care, it withered. In 1949, 59 percent of doctors in the United States were general practitioners, and that number has consistently slid lower. As of 2005 only 8 percent of medical school graduates were going into family practice. The brightest medical students were encouraged—with promise of both honor and money—to become physician scientists and find new ways of prolonging life in unusual and desperate cases. By 2010 the average specialist was earning almost twice as much as the average general practitioner.

When Wells Shoemaker, a particularly promising medical student at Stanford, told a celebrated neurosurgeon that he had decided to become a pediatrician, she said, "What a waste," as if this were the equivalent of Mozart choosing a career in automotive sales. And Shoemaker found— even after he had hurdled the discouragement of his mentors—that the economic forces were against him.

In 1981 Shoemaker set up his practice in the California farming town of Watsonville, where he worked with a mostly poor Latino population. He took special pride in giving these patients the best care possible. In most cases the diagnoses were obvious, and treatment was simple. But hidden amid the unending cases of asthma and fevers were subtle symptoms of larger threats. On one occasion Shoemaker was struck, as he examined a child who had arrived after an asthma attack, by a puzzling absence of symptoms. There was nothing physically wrong. An efficient doctor would have moved on to the next patient after dispensing some advice and perhaps a prescription. But, as was his habit, Shoemaker had examined the baby on the mother's lap, and he could see that the mother was uncharacteristically upset. He asked her to tell him what happened from the beginning, then listened patiently. As she spoke, the woman began to sob and eventually admitted that she had come to the doctor's office for shelter from an abusive husband. Despite the fact that the child was physically healthy, the boy had been in true danger, and by looking at the big picture—rather than just the quantifiable symptoms—Shoemaker had been able to help.

When one of his families went to the emergency room, Shoemaker considered it a personal failure. To prevent emergencies before they happened, he spent days every year simply educating the parents of kids with diabetes, asthma, and allergies. This worked. In the final 5 years of his practice not a single one of his patients was admitted to the hospital for complications of diabetes or asthma—a stunning achievement. But Shoemaker wasn't paid for keeping patients healthy: He was paid for treatments. There was no billing code for stopping domestic abuse before it happened. He received no reimbursement for the hours of advice he dispensed on the phone, and was paid an insignificant amount when he left a family dinner to come see a child in the office. He'd make more money if he simply told the parents to go to the emergency room and then drove in later for a quick visit. In one particularly egregious example, Shoemaker cut his own paycheck by close to $50,000 a year by teaching the parents of hemophilic children how to administer a clotting factor, rather than insisting that they come to his office every time for the procedure.

All this would have been simply annoying if Shoemaker were making a decent income, but he was barely scraping by. The problem was that most of his patients were covered by Medicaid—the insurance for low-income families—and the reimbursements he received were not high enough to support the cost of keeping the lights on and his staff paid, let alone support his family. Usually, doctors deal with this by accepting only a small percentage of poor patients and relying on the higher reimbursements from private insurance. But fewer than half of Shoemaker's patients had private insurance, and he refused to turn anyone away.

"These disparities in reimbursements are terrible," he said, "but what's worse is that it gives doctors a rational way to discriminate against the poor. It's just a facile excuse for bigotry. I couldn't do that."

Then, during the recession of the early 1990s, the money ran out. For gut-wrenching months Shoemaker agonized over the finances. He upped his hours until he was spending three nights a week in the office, and had increased his patient load by 50 percent. But more of his patients than ever were using Medicaid. The practice that Shoemaker had spent 11 years building was eroding away beneath his feet. In hindsight, he says that if he had been more mature he would have compromised to save his practice. Instead, he opted, as he put it, to "simply hammer harder, even if I were bending the nails." He drew down his line of credit to pay the rent until he reached his debt limit. He was physically haggard, emotionally spent, and his entire family was suffering. In 1992, having exhausted his resources, he abandoned his practice. He was not the only primary care doctor who had been hanging by a thread: Fifteen of the 45 doctors in Watsonville closed their doors during that recession. This kind of culling recurs periodically across the United States.

"I was financially undone by a stupid fee-for-service scheme which did not recognize or reward many of the extra good things I tried to do," Shoemaker said. "In fact, fee-for-service punished these rather severely."

Fee-for-service means that physicians are paid like mechanics: The more broken-down the customers are, the more repairs (and dollars) there are to make. It's the main mode of medical payment in the United States, though there are plenty of other systems—some doctors receive a fixed salary, some doctors are paid more if their patients stay healthier. But to those who conceive of the human body as a complex machine, an automotive pricing scheme seems most logical.

Money talks, and when it comes to health spending, it talks about the kind of medicine we believe in: We believe, it seems, in academic tertiary-care hospitals, diagnostic tests, and surgeries. The other stuff—educating patients, caring about them, and helping them change their lives—are all nice enough; but they are low on the list of economic priorities. Belief, when coupled to an economic engine, can shape reality in its image, and today most doctors can't afford to have conversations with patients, let alone serve as confidante and coach. On average, Americans spend just 30 minutes, not per visit, but per year, with their primary care doctors (less than half the time spent in comparable countries).

In many cases, the primary care clinician has been reduced to a mere barrier that patients must hurdle before proceeding to a specialist. When general practitioners relinquish their pastoral role—that is, their capacity to comprehend and care for the person as well as the patient—they become petty bureaucrats. Given the lack of time for care, it's no wonder that so many Americans demand unnecessary treatments. Perhaps this is why the words *treatment* and *care*—which, in their common English meanings, are almost antonyms—are synonyms in the realm of medicine.

POST-INDUSTRIAL SHAMANISM

Kerr White, in his study of primary care, became increasingly convinced of the importance of care, in its common meaning. In an interview near the end of his career, he respectfully acknowledged what is usually called—with a bit of a sneer—"just the placebo effect."

"I think it's the most undervalued, ubiquitous therapeutic intervention that we have," White said. "It has an all-purpose, extremely powerful effect, and it's caring. It's a manifestation of love, if you like."

This, I suspect, is what draws people to alternative medicine. When Mom visits her chiropractor, a warm and thoughtful man, they spend at least 45 minutes together. They talk during part of that time, and the rest is spent in massage. Either way, he is exquisitely attentive to her. "It's like his fingers have X-ray vision," Mom said. "He can find the painful spot in seconds, just through touch." Mom never goes expecting a cure, but always leaves feeling better.

One particularly clever method for studying this phenomena was devised by Harvard medical researcher Ted Kaptchuk, who measured the power of caring and conversation on people with irritable bowel syndrome. Kaptchuk masked the study by treating patients with sham acupuncture needles designed to telescope in on themselves and stick to the skin without penetration. The patients thought they were in a clinical trial of acupuncture, but caring was the real treatment on trial. They were divided into two groups, and when members of the first group arrived for treatment the practitioners explained that, to avoid biasing the experiment, they wouldn't talk. Then they briskly went about their work, performing the sham treatment. When the second group arrived, on the other hand, practitioners greeted them warmly and asked about their symptoms. They listened, asked for elaboration, expressed empathy, and allowed periods of silence. They inquired as to how the illness related to patients' relationships. They invited interpretation of the cause and meaning of the maladies. Only then did the practitioners perform the sham acupuncture. For this group, the reduction in symptoms was more profound than the effect of any irritable-bowel-syndrome pharmaceutical on the market. For patients in the first "efficient" group, by contrast, measures of quality of life actually fell until they were slightly worse than those on the waiting list who received no treatment.

It's important, however, not to take this too far. When it becomes apparent that an old way of thinking is insufficient to explain the way things work, Kerr White wrote, "new concepts and theories are apt to be misrepresented as claiming to explain more than the evidence supports." Which is why the excitable sometimes assert that the placebo effect proves that the mind causes, and can cure, all ills. It is this kind of shallow acceptance that makes people believe that they are at fault for their diseases, or that they can dissolve their tumors with sheer positivity, or that they are always better off without technological medicine.

The fact is that there are many ailments best treated with medical technology. When someone comes to a clinic complaining about headaches, persistent hypertension, and the sense that their heart sometimes races unaccountably, 99 percent of the time the cause will be their diet, the number of espressos they are drinking, their feelings about their job, or their failing marriage—but in rare cases the cause will be a pheochromocytoma, a tumor on the adrenal gland that may be surgically removed. The staggering challenge for clinicians is to accept both possibilities, to treat the body and care for the patient's immaterial whole, to be both physician and metaphysician.

When we spoke, Wells Shoemaker happened to mention that he'd recently had an appendectomy, and I told him the significance of my own appendicitis. In reply, he quoted a bit of doggerel he'd composed while recuperating:

"You might lie to the judge and still dodge the perjury/But appendicitis, Dude, won't go 'way without surgery." Then, just to even the score, he added, "Wouldn't it be nice if depression could be removed by surgery?"

The great failure of modern medicine is its attempt to treat the symptoms of our modern environment (our anomie, our inequity, our stress) as if they conformed to the Flexnarian model of scientific medicine—that is, as if they were diseases, each with a single, universally applicable cure. It shouldn't be surprising, Leon Eisenberg wrote, "that physicians will avoid problems they feel inadequate to manage by relying on the promiscuous prescription of tranquilizing drugs."

It shouldn't denigrate our tremendous achievements in medicine to point out that this model is outdated and simplistic. What we need now is a new model that preserves the physics of the appendectomy while embracing the ways that meaning, relationships, and coherence affect human health.

You can find a parallel to our current confusion in post-Reformation England. At that time Protestants still accepted that witchcraft caused disease, but they had rejected faith in holy water, icons, saints, and the rest of the shields against the unknown that had leaked from paganism into Catholicism. Historian Keith Thomas thinks that this is why English Protestants executed witches, while Catholics—for the most part—did not. "Protestantism," Thomas wrote, "forced its adherents into the intolerable position of asserting the reality of witchcraft, yet denying the existence of an effective and legitimate form of protection or cure."

Just as Protestants rejected the power of pagan symbols, we have divested ourselves of nonmedical methods of coping with illness and death—dismissing, as superstition, the clergy, the psychoanalysts, the shamans, and the poets. Faith in medical technology denounces suffering as illegitimate until it is expressed as physical damage. (The word *just,* in the phrase "it's just in your head," speaks volumes on this point.) As a result, people experiencing real suffering with nonphysical causes often try to shoehorn the symptoms into something recognized by the International Classification of Diseases. To paraphrase Thomas, you could say that medicalization forces us into the intolerable position of asserting the reality of these diseases, yet denying the existence of a legitimate form of protection.

When healing is reduced to a battle between technology and disease, patients lose both responsibility and control. "Medical procedures turn into black magic when, instead of mobilizing his self-healing powers, they transform the sick man into a limp and mystified voyeur of his own treatment," wrote Ivan Illich, the radical Austrian philosopher and Roman Catholic priest. "Medical procedures turn into sick religion when they are performed as rituals that focus the entire expectation of the sick on science and its functionaries instead of encouraging them to seek a poetic interpretation of their predicament or find an admirable example in some person—long dead or next door—who learned to suffer."

There's something wrong with a society that turns reflexively to its medical doctors in moments of suffering.* Now, when Francis looks back on his experience with the postmaster, he found it outrageous that he— in his capacity as a dispenser of drugs—was the person people turned to for help.

---

* Indeed, a body of science suggests that the positive health effects of strong social connections are as powerful as the negative effects of smoking, obesity, or a sedentary lifestyle.

"If we were truly a civilized society, we'd talk to each other long before we considered suicide," Francis said. "We'd have community networks. In the old days if you were even out of sorts everyone knew about it and they'd drop off a lasagna for you."

Even after learning all this, I tend to yearn for an easy technical fix when faced with the reality of illness. As I write, my 3-month-old daughter is sick for the first time in her life, and if there were some good medical solution, I'd be at the drugstore in seconds flat. It's just a cold, but she doesn't know that, and she begs for help in the only way she knows how. When she cries, her cuteness disappears and she resembles one of those bald, bloated, character actors that are cast to play Mafia goons. She looks, come to think of it, like an enraged, red-faced Paul Giamatti. She glares at me from under accusatorily tilted eyebrows and cries out in horrified, choking howls. I worry about what my neighbors might think, probably because I feel responsible for her misery. I've already done everything I can. I've suctioned out her mucus with a bulb syringe and even—when concern overcame disgust—put my mouth directly over her tiny upturned nose and sucked. But there's no cure for colds, or for the underlying discomfort they bring. And it strikes me that I react the same way when afflicted with pain and illness that I don't understand. I go to the doctors and demand relief. I become petulant when they don't deliver.

I can also get relief, however, through simple human contact, and through some basic explanation of my suffering. Accepting life, I reason over the crying, means accepting suffering. That doesn't mean anyone should seek out pain or refuse medical attempts to reduce suffering—it's only when medicine is expected to stop *all* suffering that it begins to dominate and smother life.

I don't know how to tell my daughter that this cold is an inescapable part of life, so instead, I sing to her. I sing, "Oh What a Beautiful Morning," from *Oklahoma!*, because, randomly, it seems to be her favorite, and usually she starts to squeeze her eyes into little parentheses and make winsome, dimpled smiles by the time I get to the chorus. But this time she only pauses in her sobbing for a verse. Then, she starts crying again, because that's the way life works—nothing is certain. And then, eventually, she grows quiet, and drifts off to sleep, because that is also the way life works—everything ends.

CONCLUSION

It may come as a shock to learn, after the way I've described my family's shared ideological vision, that my parents' marriage didn't last. I'd thought that perhaps I could get away with omitting that fact completely from this book—the divorce fell between chapters chronologically, and it just seemed irrelevant to the equation of nature and health. But now that I see what I've written, it's clear that the schism in my family is, in its own way, central to my inquiry.

The divorce certainly came as a shock to me. It happened, for the usual unfathomable reasons that people fall in and out of love, when I was 9—old enough to be acutely aware of what was going on and young enough that family was still the most important thing in my life. Because my parents had created such a unifying domestic mythos—founded on backpacking and wholesome food and the categorical rejection of television—the divorce felt as if it was more than the end of the marriage. It felt like the end of me being part of something exceptional. Looking back, I think I must have vaguely believed that we were a little bit of Eden in a fallen world: While everyone else's parents were getting divorced my family was holding hands around the table and singing before dinner every night. With their split I was overwhelmed by a huge, inchoate loss for the warmth and safety of home. It's taken me until now to see that I'd only lost the *idea* of home: The house and the people were still there—what was shattered was the sense that my family was special, blessed, invulnerable.

Because of the divorce, my memories from those early prelapsarian days glow with acute longing. And yet, paradoxically, something in that golden time led to its end, and that makes me doubt my ability to tell right from wrong, up from down. It makes me yearn for certainty beyond gut feeling, for universal Cartesian truths that can be trusted to remain upright when everything else falls apart.

We think of the Fall as a story that happened just once, at the beginning, but it makes more sense as personal story that keeps happening over and over: We've all been cast out, and innocence is always lost. Does that mean that that Eden never really existed, that paradise is just a childhood mirage? To a large extent, innocence is simply ignorance. But some of that childhood magic, I think, is utterly real. Clearly, the urge to get back to the garden—my parents' garden—and my contradictory skepticism that it ever existed, have guided me ever since.

These days, my parents are still inclined toward nature, though both in their own ways. They are aging gracefully on opposite sides of Nevada City, each happily remarried. When we visit, Mom tries to feed our daughter Brussels sprouts dipped in apple-cider vinegar, which (she says) is full of wonderfully healthy microbes. Dad has softened a little bit: There's usually ice cream in his freezer, and there's a big television in his living room for baseball games. But when it comes to parenting, he believes more ardently than ever in adhering to methods from a simpler past—before there were commutes, and 9 to 5 workdays, and emails to be answered.

When Beth and I bought a crib for my daughter I had to force myself to tell Dad. I knew he'd be disappointed—he thinks it's fundamentally unnatural, and thus unhealthy, for a baby to be isolated from its parent, even in sleep. It had been something of a journey for Beth and me to come to the point where we wanted a crib. I'd rolled my eyes a little at some of the things Dad said about the importance of co-sleeping, but I'd taken his ideas seriously nonetheless. Who can say that cuddling with babies doesn't feel absolutely right? I did my own research, and read the horrifying studies of SIDS (sudden infant death syndrome) and suffocation. By the time my daughter was born, I thought I'd found a sleeping arrangement that brought evidence and emotion into accord. We put our bed on the floor with a baby mattress jammed up against it. I was proud of myself: I'd weighed all the science, seen past cultural prejudice, and found a setup that was so rational and so nurturing that my baby would sleep idyllically and never cry.

As if in retribution for my hubris, she barely slept at all in her first 3 weeks. She cried inconsolably for hours on end. She would beg desperately for milk, then hyperventilate at the breast, shaking her head from side to side with her mouth open, utterly failing to drink, as if possessed by a boob goblin. There was an unfortunate backlash that came from believing my master plan would guarantee a happy baby: This belief also suggested that her distress was a sign of failure, or damage. God, I thought—she's broken. She's incapable of love. After four nights all the science, all my father's advice, and all my own plans went out the window. Beth and I were scrambling for survival, grasping at any possibility for sleep. Occasionally the baby slept on her little mattress as planned, but often she was in our bed with us, or sleeping completely on her own. And I noticed that after we gave up on theories and began to pay attention the squirming creature in front of our faces, things got easier. The flexibility freed us up to tinker our way toward solutions. We adjusted to her quirks and she to ours. Eventually, after a few months, it just made sense to get a crib. I called Dad up and presented the news cheerily, as if I didn't know that, to him, a crib was a symbol of inhumanity.

"Beth and I didn't want her to have to cry it out, but that's not really how it happened. When she wakes up at night she just kind of grumbles and yodels—it's like she's calling for us more than crying, 'Guys, hello-o, I'm awake here. Did I mention that I'm hun-gry?'"

Dad chuckled.

"She did that for about 45 minutes, and then she really did start crying, so *then* Beth fed her. After that she slept until morning, and ever since she's been sleeping through the night. It's amazing."

There was a moment of silence. "Well," Dad said, picking his words carefully, "I'm certainly happy to hear that you and Beth are getting more sleep." There was a note of anguish in his voice. It stung me to hear it.

When I'd first asked him about baby sleeping arrangements, 2 years earlier, Dad had told me there was an evolutionary argument for keeping babies and parents together. For the great apes, being left alone in infancy is a death sentence. Human babies, Dad said, feel this instinctual terror.

"When a child is left to cry it out, they go into extreme and utter panic. They think they have been abandoned and they are going to die," he said. "Forcing babies to sleep alone ends the period—starting in the womb—in which they understand themselves to be part of a larger whole. They lose that feeling of being at one with a nurturing universe—and instead feel like an isolated being fighting for survival."

The thing is, you could argue that we *are* isolated beings struggling for survival. You could also make a reasonable case that we are part of a larger whole, that nature is abundant and nurturing. And the arguments over where and how babies should sleep look completely different depending on which of these perspectives you take. If health comes from shielding against outside dangers, then a crib makes sense—it's a piece of technology that protects the baby from the parent's nighttime rolling and bedclothes tangling. If health comes instead from connections with the larger whole, then the crib looks dangerous—it separates parent and child, makes breastfeeding harder, and prevents cuddling.

These two ways of seeing, of course, are what I've been describing all along. If you see yourself as threatened by a hostile universe it makes sense to protect yourself by bringing your surroundings under your control—to build a palisade against nature's beasts. If you see yourself as part of a larger nurturing whole, then it makes sense to invite nature in and foster relationships. To the natural perspective, inhibiting connections—whether by taking antibiotics, or processing food, or putting a baby in a crib—seems risky. To the technological perspective each of these innovations is a wonderful protection against nature's chaos.

In the process of writing this book, friends would often ask me whether I was siding with nature or technology. At first I'd say that it was complex, sometimes one was right, sometimes the other, depending on the context. That's true (if dull and obvious), but in a larger sense, both are right. Nature is deadly and nurturing at the same time. The trick isn't picking a winner (in fact, the compulsion to divide by right and wrong, to see one way and not the other, is at the heart of the problem). The trick is to see the world both ways at once—with both eyes open. That sounds simple, but it's deceptively difficult because these two ways of seeing work in such different ways.

The technological perspective tends to focus narrowly on the details—which is incredibly effective, but also limiting. The concentration on the minutia has allowed us to improve our technical precision in obstetrics, but prevented us from seeing the harm those techniques are causing women over the course of their lives. In the field of food safety, the blinkered intensity with which we protect ourselves using pasteurization is matched by a failure of attention to festering farms and fragile immune systems. In nutrition, we have stared so fixedly at the molecular parts of food that we have neglected the cultural and economic milieu in which those nutrients act. In forestry and hog farming, the reductive vision for the management of trees and swine has become a self-fulfilling prophecy—we've squeezed and straightened biological complexity until the forest and the pig resemble the simple models they've been forced to fit. This has created wonderful efficiency, but it also has made the world a more ugly, brutal place.

The technological perspective tends to favor abstract theory and universal rules over individual circumstance. And although it makes perfect sense to have a one-size-fits-all rule for the speed of light or the molecular weight of cesium, it makes less sense when trying to impose laws on humanity. It can cause problems when the rules imposed by authorities override the guidance of an individual's own experience. In nutrition there's a problem with the way the sensory experience of food has been trumped by abstractions like "good cholesterol." (The labels we place on foods have made it more difficult to actually taste them: Both the literal nutrition labels, and figurative labels that categorize foods as either healthy or unhealthy, are often more persuasive than how the food makes us *feel*.) In healthcare, there's a problem with the way medicine has specialized in the algorithmic matching of diagnosis to treatment at the expense of those skills needed to care for the unique contingencies of an individual. (As Franz Kafka's country doctor puts it, "To write prescriptions is easy but to come to an understanding with people is hard.") And specifically in obstetrics, there's a problem with the view of birth as a surgical procedure to be performed on a woman, rather than a physical (and psychological) act to be performed by her. * Too much reliance on authority (which depends on knowledge that is abstract, universal, and timeless) leads to failures in those cases where personal attention (which brings knowledge of the particular, the timely, and the local) is of paramount importance.

Despite its faults, the narrow technological perspective is an essential tool. It gives us control. The reductive stare allows us to break nature down to pieces that may be studied with precision. I want obstetricians innovating to make C-sections safer. I want scientists working on a molecular understanding of food. I want those clinical algorithms that keep doctors from making mistakes. The problems only begin to arise when these things become ends unto themselves, when they limit our ability to see and judge the world in all its wonderfully messy fullness.

There are also ways in which an inclination toward nature leads people astray. The suspicions that spring from the bodily fear of vaccination needles are almost all misleading. The belief that people with immune deficiencies or cancer will be cured by raw milk is totally false. The temptation to buy the cheese marked "natural," even when I have no idea what this means for that particular cheddar, frequently causes me to waste my money. But this natural perspective, because it is rooted in bodily sensation rather than faith in authority, can be swayed by evidence and observation.

There's something more complicated going on with those who trust in nature, but cannot be swayed. There are people who see the world

---

* The shift of power away from lived experience to abstract expert knowledge can also lead to a failure of personal responsibility. This may provoke medical litigation: When people feel powerless to do anything about their own suffering it only makes sense for them to blame others. Perhaps this is why obstetrics is one of the most sued medical specialties while midwives, who focus on empowering and coaching, are hardly ever sued.

with the black-and-white certainty of the technological gaze, but vote for nature rather than technology. Those who become fixated on a particular form of alternative medicine, or obsessed with toxic fumes, or convinced that vaccines must cause autism—though they may initially have been guided by their gut feelings and personal experience—display all the hallmarks of the narrow technological perspective: a blinkered insistence on a single point of danger (or cure), a focus on small mechanical explanations rather than large relational ones, and a prioritization of theory over evidence. At the extreme, these people will grow paranoid and devise ever more intricate conspiracy theories to justify a position that increasingly contradicts reality.

In the process of writing this conclusion I happened to pick up Iain McGilchrist's book, *The Master and His Emissary*. McGilchrist has made the case that these two ways of thinking—the technological view and the natural one—are, in fact, the product of the two hemispheres of the brain. The division between the sides of the brain is profound. Sever the corpus callosum—the bundle of neurons through which the hemispheres communicate—and the organ will fall open in your hands at the fracture down the middle. The brain evolved this split, McGilchrist says, to allow for a dual perspective on the world. The qualities that McGilchrist ascribes to each half of the brain are utterly consistent with what I've described here. The left brain generates a narrow beam of attention, directed by our needs, mainly for the purpose of consumption and control (I have called this the technological perspective). The right brain generates a broad sphere of attention directed by whatever is going on in our environment besides ourselves (the all-natural perspective). The left hemisphere allows the bird, for instance, to maintain intense focus on the problem of cracking open a nut and gobbling up the scattered pieces, while the right maintains a broad sense of the creature's relationship to the ecosystem surrounding it—vigilant for dangers and opportunities outside the left's narrow field of focus. (Birds, in fact, divide these two types of attention so that the eye associated with the right hemisphere may maintain a broad awareness of its environment while the other eye is trained on some morsel.) The right sees the whole, and the left sees the parts. The right looks for relationships, the left focuses on control. The right is open to new stimulus and sensation from the outside, while the left focuses on the task at hand. The cooperation of these two entities, McGilchrist maintains, is essential for making meaning of the world:

> Experience is forever in motion, ramifying and unpredictable. In order for us to *know* anything at all, that thing must have enduring properties. If all things flow, and one can never step in the same river twice . . . one will always be taken unawares by experience, since nothing being ever repeated, nothing can ever be known. We have to find a way of fixing it as it flies, stepping back from the immediacy of the experience, stepping outside the flow. Hence the brain has to attend to the world in two completely different ways, and in so doing, bring two different worlds into being. In one, we *experience*—the live, complex, embodied, world of individual, always unique beings, forever in flux, a net of interdependencies, forming and reforming wholes, a world with which we are deeply connected. In the other we 'experience' our experience in a special way: a 're-presented' version of it, containing static, separable, bounded, but essentially fragmented entities, grouped into classes, on which predictions can be based. This kind of attention isolates, fixes and makes each thing explicit by bringing it under the spotlight of attention. In doing so it renders things inert, mechanical, lifeless. But it also enables us for the first time to know, and consequently to learn and to make things. This gives us power.

McGilchrist is most worried about the problems that arise when the (technological) left dominates the (natural) right because the narrowly focused mind cannot comprehend the possibility of an alternative perspective. Experiments in which the right hemisphere is deactivated, he writes, suggest that "not only does . . . the left hemisphere tend to insist on its theory at the expense of getting things wrong, but it will later cheerfully insist that it got it right." A system of logic, as long as it remains inward looking and self-consistent, cannot accept outside contradictions. This sort of intransigence generates paradoxes—conditions that, according to the orthodoxy (correct thinking), cannot exist. You can see this in computer programs and bureaucracies, which operate with perfect consistency according to their own internal logic, but with remarkable absence of common sense.

It's not so terrible when the all-natural, right-brained reflex guides us toward phony alternative medical practitioners, or overpriced groceries. Sure, people (or more often pocketbooks) are harmed by a credulous assumption of natural goodness, but the number of people seriously hurt by these things is relatively low. I'm more concerned with the problems that arise when the technological, left-brained gaze fixes tenaciously on a perceived problem while ignoring any larger, systematic problems that might exist. The gravest dangers we face, in my opinion, stem from our tendency to grasp desperately at control where none is available; they stem from our tendency to focus so intently on small technical solutions that we lose sight of the whole and the holy. Give nature its due and I think we'd start solving our most frustratingly intransigent problems. There would be fewer blind-spot oversights because we'd see the value in stepping back to check reality against theory. People would be less prone to crackpot theories and denialism. We'd be more humble. We'd better understand those who disagreed with us. We'd have a more civil culture.

And can nature make us healthier? I started this inquiry with a story of walking in Yosemite, and feeling as if the beauty of the place was seeping into my bones, and though I've circled around it I haven't addressed this directly. Since those mountain memories launched this book, it seems appropriate to return to them here. To start with the left brain's analytic view, there is some evidence that when we try to bring nature under our control the left hemisphere of the brain dominates. This is true in animals as well as humans: Researchers have observed that crows engaged in tool use turn their head to favor their right eye (associated with the left hemisphere) even when it makes their task more difficult. When humans use tools to transform their environment it's usually to plane nature's complexity down to Cartesian simplicity: to plow a riotous field into furrows, to break a tangled forest down to regular boards—then build it up again as a grid of perpendicular walls. The left brain tends to transform the world into its own mechanistic image, McGilchrist writes. These transformations, which create straight lines and industrial uniformity, "in turn help to influence the workings of the brain in a mutually reinforcing, self perpetuating way. This would suggest that . . . the modern Western urban environment may be exaggerating the tendencies that the left hemisphere has projected there, as well as suggesting one reason why the natural environment is felt to have such a healing influence."

Leave the city, in other words, and the right hemisphere has a chance to breathe. Anyone who moves between a built and natural environment will recognize a certain relaxation, a melting away of problems that had previously seemed all-important, as they step out into the wilderness. Kayakers, mountain bikers, surfers, and anyone who finds themselves moving through the natural world too quickly for rational thought, will be familiar with the release that comes with abandoning logic, and accepting the flow of intuitive movement.

There is some scattered science to back up this impression. Schizophrenia (which, interestingly, may be related to left-brain dominance) is twice as common among urban residents compared to those who live in the country. People who spend much of their time outdoors (especially hunters) tend to have sharper senses. And, researchers have suggested that the rise in nearsightedness is related to increased time spent inside. People rate their stress levels lower when in natural areas, and studies of real estate prices reveal that buyers are willing to spend thousands of dollars more for environments (or simply views) that include water, trees, or vegetation. In Portland, women living in neighborhoods with lots of trees were less likely to have low-birth-weight babies, even after controlling for their economic status. A famous study of gallbladder-surgery patients found that those whose windows faced a brick wall took longer to recover than those with windows opening onto leafy foliage. The patients with a view had less trouble with headaches or nausea, and mostly required only over-the-counter painkillers. Greater numbers of the patients with a view of the wall required more potent medication. Finally, and most frivolously, the fact that Albert Einstein and Kurt Gödel would make time each day to walk through the trees at Princeton, seems to anecdotally link high brain function with exposure to nature. In this last example, however, it's not clear which way the arrow of causality points: Did nature make these geniuses smarter, or did they seek out nature because they were smart enough to realize it made them happier? I think it's a mistake to focus too tightly on nature as the solution, to think of wilderness as a sort of pill that can boost health. My personal experience in Yosemite (to give the natural perspective its due now) suggests that it was the beauty of the surroundings, yes, but there were even more important elements of that moment that made me feel so good.

Though I frequently went back to those wild places as I grew older, it became harder for me to recapture that childhood sense of something put aright. At first I suspected my companions were the problem: In high school I started working with white water guides, men who sweated equal parts alcohol and testosterone, who had no patience for reverence. Going to beautiful places with these guys was an utterly different experience from visiting them with my family. But that wasn't exactly it. I was right that companionship was at the core of the problem, but in a different way than I'd thought. It was only when I found myself alone in the wilderness with more than enough time for reverent contemplation that I understood what had changed.

I remember the precise moment of this epiphany: I was perched high on a slope, with a view of Denali National Park. It was a week after the summer solstice and the sunset was merging into sunrise. I'd hitchhiked from Anchorage that day, and for dinner I'd eaten a little cornmeal and two firm spears of salmon flesh from a mason jar (a gift from a Juneau family that had taken me in earlier on the trip). As I looked out on the Alaskan splendor, instead of experiencing fulfillment, the feeling that engulfed me was one of crushing isolation. I began bargaining with myself: I would trade this view—along with the roll of bills in the side-pocket of my backpack, and my left pinky toe if necessary—for one night spent playing poker with a few raft guides in a grungy boathouse. I chalked up my forlornness to lack of character.

I might have felt better if I'd known there was a whole tribe of lost boys like me searching the lonely lands for something that they'd felt there once. At that moment, I'd later learn, I was separated—by just a few miles and fewer years—from another young hitchhiker named Christopher McCandless, whose story Jon Krakauer had told in *Into the Wild*. Off in the direction of the sun from where I sat was the abandoned bus where he'd died, and where, in the margin of *Doctor Zhivago,* he'd written one of his last realizations in capital letters: "HAPPINESS ONLY REAL WHEN SHARED."

It wasn't the Yosemite sunsets that had filled me with such hale energy as a child, it was watching those sunsets with my family, the four of us huddled together, windbreaker against windbreaker. It wasn't the close clarity of the stars, but Mom pointing out the Milky Way, that gave me the vertiginous feeling of falling into the vast heart of our galaxy. It was not only the place that mattered, but the fact that in that place the family was together and uninterrupted. I'd gone looking for Eden in the places where human fingerprints disappeared, but paradise was empty without the human touch. The technological perspective tends to insist on naming winners and losers, but I can argue neither for nature or technology, only for reunification.

ACKNOWLEDGMENTS

Whenever I do any reporting I rely on extremely busy people—with much more important things to do—to carve out the time to give me a personalized education. I offer very little in return—I can't promise that I'll fully flesh out their stories, come to conclusions that they will agree with, or even present them in a positive light. So I'm grateful first and foremost to the many sources who let me into their lives, to all the scientists who indulged, advised, and corrected me even when my topic only touched tangentially on their areas of interest. Their names appear in the notes.

When I first started working as a writer I had this crazy idea that my editors would be artistic collaborators who would read with the care of a generous critic, help me grapple with the creative process, and—in the end—sprinkle a little magic fairy dust over the work to make it come alive. In reality, of course, most editors don't have the time, let alone the fairy dust. But my editor Alex Postman made the time, incisively locating problems, gently breaking the news to me, then stepping back to let me find solutions.

My agent David Kuhn patiently coached me through the process of turning a vague sense of something out there into a book. Colin Dickerman saw the potential in this strange mix of essayistic memoir and science writing from an unknown writer.

I profited from the generosity of the Mesa Refuge, which gave me 2 weeks of my most productive work in a place completely free of distractions, except for the raptors, sea birds, and the breathtaking view. I also owe something to Porteños in general, and the cafés of Buenos Aires where I spent 3 months writing.

I'm thankful to Josh Berezin and Bonnie-Sue Hitchcock, who read early versions of the manuscript and offered trenchant literary direction.

I also owe thanks to Catherine Price, Jennifer Kahn, Bill Wasik, and Jennifer Block who read portions of this and kept me sane by hashing out my picayune concerns.

My debt to Michael Pollan is impossible to quantify. His instruction at the UC Berkeley Graduate School of Journalism, his continuing mentorship, and more than anything else, the example of his work, has been absolutely fundamental in showing me what sort of writer, and what sort of human being, I'd like to be.

Other editors helped me with pieces of this book that were previously published elsewhere. Roger Hodge and Ben Austen sharpened my writing for the greater part of the chapters on hogs and raw milk respectively when those pieces were published in *Harper's*. David Bunnell helped guide me to write about Dr. Francis by publishing a story on assisted death in Eldr, and Filip Zalewski gave me the opportunity to shape my ideas about modern birth by buying an early version of Michelle Niska's story for *Assembly*. Gail Rudd Entrekin published a version of my Lake Vera story in the collection *Sierra Songs and Descants*.

Most of all, I'm thankful to my wife, Beth Goldstein, who brings me food when I forget to eat and lets me take up the entire couch when I write at night, who keeps me honest, brings me down to earth, shows me by example how to laugh at myself, and reminds me constantly of what's important in life.

ENDNOTES

Listed below are the sources I've called upon, divided by chapter, aside from those people and publications adequately identified in the text.

INTRODUCTION

Carson, Rachel. *Silent Spring* (Houghton Mifflin, 2002); Gould, Stephen Jay. *Bully for Brontosaurus* (W. W. Norton & Company, 1992); Holmes, Richard. *The Age of Wonder* (Vintage Books, 2010); Montaigne, Michel de. *The Complete Works* (Everyman's Library, 2003); Norgaard, Richard. *Development Betrayed* (Routledge, 1994); Toulmin, Stephen. *Cosmopolis* (University of Chicago Press, 1992); Wilson, Edward Osborne. *Consilience* (Vintage Books, 1999). **On dieting and weight gain:** See Chapter 3 and Pollan, Michael. *In Defense of Food* (Penguin Press, 2008); Taubes, Gary. *Good Calories, Bad Calories* (Anchor, 2008). **Paradoxes: On increasing maternal mortality and morbidity:** See Chapter 1. **On autoimmunity and our increasing susceptibility to disease:** See discussion of autoimmunity in Chapter 2, and of polio in Chapter 4. **On iatrogenesis versus deaths from lack of healthcare in the United States:** See Chapter 7. **On depression and antidepressants:** Angell, Marcia. "The Epidemic of Mental Illness: Why?" *New York Review of Books* (June 23, 2011); Hensly, Scott. "1 in 10 Americans Takes Antidepressants." NPR (Oct. 10, 2011).

CHAPTER 1

I'm indebted to Christine Morton, a sociologist at the California Maternal Quality Care Collaborative, who first let the cat out of the bag by telling me that it looked like maternal morbidity and mortality rates were rising, and then spent hours on the phone giving me referrals and citations. Debra Bingham, now at the Association of Women's Health, Obstetric & Neonatal Nurses, was crucial in bringing me up to speed on the state of the science and correcting my errors in thinking (any that remain are mine alone). In addition to those mentioned in the text, the obstetricians David LaGrew, Brian Schaffer, Tracy Flanagan, Jeffrey Phelan, and Jeanne Conry also gave generously of their time to provide me with perspectives of the way things work in labor and delivery units. Susan Jenkins with the Big Push for Midwives gave me the lay of the land and introductions when I was getting started. I also profited from conversations with Sister Angela Murdaugh of the American College of Nurse Midwives, Carol Sakala of Childbirth Connection, and Susan Stone of the Frontier School of Midwifery and Family Nursing. **On views of natural childbirth around the time I was born:** Arms, Suzanne. *Immaculate Deception: A New Look at Women and Childbirth in America* (Bantam, 1977); Leboyer, Frédérick. *Birth without Violence* (Knopf, 1975); Wilson, Sloan. "The

American Way of Birth." *Harper's* (July 1964): 48–54. **Lewis Mehl's (now Mehl-Madrona) early work on home birth:** Mehl, L.E., et al. "Outcomes of Elective Home Births: a Series of 1,146 Cases." *Journal of Reproductive Medicine* 19, no. 5 (Nov. 1977): 281–290. **On improvements in maternal mortality rates and the industrialization of birth:** "Achievements in Public Health, 1900–1999: Healthier Mothers and Babies." *Morbidity and Mortality Weekly Report (MMWR)* 48 no. 38 (Oct. 1, 1999): 849–858; Gawande, Atul. "The Score." *New Yorker* (Oct. 9, 2006): 58–67. **On reasons for the rising C-section rate:** Birnbaum, Cara. "What Doctors Don't Tell You About C-sections." *Health.com* (Nov. 11, 2009); Johnson, Nathanael. "More Women Dying from Pregnancy Complications; State Holds on to Report." *California Watch* (Feb. 2, 2010); Declercq, E.R., et al. "Listening to Mothers II." *Childbirth Connection* (Oct. 2006). **On trends in infant mortality and morbidity:** Lisonkova, Sarka, et al. "Temporal Trends in Neonatal Outcomes Following Iatrogenic Preterm Delivery." *BMC Pregnancy and Childbirth* 11 (2011): 39; Macdorman, Marian, and T.J. Mathews. "Recent Trends in Infant Mortality in the United States." National Center for Health Statistics (NCHS) Data Brief, no. 9 (Oct. 2008). **On trends in maternal mortality and morbidity:** Hoyert, Donna L. "Maternal Mortality and Related Concepts." National Center for Health Statistics (NCHS). *Vital and Health Statistics*. Series 3, Analytical and Epidemiological Studies, no. 33 (Feb. 2007); Kuklina, Elena, et al. "Severe Obstetric Morbidity in the United States: 1998–2005." *Obstetrics and Gynecology* 113, no. 2 pt. 1 (Feb. 2009): 293–299; The California Pregnancy-Associated Mortality Review. "Report from 2002 and 2003 Maternal Death Reviews." (California Department of Public Health, Maternal Child and Adolescent Health Division, 2011). **On improvements in the health corresponding to C-section rates:** Sakala, Carol. "Evidence-based Maternity Care: What It Is and What It Can Achieve." (Milbank Memorial Fund 2008); Main, Elliott, et al. "Cesarean Deliveries, Outcomes, and Opportunities for Change in California." (California Maternal Quality Care Collaborative, 2011). **On continuous fetal heart monitoring:** Alfirevic, Z., et al. "Continuous Cardiotocography as a Form of Electronic Fetal Monitoring for Fetal Assessment During Labour." Cochrane Database of Systematic Reviews (online), no. 3 (2006); Haggerty, L.A. "Continuous Electronic Fetal Monitoring: Contradictions Between Practice and Research." *Journal of Obstetric, Gynecologic, and Neonatal Nursing* 28, no. 4 (Aug. 1999): 409–416. **On the value of allowing mothers and babies to stay together:** Crenshaw, Jeannette. "Care Practice #6: No Separation of Mother and Baby, with Unlimited Opportunities for Breastfeeding." *Journal of Perinatal Education* 16, no. 3 (2007): 39–43. **On babies routinely separated from mothers:** Declercq, E.R., et al. "Listening to Mothers II." *Childbirth Connection* (Oct. 2006). **On the evidence behind clinical guidelines in obstetrics:** Block, Jennifer. *Pushed* (Da Capo Press, 2008); Wright, Jason, et al. "Scientific Evidence Underlying the American College of Obstetricians and Gynecologists' Practice Bulletins." *Obstetrics and Gynecology* 118, no. 3 (Sept. 2011): 505–512. **The newspaper story about Michelle Niska:** Kaner, Elyse. "Mother, Teacher, Daughter Saved by 'Invisible' Angels." *Anoka County Union* (Sept. 26, 2007). **On the placenta:** Cunningham, F., et al. *Williams Obstetrics*, 23rd ed.

(McGraw-Hill, 2009). *On freedom of movement during labor:* Declercq, E.R., et al. "Listening to Mothers II" *Childbirth Connection* (Oct. 2006). *On the inherent mystery of reproduction:* Paglia, Camille. *Sexual Personae* (Vintage Books, 1991): 12. *On this history of the Caesarean:* Sewell, Jane. "Caesarean Section—A Brief History." *National Library of Medicine* (1993); Harris, Robert. "Cattle-horn Lacerations of the Abdomen and Uterus in Pregnant Women." *American Journal of Obstetrics and Diseases of Women and Children* 20, no. 7 (July 1887): 673–685. *On the safety of modern Cesareans:* "NIH State-of-the-Science Conference Statement on Cesarean Delivery on Maternal Request." National Institutes of Health Consensus and State-of-the-Science Statements 23, no. 1 (March 27, 2006): 1–29. *On Caesarean recovery time:* Declercq, E.R., et al. "Listening to Mothers II." *Childbirth Connection* (Oct. 2006). *On infections of the Caesarean wound:* Main, Elliott, et al. "Cesarean Deliveries, Outcomes, and Opportunities for Change in California." (California Maternal Quality Care Collaborative, 2011). *On adhesions:* Alpay, Zeynep, et al. "Postoperative Adhesions." Seminars in Reproductive Medicine 26, no. 4 (July 2008): 313–321; Berman, Jay M. "Intrauterine Adhesions." Seminars in Reproductive Medicine 26, no. 4 (July 2008): 349–355. *On Caesareans and the infant's health:* Tita, Alan, et al. "Timing of Elective Repeat Cesarean Delivery at Term and Neonatal Outcomes." *New England Journal of Medicine* 360, no. 2 (Jan. 8, 2009): 111–120; Sinha, Anjita, et al. "Myth: Babies Would Choose Prelabour Caesarean Section." Seminars in Fetal and Neonatal Medicine 16, no. 5 (Oct. 2011): 247–253; Kamath, Beena, et al. "Neonatal Outcomes after Elective Cesarean Delivery." *Obstetrics and Gynecology* 113, no. 6 (June 2009): 1231–1238; Villar, José, et al. "Maternal and Neonatal Individual Risks and Benefits Associated with Caesarean Delivery." *BMJ* (clinical research ed.) 335, no. 7628 (Nov. 17, 2007): 1025. *On Caesarean-scar ectopic pregnancy:* Sadeghi, Homayoun, et al. "Cesarean Scar Ectopic Pregnancy: Case Series and Review of the Literature." *American Journal of Perinatology* 27, no. 2 (Feb. 2010): 111–120. *On stillbirth after Caesareans:* Kennare, Robyn, et al. "Risks of Adverse Outcomes in the Next Birth after a First Cesarean Delivery." *Obstetrics and Gynecology* 109, no. 2 pt. 1 (Feb. 2007): 270–276; Gray, R., et al. "Caesarean Delivery and Risk of Stillbirth in Subsequent Pregnancy." *BJOG* 114, no. 3 (March 2007): 264–270. *On placenta accreta and related conditions:* Clark, S.L., et al. "Placenta Previa/accreta and Prior Cesarean Section." *Obstetrics and Gynecology* 66, no. 1 (July 1985): 89–92; Clark, Erin, and Robert Silver. "Long-term Maternal Morbidity Associated with Repeat Cesarean Delivery." *American Journal of Obstetrics and Gynecology* 205, no. 6 (Dec. 2011): S2–10; Wu, Serena, et al. "Abnormal Placentation: Twenty year Analysis." *American Journal of Obstetrics and Gynecology* 192, no. 5 (May 2005): 1458–1461. *On factors contributing to maternal mortality:* The California Pregnancy-Associated Mortality Review. "Report from 2002 and 2003 Maternal Death Reviews" (California Department of Public Health, Maternal Child and Adolescent Health Division, 2011). *On international comparisons of maternal heath:* Lozano, Rafael, et al. "Progress Towards Millennium Development Goals 4 and 5 on Maternal and Child Mortality." *Lancet* 378, no. 9797 (Sept. 24, 2011): 1139–1165. *On pelvic floor damage:* Albers, Leah, and Noelle

Borders. "Minimizing Genital Tract Trauma and Related Pain Following Spontaneous Vaginal Birth." *Journal of Midwifery and Women's Health* 52, no. 3 (June 2007): 246–253; Bosomworth, A., and J. Bettany-Saltikov. "Just Take a Deep Breath." *MIDIRS Midwifery Digest* 16, no. 2 (2006): 157–165; O'Boyle, Amy, et al. "Informed Consent and Birth." *American Journal of Obstetrics and Gynecology* 187, no. 4 (Oct. 2002): 981–983. **On Ignaz Semmelweis:** Semmelweis Society International. Dr. Semmelweis Biography. (Jan. 2009) http://semmelweis.org/about/dr-semmelweis-biography/. **On iatrogenesis in early 20th-century obstetrics:** "Achievements in Public Health, 1900–1999: Healthier Mothers and Babies." *MMWR: Morbidity and Mortality Weekly Report* 48 no. 38 (Oct. 1, 1999): 849–858. **On the evolution of pregnancy and birth:** Markow, T.A., et al. "Egg Size, Embryonic Development Time and Ovoviviparity in Drosophila Species." *Journal of Evolutionary Biology* 22, no. 2 (Feb. 2009): 430–434; Carter, A.M. "What Fossils Can Tell Us About the Evolution of Viviparity and Placentation." *Placenta* 29, no. 11 (Nov. 2008): 930–931. **On the spotted hyena:** Judson, Olivia. *Dr. Tatiana's Sex Advice to All Creation* (Metropolitan, 2003): 204–211. **On human birth, bipedalism, and feelings:** Lewin, Roger. *Human Evolution* (Blackwell Science, 1999): 93–98; Rosenberg, Karen, and Wenda Trevathan. "Bipedalism and Human Birth." *Evolutionary Anthropology* 4, no. 5 (1995): 161–168; Trevathan, Wenda. *Human Birth* (Transaction Publishers, 2011); Trevathan, Wenda, et al. *Evolutionary Medicine* (Oxford University Press, 1999). **On tall women and difficulty of labor:** This comes from the midwife Faith Gibson. **On the benefits of company during labor:** Hodnett, Ellen, et al. "Continuous Support for Women during Childbirth." Cochrane Database of Systematic Reviews, no. 2 (2011). **On oxytocin and nipple stroking:** Gaskin, Ina May. *Spiritual Midwifery*. 4th ed. (Book Publishing Company, 2002); American College of Obstetricians and Gynecologists. "Induction of Labor." ACOG practice bulletin; no. 107 (Aug. 2009). **On hyaline membrane disease:** Groopman, Jerome. "A Child in Time." *New Yorker* (Oct. 24, 2011). **On shoulder dystocia:** Baxley, Elizabeth, et al. "Shoulder Dystocia." *American Family Physician* 69, no. 7 (April 1, 2004): 1707–1714; Cunningham, F., et al. *Williams Obstetrics*, 23rd ed. (McGraw-Hill, 2009). **On birth statistics at the Farm, on the Navajo Nation, and at the Family Health and Birth Center:** Gaskin, Ina May. *Birth Matters* (Seven Stories Press, 2011); Grady, Denise. "Lessons at Indian Hospital about Births." *New York Times* (Mar. 6, 2010): A20; Ly, Phuong. "A Labor without End." *Washington Post Magazine* (May 27, 2002). **On Mary Breckinridge and the history of the Frontier Nursing Service:** Bartlett, Mary. *The Frontier Nursing Service* (McFarland, 2008); Breckinridge, Mary. *Wide Neighborhoods* (University Press of Kentucky, 1981). "[T]here would be a saving of 10,000 mothers" quoted in: Kalisch, P.A., and B.J. Kalisch. *The Advance of American Nursing*. (Little, Brown and Company, 1978): 388. **On the maternal mortality rates in the 1920s:** National Office of Vital Statistics. *Vital Statistics Rates in the United States, 1900–1940* (GPO, 1947). **On the difficulty of seeing the mother in obstetrical science:** Wendland, Claire L. "The Vanishing Mother." *Medical Anthropology Quarterly* 21, no. 2 (June 2007): 218–233. **On further Caesarean risks in later pregnancies:** Smith, Gordon, et al. "Caesarean Section and Risk of Unexplained Stillbirth in Subsequent

Pregnancy." *Lancet* 362, no. 9398 (Nov. 29, 2003): 1779–1784; Solheim, Karla, et al. "The Effect of Cesarean Delivery Rates on the Future Incidence of Placenta Previa, Placenta Accreta, and Maternal Mortality." *Journal of Maternal-Fetal and Neonatal Medicine* 24, no. 11 (Nov. 2011): 1341–1346. **On ultrasounds:** Abramowicz, J.S., et al. "[Obstetrical Ultrasound: Can the Fetus Hear the Wave and Feel the Heat?]" *Ultraschall in Der Medizin* (Stuttgart, Germany: 1980) 33, no. 3 (June 2012): 215–217; Bricker, L., et al. "Ultrasound Screening in Pregnancy." *Health Technology Assessment* 4, no. 16 (2000): i–vi, 1–193; Salomon, L., et al. "Practice Guidelines for Performance of the Routine Midtrimester Fetal Ultrasound Scan." *Ultrasound in Obstetrics and Gynecology* 37, no. 1 (2011): 116–126. **On Intermountain Health Care:** James, Brent, and Lucy Savitz. "How Intermountain Trimmed Health Care Costs through Robust Quality Improvement Efforts." *Health Affairs* 30, no. 6 (June 2011): 1185–1191. **On the risks and benefits of inducing labor:** Caughey, Aaron, et al. "Maternal and Neonatal Outcomes of Elective Induction of Labor." *Evidence Report/Technology Assessment*, no. 176 (March 2009); Johnson, Nathanael. "As Early Elective Births Increase So Do Health Risks for Mother, Child." *California Watch* (Dec. 26, 2010); Main, Elliott, et al. "Elimination of Non-medically Indicated (Elective) Deliveries before 39 Weeks Gestational Age" (March of Dimes, July 2010).

CHAPTER 2

Burkhard Bilger's story "Raw Faith" taught me that milk and microbes could yield compelling literary material. Stephanie Nani and Kari Way filled me in on sicknesses that arose in their households after drinking Organic Pastures milk. The journalist David Gumpert was a good reference when I went looking for stories about the milk wars and science about raw milk that defied conventional wisdom. I owe my education on Dannon's yogurt making to the good people at the Fort Worth processing plant, including J. Erskin, Duc Nguyen, and Michael Neuwirth. Conversations with David Relman at Stanford and Jeffrey Gordon at Washington University in St. Louis aided me in my research on gut microbes. **On Rolfing:** Rolf, Ida Pauline. *Rolfing: The Integration of Human Structures* (Dennis-Landman, 1977). **On the hygiene hypothesis and interspecies exchange:** Strachan, David. "Hay Fever, Hygiene, and Household Size." *BMJ* 299, no. 6710 (Nov. 18, 1989): 1259–1260; Sadeharju, K., et al. "Maternal Antibodies in Breast Milk Protect the Child from Enterovirus Infections." *Pediatrics.* 2007; 119(5):941–946. **On the evolving perspectives on IgA antibodies:** Dunn, Rob. *The Wild Life of Our Bodies* (Harper, 2011): 100–103. Dunn's book also addresses **the domestication of aurochs and beginnings of human dairying.** Anne Mendelson discusses this period as well in her lovely book *Milk* (Knopf, 2008). **On lactose intolerance, lactase persistence, and dairying:** Itan, Yuval, et al. "The Origins of Lactase Persistence in Europe." *PLoS Comput Biol* 5, no. 8 (2009): e1000491. **On Louis Pasteur:** Frankland, Percy, and Mrs. Percy Frankland. *Pasteur* (Macmillan, 1898); the story of Pasteur's deathbed confession first appears (in English at least) in *The Stress* *of Life* (McGraw-Hill, 1984) by Hans Selye, but Selye, writing 83 years after Pasteur's death, gives no citation. Curiously, some raw-milk advocates replace Bernard's name in this story with that of Antoine Béchamp—another scientist with ideas related to Bernard's—perhaps because there was more conflict between Pasteur and Béchamp. **On the milk wars:** Jones, Robert A. "Raw Milk: A Holy War over Health." *Los Angeles Times* (Aug. 31, 1984). **Evidence of an increase in autoimmune disorders:** Bach, Jean-François. "Infections and Autoimmune Diseases." *Journal of Autoimmunity* 25 Suppl (2005): 74–80; Bodansky, H.J., et al. "Evidence for an Environmental Effect in the Aetiology of Insulin Dependent Diabetes in a Transmigratory Population." *BMJ* 304, no. 6833 (April 18, 1992): 1020–1022; Conradi, Silja, et al. "Environmental Factors in Early Childhood Are Associated with Multiple Sclerosis." *BMC Neurology* 11 (2011): 123; Correale, Jorge, and Mauricio F. Farez. "The Impact of Environmental Infections (Parasites) on MS Activity." *Multiple Sclerosis* (Houndmills, Basingstoke, England) 17, no. 10 (Oct. 2011): 1162–1169; Cosnes, Jacques, et al. "Epidemiology and Natural History of Inflammatory Bowel Diseases." *Gastroenterology* 140, no. 6 (May 2011): 1785–1794; Gale, Edwin. "The Rise of Childhood Type 1 Diabetes in the 20th Century." *Diabetes* 51, no. 12 (Dec. 2002): 3353–3361; Holgate, Stephen. "The Epidemic of Asthma and Allergy." *Journal of the Royal Society of Medicine* 97, no. 3 (March 2004): 103–110; finally, this study is of interest because it suggests that those in white-collar professions have a greater risk of MS than those in the lower classes: Russell, W.R. "Multiple Sclerosis: Occupation and Social Group at Onset." *Lancet* 2, no. 7729 (Oct. 16, 1971): 832–834. **On the raw-milk raids:** The details of the raw-milk busts of 2005–2006 come from interviews with Richard Hebron, Carol Schmitmeyer, members of Gary Oakes's cow share, as well as press releases from the Ohio Department of Agriculture. And from Tullis, Matt. "ODA: Farmer Didn't Follow Law." *Daily Record* (March 17, 2006). The description of the raid on Michael Schmidt's farm comes from a video recorded by Schmidt and from reports by the agents. The history comes from Schmidt, and was confirmed by his ex-wife and several neighbors. **The estimates of raw-milk illnesses and raw-milk drinkers comes from** Langer, Adam, et al. "Nonpasteurized Dairy Products, Disease Outbreaks, and State laws-United States, 1993–2006." *Emerging Infectious Diseases* 18, no. 3 (March 2012): 385–391; *Foodborne Active Surveillance Network Population Survey Atlas of Exposures* (Centers for Disease Control and Prevention, 2006–2007). **On the Organic Pastures recall:** "Organic Pastures Raw Milk Recall Announced by CDFA." California Department of Food and Agriculture (Sept. 21, 2006); Arax, Mark. *West of the West* (PublicAffairs, 2009): 229–260; "Escherichia Coli 0157:H7 Infections in Children Associated with Raw Milk and Raw Colostrum from Cows-California, 2006." *Morbidity and Mortality Weekly Report* (June 13, 2008). **On the behavior of O157:H7 in contact with antibiotics:** Wong, C.S., et al. "The Risk of the Hemolytic-uremic Syndrome after Antibiotic Treatment of Escherichia Coli O157:H7 Infections." *New England Journal of Medicine* 342, no. 26 (June 29, 2000): 1930–1936. **On the date of the first pasteurization laws:** "Milestones of Milk." International Dairy Foods Association. http://www.idfa.org/

news—views/media-kits/milk/milestones/. *On the condition of dairies at the turn of the century:* Schmid, Ronald. *The Untold Story of Milk* (New Trends Pub., 2003). *The guidelines limiting bacteria in milk:* U.S. Dept. of Health and Human Services, Public Health Service and Food and Drug Administration. Grade "A" Pasteurized Milk Ordinance (2009 Revision). *On cows digesting grass and corn:* Pollan, Michael. *The Omnivore's Dilemma* (Penguin Press, 2007); Russell, J.B., and J.L. Rychlik. "Factors That Alter Rumen Microbial Ecology." *Science* 292, no. 5519 (May 11, 2001): 1119–1122. *On problems resulting from high-energy, low-fiber feeds in dairy cows:* Shaver, R.D. "Nutritional Risk Factors in the Etiology of Left Displaced Abomasum in Dairy Cows." *Journal of Dairy Science* 80, no. 10 (Oct. 1997): 2449–2453. *On the prevalence of pathogens on dairy farms:* USDA, Veterinary Services. "E. coli O157:H7 on U.S. Dairy Operations" (Centers for Epidemiology and Animal Health, Dec. 2003); USDA, Veterinary Services. "Salmonella and Campylobacter on U.S. Dairy Operations" (Centers for Epidemiology and Animal Health, Dec. 2003). *On the longevity of industrial dairy cows:* Norman, H.D., E. Hare. "Historical Examination of Culling of Dairy Cows from Herds in the United States." *Journal of Dairy Science* 88, no. 7 Suppl 1 (July 24, 2005): 122. *On the false-advertising lawsuit against Dannon:* Olivarez-Giles, Nathan. "Dannon Settles False Advertising Lawsuit over Activia, DanActive Yogurt." *Los Angeles Times* (Sept. 19, 2009). *On the reign of microbes:* Gould, Stephen Jay. *Full House: The Spread of Excellence from Plato to Darwin* (Harmony Books, 1996): 175–192. *On humans as superorganisms:* Gill, Steven, et al. "Metagenomic Analysis of the Human Distal Gut Microbiome." *Science* 312, no. 5778 (June 2, 2006): 1355–1359. Bruce German told me about *milk ecology.* Another interesting fact is that the milk-fat-globule membrane is essentially processed out of pasteurized dairy products. Both human and bovine mammary glands assemble this incredibly complex membrane for holding fat globules. There's no proof that the membrane is useful, but the mechanism that makes it is so elaborate that German suspects it must confer some kind of evolutionary advantage. *On development of epithelial cells in the crypts of Lieberkühn:* Savage, D.C., and D.D. Whitt. "Influence of the Indigenous Microbiota on Amounts of Protein, DNA, and Alkaline Phosphatase Activity Extractable from Epithelial Cells of the Small Intestines of Mice." *Infection and Immunity* 37, no. 2 (Aug. 1982): 539–549. *On the evolution of the hygiene hypothesis:* Hyde, Rob. "Erika Von Mutius: Reshaping the Landscape of Asthma Research." *Lancet* 372, no. 9643 (Sept. 20, 2008): 1029; Rook, G.A., and L.R. Brunet. "Microbes, Immunoregulation, and the Gut." *Gut* 54, no. 3 (March 2005): 317–320. *On farm children being less likely to develop asthma and allergies:* Perkin, M.R. "Unpasteurized Milk: Health or Hazard?" *Clinical and Experimental Allergy* 37, no. 5 (May 2007): 627–630. Von Mutius, E. "99th Dahlem Conference on Infection, Inflammation and Chronic Inflammatory Disorders." *Clinical and Experimental Immunology* 160, no. 1 (April 2010): 130–135; Perkin, Michael, and David Strachan. "Which Aspects of the Farming Lifestyle Explain the Inverse Association with Childhood Allergy?" *Journal of Allergy and Clinical Immunology* 117, no. 6 (June 2006): 1374–1381; Waser, M., et al. "Inverse

Association of Farm Milk Consumption with Asthma and Allergy in Rural and Sub-urban Populations Across Europe." *Clinical and Experimental Allergy* 37, no. 5 (May 2007): 661–670. **On O157:H7 dwindling in raw milk:** The science on O157:H7 spe-cifically shows that it can die off in milk, though it can also (less frequently) increase. Lactic acid bacteria may also prevent the *E. coli* from attaching or releasing poisons. Leblanc et al. "Induction of a Humoral Immune Response Following an Escherichia Coli O157:H7 Infection with an Immunomodulatory Peptidic Fraction Derived from Lactobacillus Helveticus-fermented Milk." *Clinical and Diagnostic Laboratory Immu-nology* 11, no. 6 (Nov. 2004): 1171–1181; de Sablet, Thibaut, et al. "Human Microbiota-secreted Factors Inhibit Shiga Toxin Synthesis by Enterohemorrhagic Escherichia Coli O157:H7." *Infection and Immunity* 77, no. 2 (Feb. 2009): 783–790. **On gaining immunity through milk consumption:** There are mountains of anecdotal evidence that people gain immunity to pathogens in raw milk. Nearly every industrial dairy farmer I've talked to drinks raw milk from his bulk tank on a regular basis. Blaser, M.J., et al. "The Influence of Immunity on Raw Milk." *JAMA* 257, no. 1 (Jan. 2, 1987): 43–46. **On the emergence of O157:H7:** Roan, Shari. "Battling an Elusive Bacterium." *Los Angeles Times* (July 11, 1990); Kolata, Gina. "Detective Work and Science Reveal a New Lethal Bacteria." *New York Times* (Jan. 6, 1998). There is some evidence that *feeding cattle grass reduces the number of pathogens:* Hutchison, M.L., et al. "Analy-ses of Livestock Production, Waste Storage, and Pathogen Levels and Prevalences in Farm Manures." *Applied and Environmental Microbiology* 71, no. 3 (March 2005): 1231–1236. But at least one large outbreak has been traced to a ranch where cattle were exclusively grass-fed: California Food Emergency Response Team. "Investiga-tion of an Escherichia coli O157:H7 outbreak associated with Dole pre-packaged spinach" (California Department of Health Services, FDA, 2007). It does seem that many forms of *E. coli*, including O157:H7, gain acid resistance when living in acidic rumens: Diez-Gonzalez, F., et al. "Grain Feeding and the Dissemination of Acid-resistant Escherichia Coli from Cattle." *Science* 281, no. 5383 (Sept. 11, 1998): 1666–1668. But **acid-resistant E. coli of the O157:H7 type can also be found in grass-fed cows:** Garber, L., et al. "Factors Associated with Fecal Shedding of Verotoxin-produc-ing Escherichia Coli O157 on Dairy Farms." *Journal of Food Protection* 62, no. 4 (April 1999): 307–312; Grauke, L.J., et al. "Acid Resistance of Escherichia Coli O157:H7 from the Gastrointestinal Tract of Cattle Fed Hay or Grain." *Veterinary Microbiology* 95, no. 3 (Sept. 1, 2003): 211–225; Van Baale, M.J., et al. "Effect of Forage or Grain Diets with or without Monensin on Ruminal Persistence and Fecal Esche-richia Coli O157:H7 in Cattle." *Applied and Environmental Microbiology* 70, no. 9 (Sept. 2004): 5336–5342. **On immunity to pathogenic E. coli in Brazil:** Palmeira, Patricia, et al. "Colostrum from Healthy Brazilian Women Inhibits Adhesion and Contains IgA Antibodies Reactive with Shiga Toxin-producing Escherichia Coli." *European Journal of Pediatrics* 164, no. 1 (Jan. 2005): 37–43; Palmeira et al. "Passive Immunity Acquisition of Maternal Anti-enterohemorrhagic Escherichia Coli O157:H7 IgG Antibodies by the Newborn." *European Journal of Pediatrics* 166, no. 5

(May 2007): 413–419; Zapata-Quintanilla, L.B., et al. "Systemic Antibody Response to Diarrheagenic Escherichia Coli and LPS O111, O157 and O55 in Healthy Brazilian Adults." *Scandinavian Journal of Immunology* 64, no. 6 (Dec. 2006): 661–667. *On the Los Angeles County Milk Commission:* Simon, Richard. "County Milk Board May Lose Authority." *Los Angeles Times* (Aug. 25, 1989). *On Paul Fleiss:* Hubler, Shawn. "Did Father Know Best? Paul Fleiss." *Los Angeles Times Magazine* (1995 April 9). *On the evidence that Alta Dena milk caused illness:* Linnan, M.J., et al. "Epidemic Listeriosis Associated with Mexican-style Cheese." *New England Journal of Medicine* 319, no. 13 (Sept. 29, 1988): 823–828; Werner, S.B., et al. "Association between Raw Milk and Human Salmonella Dublin Infection." *BMJ* 2, no. 6184 (July 28, 1979): 238–241; Puzo, Daniel. "Study Urges Warning Label on Raw Milk." *Los Angeles Times* (April 1, 1986).

CHAPTER 3

Several of Bruce German's colleagues and graduate students helped answer various questions, including David Mills, Carlito Lebrilla, Bruce Hammock, Xi Chen, Katie Hinde, Hyeyoung Lee, Sara Schaefer, and Jennifer Smilowitz. Barb Stuckey at Mattson told me about the lazy American palate. Information on the International Life Sciences Institute comes from interviews with Kelly Brownell at Yale, Geoffrey Cannon of the World Public Health and Nutrition Association, Carlos Camargo at Harvard, Michael Jacobson at the Center for Science in the Public Interest, Jennifer Sass at the National Resource Defense Council, Michele Simon of Eat Drink Politics, Amalia Waxman formerly at the World Health Organization, and Derek Yach then at Yale. *On the errors of nutrition science:* Taubes, Gary. *Good Calories, Bad Calories* (Anchor, 2008). *On the confusion over cholesterol:* Lehrer, Jonah. "Trials and Errors: Why Science Is Failing Us." *Wired* (Jan. 2012). *On sugar myths:* Anderson, C.A., et al. "Sucrose and Dental Caries." *Obesity Reviews: An Official Journal of the International Association for the Study of Obesity* 10 Suppl 1 (March 2009): 41–54; Hoover, D.W., and R. Milich. "Effects of Sugar Ingestion Expectancies on Mother-child Interactions." *Journal of Abnormal Child Psychology* 22, no. 4 (Aug. 1994): 501–515; Jeukendrup, Asker E., and Sophie C. Killer. "The Myths Surrounding Pre-exercise Carbohydrate Feeding." *Annals of Nutrition and Metabolism* 57 Suppl 2 (2010): 18–25; Newbrun, E. "Sugar and Dental Caries." *Science* 217, no. 4558 (July 30, 1982): 418–423; Painter, Kim. "Does a Spoonful of Sugar Help the Flu Take Hold?" *USA Today* (Oct. 5, 2009); Wolraich, M.L., et al. "The Effect of Sugar on Behavior or Cognition in Children." *JAMA* 274, no. 20 (Nov. 22, 1995): 1617–1621. *On recommendations to eat a diet low in protein, carbs, and fats (respectively):* Campbell, Colin, and Thomas Campbell. *The China Study* (BenBella Books, 2006); Ornish, Dean. *Eat More, Weigh Less* (HarperCollins, 2000); Taubes, Gary. *Why We Get Fat* (Random House, 2011). *On Kellogg:* Kellogg, John Harvey. *Colon Hygiene* (Good Health Publishing Company, 1915); Kellogg, John Harvey. *Plain Facts for Old and Young* (Segner & Condit, 1881): 382. *On Liebig and the pattern of nutritional presumption:* Pollan, Michael. *In Defense of Food* (Penguin Press, 2008); McGee, Harold.

On Food and Cooking (Simon & Schuster, 2004). **On the rise in obesity and diabetes:** Narayan, K., et al. "Lifetime Risk for Diabetes Mellitus in the United States." *JAMA* 290, no. 14 (Oct. 8, 2003): 1884–1890; Olshansky, S., et al. "A Potential Decline in Life Expectancy in the United States in the 21st Century." *New England Journal of Medicine* 352, no. 11 (March 17, 2005): 1138–1145. **On the insights provided by milk science:** German, Bruce, et al. "Metabolomics: Building on a Century of Biochemistry to Guide Human Health." *Metabolomics* 1, no. 1 (March 2005): 3–9; Ahmed, A., et al. "Effect of Milk Constituents on Hepatic Cholesterol-genesis." *Atherosclerosis* 32, no. 4 (April 1979): 347–357. **On breast milk variation for male and female infants:** Katherine Hinde quoted in: Williams, Florence. *Breasts* (W. W. Norton, 2012): 190–191. **On infant flavor preferences:** Forestell, Catherine, and Julie Mennella. "Early Determinants of Fruit and Vegetable Acceptance." *Pediatrics* 120, no. 6 (Dec. 2007): 1247–1254; Forestell, Catherine, Julie Mennella. "Food, Folklore, and Flavor Preference Development," in *Handbook of Nutrition and Pregnancy*, edited by Carol Lammi-Keefe (Humana Press, 2008). **On sugarphobia:** Dufty, William. *Sugar Blues* (Warner Books, 1976); Haley, S., et al. "Sweetener Consumption in the United States." *ERS: Outlook Report Series* (2005); Putnam, Judith, and Steven Haley. "Indicators: Behind the Data." *Economic Research Service: Amber Waves* (2003). **On Richard Lustig:** Lustig, Richard. "Sugar: The Bitter Truth." Speech presented at UC San Francisco's Mini Medical School for the Public (2009). http://uctv.tv/shows/Sugar-The-Bitter-Truth-16717; Taubes, Gary. "Is Sugar Toxic?" *New York Times Magazine* (April 13, 2011). **On the sociological power of sugar see:** Mintz, Sidney. *Sweetness and Power* (Penguin Press, 1986). **On ILSI:** McGarity, Thomas, and Wendy Wagner. *Bending Science* (Harvard University Press, 2010); Powys, Betsan. "The Trouble with Sugar." *Panorama*, BBC One. Transcript (2004); "The Tobacco Industry and Scientific Groups, ILSI." Tobacco Free Initiative, World Health Organization (2001), www.who.int/tobacco/media/en/ILSI.pdf; Yach, Derek, and Stella Bialous. "Junking Science to Promote Tobacco." *American Journal of Public Health* 91, no. 11 (Nov. 2001): 1745–1748; **On Alfy Fanjul:** Brenner, Marie. "In the Kingdom of Big Sugar." *Vanity Fair* (Feb. 2001). **On the etymology of sweet:** Tietz, Joan Ann. *A Thousand Years of Sweet* (Peter Lang, 2001). **On wanting versus liking:** Berridge, Kent, et al. "Taste Reactivity Analysis of 6-hydroxydopamine-induced Aphagia: Implications for Arousal and Anhedonia Hypotheses of Dopamine Function." *Behavioral Neuroscience* 103, no. 1 (Feb. 1989): 36–45; "Pleasures of the Brain." *Brain and Cognition* 52, no. 1 (June 2003): 106–128; Heath, R.G. "Pleasure and Brain Activity in Man." *Journal of Nervous and Mental Disease* 154, no. 1 (Jan. 1972): 3–18; Kessler, David. *The End of Overeating* (Rodale, 2009). Rada, P., et al. "Daily Bingeing on Sugar Repeatedly Releases Dopamine in the Accumbens Shell." *Neuroscience* 134, no. 3 (2005): 737–744. **On the links between work, consumption, and dopamine:** Sapolsky, Robert. "Are Humans Just Another Primate?" Speech presented at the California Academy of Sciences (2011). Available online at fora.tv. **On the taste of nations:** Fisher, M.F.K. *Serve It Forth* (North Point Press, 2002). Julie Mennella introduced me to the Lin Yutang's epigram on patriotism and taste.

CHAPTER 4

This chapter relied on numerous interviews with Peter Spencer, who is engaged in the utterly serious business of finding ways to understand neurodegeneration; nonetheless, he generously indulged my somewhat fanciful interest in his work. *On the way various cultures deal with the problem of ignorance:* Nader, Laura, ed. *Naked Science* (Routledge, 1996). *On the number and regulation of new chemicals introduced to the market:* Williams, Florence. *Breasts* (W. W. Norton, 2012): 98. *On acting without certainty:* Berry, Wendell. *Life Is a Miracle.* (Counterpoint, 2001). *On vaccine making being something like the witch's brew in Macbeth:* Warren, Joel. "Industrial Production of Primary Tissue Cultures," in *Cell Cultures for Virus Vaccine Production,* NCI Monograph 29 (1968): 35–43. *On parents who refuse or delay shots:* Smith, Philip, et al. "Parental Delay or Refusal of Vaccine Doses, Childhood Vaccination Coverage at 24 Months of Age, and the Health Belief Model." *Public Health Reports* 126, Suppl 2 (2011): 135–146; "The 2009 National Immunization Survey." U.S. Dept. of Health and Human Services, National Center for Health Statistics (Centers for Disease Control and Prevention, 2010). *On toxins in edible plants:* "Cruciferous Plants: Phytochemical Toxicity Versus Cancer Chemoprotection." *Mini Reviews in Medicinal Chemistry* 9, no. 13 (Nov. 1, 2009): 1470–1478; Beier, R.C. "Natural Pesticides and Bioactive Components in Foods." *Reviews of Environmental Contamination and Toxicology* 113 (1990): 47–137; Chai, Weiwen, and Michael Liebman. "Effect of Different Cooking Methods on Vegetable Oxalate Content." *Journal of Agricultural and Food Chemistry* 53, no. 8 (April 20, 2005): 3027–3030; Champ, Martine. "Non-nutrient Bioactive Substances of Pulses." *British Journal of Nutrition* 88 Suppl 3 (Dec. 2002): s307–319; Giannetti, B., et al. "Efficacy and Safety of Comfrey Root Extract Ointment in the Treatment of Acute Upper or Lower Back Pain." *British Journal of Sports Medicine* 44, no. 9 (July 2010): 637–641. *On the Guam disease:* Goldwyn, Edward. "The poison that waits?" BBC, Horizon (1988); Sacks, Oliver. *The Island of the Colorblind and Cycad Island* (Knopf, 1997); Spencer, Peter. "Are Neurotoxins Driving Us Crazy? Planetary Observations on the Causes of Neurodegenerative Diseases of Old Age," in *Behavioral Measures of Neurotoxicity,* eds. Russell, Flattau, and Pope (National Academies Press, 1990); Whiting, Marjorie. *Toxicity of Cycads.* Third World Medical Research Foundation and Lyon Arboretum (University of Hawaii, 1988); The Marjorie Grant Whiting Papers at the University of Hawaii at Manoa. *On the implications of the Guam evidence:* Cucchiaroni, Maria, et al. "Metabotropic Glutamate Receptor 1 Mediates the Electrophysiological and Toxic Actions of the Cycad Derivative beta-N-Methylamino-L-alanine on Substantia Nigra Pars Compacta DA-ergic Neurons." *Journal of Neuroscience* 30, no. 15 (April 14, 2010): 5176–5188; Galasko, D., et al. "Prevalence of Dementia in Chamorros on Guam." *Neurology* 68, no. 21 (May 22, 2007): 1772–1781; Pablo, J., et al. "Cyanobacterial Neurotoxin BMAA in ALS and Alzheimer's Disease." *Acta Neurologica Scandinavica* 120, no. 4 (Oct. 2009): 216–225; Steele, John C., and Patrick L. McGeer. "The ALS/PDC Syndrome of Guam and the Cycad Hypothesis." *Neurology* 70, no. 21 (May 20, 2008): 1984–1990.

Evidence of toxins in blue-green algae nutritional supplements: Dietrich, Fischer, et al. "Toxin mixture in cyanobacterial blooms," in *Cyanobacterial Harmful Algal Blooms*, edited by Hudnell and Dortch, *Advances in Experimental Medicine and Biology*, 619 (Springer, 2008): 885–912; Draisci, R., et al. "Identification of Anatoxins in Blue-green Algae Food Supplements Using Liquid Chromatography-tandem Mass Spectrometry." *Food Additives and Contaminants* 18, no. 6 (June 2001): 525–531.*On Australian cycad preparation:* Beck, Wendy, et al. "Archaeology from Ethnography: the Aboriginal Use of Cycads," in *Archaeology with Ethnography*, edited by Meehan and Jones (Australian National University, 1988); Beck. "Aboriginal Preparation of Cycas Seeds in Australia." *Economic Botany* 46, no. 2 (1992): 133–147. *On dreams and visions advancing science:* Abumrad, Jad. "Yellow Fluff and Other Curious Encounters." *Radiolab*, season 5, episode 5; Roberts, Royston M. *Serendipity* (Wiley, 1989): 123–125; Valenstein, Elliot. *The War of the Soups and the Sparks* (Columbia University Press, 2005): 57–59; Broad, William. "For Delphic Oracle, Fumes and Visions." *New York Times* (March 19, 2002); Watson, P.L., et al. "The Ethnopharmacology of Pituri." *Journal of Ethnopharmacology* 8, no. 3 (Sept. 1983): 303–311. *On evolution and cooking:* Wrangham, Richard. *Catching Fire* (Basic Books, 2010). The fact about chimps preferring cooked food also comes from page 90: "Evolutionary anthropologists Victoria Wobber and Brian Hare tested chimpanzees and other apes in the United States, Germany, and Tchimpounga, a Congolese sanctuary. Across the different locations, despite different diets and living conditions, the apes responded similarly. No apes preferred any raw food." *On the muscle-bound cranium hypothesis:* McCollum, Melanie, et al. "Of Muscle-bound Crania and Human Brain Evolution." *Journal of Human Evolution* 50, no. 2 (Feb. 2006): 232–236; Perry, George, et al. "Comparative Analyses Reveal a Complex History of Molecular Evolution for Human MYH16." *Molecular Biology and Evolution* 22, no. 3 (March 2005): 379–382. *On natural endocrine disruptors:* Henley, Derek, et al. "Prepubertal Gynecomastia Linked to Lavender and Tea Tree Oils." *New England Journal of Medicine* 356, no. 5 (Feb. 1, 2007): 479–485. *On evidence against vaccines:* Kirby, David. *Evidence of Harm: Mercury in Vaccines and the Autism Epidemic: A Medical Controversy* (St. Martin's Griffin, 2006). *On Edward Jenner:* Allen, Arthur. *Vaccine* (W. W. Norton, 2007): 46–50. *On polio incidence 1952–1993:* "Polio Vaccine and Immunization Information." The National Network for Immunization Information. http://www.immunizationinfo.org /vaccines/polio. *On the vaccine controversy circa 2005:* Kennedy, Robert F., Jr. "Deadly Immunity." *Rolling Stone* (July 14, 2005); Murch, Simon, et al. "Retraction of an Interpretation." *Lancet* 363, no. 9411 (March 6, 2004): 750; Wakefield, Andrew, et al. "Ileal-lymphoid-nodular Hyperplasia, Non-specific Colitis, and Pervasive Developmental Disorder in Children." *Lancet* 351, no. 9103 (Feb. 28, 1998): 637–641; Mnookin, Seth. *The Panic Virus* (Simon & Schuster, 2011). *On swine flu deaths:* Brown, David. "CDC Reports 28 Swine Flu Deaths among pregnant Women." *Washington Post* (Oct. 2, 2009). *On weighing risks:* Cooper, Mary Ann. "Medical Aspects of Lightning." National Weather Service Lightning Safety, n.d. http://www.lightningsafety.noaa.gov/medical. htm; Demicheli, V., et al. "Vaccines for Measles, Mumps and Rubella in Children."

Cochrane Database of Systematic Reviews, no. 4 (2005); Institute of Medicine. *Adverse Effects of Vaccines*, edited by Ford, Stratton, and Rusch (National Academies Press, 2012); "Some Common Misconceptions." www.cdc.gov (Feb. 18, 2011) http://www.cdc.gov/vaccines/vac-gen/6mishome.htm#risk; "VAERS Data." Vaccine Adverse Event Reporting System (July 13, 2012) http://vaers.hhs.gov/data/index. **On the comparison to homicides:** "Ten Leading Causes of Death and Injury." Centers for Disease Control and Prevention (2007) http://www.cdc.gov/injury/wisqars/LeadingCauses.html. These data show that there were 290 homicide victims under one year of age in 2007, or a little more than five per week. Infants generally have five rounds of immunizations in the first year, which means that there are 10 weeks during which coincidental deaths could occur, and—on average—during which 56 infant homicides would occur. I compared that to the 59 infant deaths per year reported to VAERS. **On parental concern about vaccination:** Kennedy, Allison, et al. "Confidence about Vaccines in the United States." *Health Affairs* 30, no. 6 (June 2011): 1151–1159. **On pertussis:** Cherry, James. "Historical Perspective on Pertussis and Use of Vaccines to Prevent It." *Microbe Magazine* (March 2007); Thompson, Lea. "Vaccine Roulette." (WRC-TV, 1982); Tsouderos, Trine. "Whooping Cough: Why Is Pertussis Making a Comeback?" *Chicago Tribune* (Jan. 6, 2012). **On the fraud behind the autism hypothesis:** Allen, Arthur. *Vaccine* (W. W. Norton, 2007); Deer, Brian. "How the Case against the MMR Vaccine Was Fixed." *BMJ* 342 (2011): c5347; Deer, Brian. "Secrets of the MMR Scare." *BMJ* 342 (2011): c5258; "Retraction—Ileal-lymphoid-nodular Hyperplasia, Non-specific Colitis, and Pervasive Developmental Disorder in Children." *Lancet* 375, no. 9713 (Feb. 6, 2010): 445; Verstraeten, Tom. "Scientific Review of Vaccine Safety Datalink Information," transcript (Norcross, Georgia, June 7–8, 2000). **On the history of immunization scandals:** Allen, Arthur. *Vaccine* (W. W. Norton, 2007) (injuries and missteps: 70–111, typhus: 141, Cutter: 196–205); Willrich, Michael. *Pox: An American History* (Penguin Press, 2011); Willrich, Michael. "Why Parents Fear the Needle." *New York Times* (Jan. 20, 2011). **On hepatitis and chicken pox vaccines for babies:** Allen, Arthur. *Vaccine* (W. W. Norton, 2007): 294–326. **On Bob Sears:** Sears, Robert. *The Vaccine Book: Making the Right Decision for Your Child* (Little, Brown and Company, 2011); Offit, Paul, and Charlotte Moser. "The Problem with Dr. Bob's Alternative Vaccine Schedule." *Pediatrics* 123, no. 1 (Jan. 2009): e164–169. **On vaccines and the immune system:** Hviid, Anders, and Mads Melbye. "Measles-mumps-rubella Vaccination and Asthma-like Disease in Early Childhood." *American Journal of Epidemiology* 168, no. 11 (Dec. 1, 2008): 1277–1283; Orbach, Hedi, et al. "Vaccines and Autoimmune Diseases of the Adult." *Discovery Medicine* 9, no. 45 (Feb. 2010): 90–97; Rook, Graham. "Review Series on Helminths, Immune Modulation and the Hygiene Hypothesis." *Immunology* 126, no. 1 (Jan. 2009): 3–11; Schmitz, Roma, et al. "Vaccination Status and Health in Children and Adolescents: Findings of the German Health Interview and Examination Survey for Children and Adolescents (KiGGS)." *Deutsches Ärzteblatt International* 108, no. 7 (Feb. 2011): 99–104. **On polio's rise:** Smallman-Raynor, Matthew, and A. Cliff. *Poliomyelitis* (Oxford University Press, 2006). **On ancient inoculation:** Hopkins, Donald. *The Greatest Killer* (University of Chicago Press,

2002): 140; Needham, Joseph. *Science and Civilisation in China, Vol. 6, Biology and Biological Technology* (Cambridge University Press, 2000): 155.

CHAPTER 5

The jumping-off point for this chapter was Michael Pollan's *Second Nature* (Delta, 1993), and discussions with him that started in his class in journalism school and continued after my graduation. Diligent readers will find his fingerprints all over the book, but especially in this chapter. I profited from conversations with various Nevada County naturalists, including Ralph Cutter, Ted Beedy, Bob Erickson, and Liese Greensfelder. I owe a great deal of my understanding of forestry to people who work with trees. Ann Camp, at the Yale School of Forestry; Charles Brown, forester with Fruit Growers Supply Company; Wade Mosby, with Collins Company; Irv Penner, with the Ecoforestry Institute; and Richard Waring, emeritus at the Oregon State College of Forestry; all answered questions about the business and science of growing trees. Michael Barbour, professor emeritus at the University of California at Davis, told me about "backwards" succession in Alaska, and the decline of songbird diversity in some mature forests. **On environmental thinking:** Berry, Wendell. *The Unsettling of America* (Sierra Club Books, 1996); Botkin, Daniel. *Discordant Harmonies* (Oxford University Press, 1990); Budiansky, Stephen. *Nature's Keepers* (The Free Press, 1995); Emerson, Ralph Waldo. *The Essential Writings of Ralph Waldo Emerson*, edited by Brooks Atkinson (Modern Library, 2000); Kennedy, Roger. *Wildfire and Americans* (University of Nebraska Press, 2008); Latour, Bruno. *Politics of Nature*, translated by Catherine Porter (Harvard University Press, 2004); McKibben, Bill. *The End of Nature* (Random House, 2006); Nash, Roderick. *The Rights of Nature* (University of Wisconsin Press, 1989); Thoreau, Henry David. *Walden* (Project Gutenberg, 1995); Wilshire, Howard, Jane Nielson, and Rick Hazlett. *The American West at Risk* (Oxford University Press, 2008); Worster, Donald. *Nature's Economy* (Random House, 1982). **On humanity going bad with agriculture:** Manning, Richard. *Against the Grain* (North Point Press, 2005); Quinn, Daniel. *Ishmael* (Bantam, 1995). **On the San Francisco Bay:** Rubissow, Okamoto Ariel, and Kathleen Wong. *Natural History of San Francisco Bay* (University of California Press, 2011); Smith, Rich, and Bruce Jaffe. "San Francisco Bay Bathymetry." *US Geological Survey* (Dec. 13, 2007). http://sfbay.wr.usgs.gov/sediment/sfbay/index.html. **On the history of the land around Nevada City:** Bancroft, Hubert Howe. *The Works of Hubert Howe Bancroft*, vol. 23 (A.L. Bancroft & Company, 1888): 470. Hittell, Theodore Henry. *History of California*, vol. 3 (N.J. Stone, 1898). Holliday, J.S. *Rush for Riches* (University of California Press, 1999). Hittell, John. *Hittel on Gold Mines and Mining* (Desbarats, 1864). **On ecological succession and climax:** Nebel, Bernard, and Richard Wright. *Environmental Science* (Prentice Hall, 1993). **On the Yuba River watershed:** Boyd, Bruce, and Liese Greensfelder. *The Nature of This Place* (Comstock Bonanza Press, 2010). **On Forest Service costs and profits:** "Overview of Fiscal Year 2010 Budget Justification" (USDA Forest Service, 2009). Prestemon et al. "Forest Service Suppression Cost

Forecasts and Simulation Forecast for FY 2010" (USDA, Forest Service, 2009); Voss, R. "Taxpayer Losses from Logging Our National Forests." The John Muir Project (Earth Island Institute, 2005). *On early human management of forests:* Bonnicksen, Thomas. *America's Ancient Forests* (Wiley, 2000); Bowman, David, et al. "The Human Dimension of Fire Regimes on Earth." *Journal of Biogeography* 38, no. 12 (2011): 2223–2236; Mann, Charles. *1491* (Vintage Books, 2006); Platt, Rutherford, et al. "Are Wildfire Mitigation and Restoration of Historic Forest Structure Compatible?" *Annals of the Association of American Geographers* 96, no. 3 (2006): 455–470. *On Thomas Derham and Aristotle:* Botkin, Daniel. *Discordant Harmonies* (Oxford University Press, 1990) 81–84. *On William Libby:* Libby, William. "Local and Global Considerations of Sustainability." A conversation about the forest—a lecture recorded on video by the Yuba Watershed Institute (Nevada City, California: Jan. 26, 2002). *On historical perceptions of forests:* Mayr, Ernst. *The Growth of Biological Thought* (Harvard University Press, 1982): 330; Thomas, Keith. *Man and the Natural World* (Penguin Press, 1983): 203, 213. *On the value of water and timber from the Yuba River watershed:* Steward, William. "Sierra Nevada Ecosystem Project: Final Report to Congress, vol. III, Assessments and scientific basis for management options" (University of California, Centers for Water and Wildland Resources, 1996); "Timber Yield Tax and Harvest Values Schedules." California State Board of Equalization, California Timber Harvest by County 1994–2009. http://www.boe.ca.gov/proptaxes/timbertax.htm. Sixty-six million dollars is a very conservative estimate for power, based on a rate of 2.5 cents per kilowatt-hour. In 2010 timber receipts from Nevada, Sierra, and Yuba counties were less than $20 million. In 1994, when timber prices peaked, receipts from those three counties were $43 million. This is an overestimate because significant timber areas in these counties lie in the Truckee River and Feather River watersheds. *On the history of Prussian forestry:* Lowood, Henry. "The Calculating Forester" in *The Quantifying Spirit in the 18th Century,* edited by Frängsmyr and Heilbron (University of California Press, 1990): 332, 334; Maser, Chris. *The Redesigned Forest* (Miles & Miles, 1988): 70–82. Scott, James. *Seeing like a State* (Yale University Press, 1999): 11–52. *On Biosphere 2:* Cohen, J.E., and D. Tilman. "Biosphere 2 and Biodiversity: The Lessons So Far." *Science* 274, no. 5290 (Nov. 15, 1996): 1150–1151; Mitsch, William. "Editorial in Biosphere 2," edited by Marino and Odum. *Ecological Engineering* 13, no. 1 (Elsevier Science, 1999); Poynter, Jane. *The Human Experiment* (Thunder's Mouth Press, 2006): 191; Reider, Rebecca. *Dreaming the Biosphere* (University of New Mexico Press, 2009). *The tragedy of the commons:* Hardin, Garrett. "The Tragedy of the Commons." *Science* 162, no. 5364 (Dec. 13, 1968): 1243–1248. *On the arguments for protecting diversity:* May, Robert. "The future of biological diversity in a crowded world." *Current Science* 82, no. 11 (2002): 1325–1331. *The statement that all humus is unique* is from soil scientist James Rice, quoted in: Logan, William Bryant. *Dirt* (W. W. Norton, 2007). *On alternatives to the tragedy of the commons:* Ostrom, Elinor. *Governing the Commons* (Cambridge University Press, 1990). *On the 'Inimim Forest:* "'Inimim Forest Management Plan," Yuba Watershed Institute, Timber Framer's Guild of North America, and the Bureau of Land

Management (1996). *On commons and community:* Snyder, Gary. *Practice of the Wild* (North Point Press, 1990). *On San Francisco's carbon reductions:* Cote, John. "Green Efforts Best in the Country, but Not Good Enough." *San Francisco Chronicle*, City Insider (Oct. 19, 2011).

CHAPTER 6

This chapter was informed by conversations with Ron Bates, professor of swine genetics at Michigan State; Steve Bjerklie, editor of *Meat Processing Magazine*; Don Butler at Murphy Brown LLC, Smithfield Foods; Al Christian at Iowa State; Andrew Coates at the Pig Improvement Company; the aptly named Cindy Cunningham at the National Pork Board; Bruce Friedrich at PETA; Marlene Halverson of the Animal Welfare Institute; Dan Hamilton at Genetiporc; Mary Hendrickson, extension assistant professor of rural sociology at the University of Missouri; Jen Holtkamp at the Iowa Pork Producers Association; John Ikerd, professor emeritus at the University of Missouri–Columbia; John Mabry, professor at Iowa State; Pramod Mathur at the Canadian Centre for Swine Improvement; Brian Mauldwin at Circle 4 Farms; Larry Rasch at Hormel Food Corp.; dairy farmer Randy Robinson; and hog farmer Chuck Wirtz. Tara Smith at Iowa State briefed me on antibiotics. I'm thankful for the help of Timbri Hurst and Melissa Price in the Cassia County offices. *I referred to the following books for background:* Schell, Orville. *Modern Meat* (Vintage Books, 1985); Scully, Matthew. *Dominion* (St. Martin's Griffin, 2003); Sinclair, Upton. *The Jungle* (Penguin Classics, 1985); Singer, Peter. *Animal Liberation* (Ecco Press, 2001). *On meth in rural America:* Reding, Nick. *Methland: The Death and Life of an American Small Town* (Bloomsbury, 2009). *On the rise of artificial insemination:* Foote, R. "The History of Artificial Insemination" (American Society of Animal Science, 2002); Schneider, J.F. "Evolution of Breeding Companies as Seedstock Suppliers in the USA" (National Swine Improvement Federation Conference, 2004); "Swine Mating Practices," APHIS Infosheet. Veterinary Services (Centers for Epidemiology and Animal Health, Sept. 2002). *On uniformity during slaughter:* Hennessy, David. "Slaughterhouse Rules." Center for Agricultural and Rural Development, Iowa State University, (2003). *On biosecurity:* "Biosecurity and Health Management on U.S. Swine Operations." APHIS Infosheet. Veterinary Services. (Centers for Epidemiology and Animal Health, 2003); Horwitz, Richard. *Hog Ties* (St. Martin's Press, 1998): 81. *On subtherapeutic antibiotics:* A large portion of the antibiotics given to animals are ionophores, which are generally not used in human medicine because they are hard on the heart. Still, a huge amount of conventional human antibiotics are utilized in agriculture. Hanson, B.M., et al. "Prevalence of Staphylococcus Aureus and Methicillin-resistant Staphylococcus Aureus (MRSA) on Retail Meat in Iowa." *Journal of Infection and Public Health* 4, no. 4 (Sept. 2011): 169–174; Waters, Andrew, et al. "Multidrug-Resistant Staphylococcus Aureus in US Meat and Poultry." *Clinical Infectious Diseases* (April 15, 2011). *On Henry Ford and the disassembly line:* Encyclopædia Britannica Online, s.v. "History of the Organization of

Work," accessed Oct. 2008, http://www.britannica.com/EBchecked/topic/648000/history-of-work-organization. *On manure pit gases:* "Treat Foaming Manure Pits Carefully to Avoid Explosions." Penton Media (Dec. 14, 2009); "Avoid Manure Pit Explosions." Penton Media (Nov. 9, 2009). *On Circle 4 Farms:* Dalrymple, Jim. "Let's Put Livestock Manure Production in Its Proper Perspective." *Better Pork* (June 2003) http://www.betterfarming.com/bp/jj03_stor3.htm; Israelson, Brent. "Circle Four Workers Quit, Decry 'Inhumane' Conditions in Utah Hog Production Factory." *Salt Lake Tribune* (Jan. 23, 2003). *On the decline of small hog farms:* Benjamin, Gary. "Industrialization in Hog Production." *Economic Perspectives*, 21 no. 1 (Jan. 1997): 2–13; McBride, William, and Nigel Key. *Economic and Structural Relationships in U.S. Hog Production* (Economic Research Service, Feb. 2003). *On show pigs:* "Lean Value Sires 2003 Sire Directory." The Syndicate-Lean Value Sires; Mabry, John. "Evolution of the Independent Purebred Seedstock Industry in the USA" (National Swine Improvement Federation Conference 2004). *On how to "be the boar":* Pig Improvement Corporation. "6 Habits of Highly Effective Inseminators" (instructional booklet). *On Smithfield Foods and the rise of the megafarm:* Agricultural Statistics, 2004, Chapter VII. USDA; "Annual Report Pursuant to Section 13 or 15(D) of the Securities Exchange Act." Smithfield Foods (2011); "History of Smithfield Foods." Understanding Smithfield. http://www.smithfieldfoods.com/Understand/History/; "Hogs: Number of Operations by Year, 1979-2004." US National Agricultural Statistics Service (USDA, 2006); Barboza, David. "Goliath of the Hog World," *New York Times* (April 7, 2000); Miller, Dale. "Straight Talk from Smithfield's Joe Luter." *National Hog Farmer* (May 1, 2000). *On Tylan:* "Minimizing Attrition." Elanco Animal Health. Advertising package (2004). *On improvements in swine genetics:* Numbers come from the Canadian Centre for Swine Improvement. *On pale, soft, exudative pork and stressed pigs:* Christian, Lauren. "Clarifying the Impact of the Stress Gene." *National Hog Farmer* (June 1995); Martinez, Steve, and Kelly Zering. "Pork Quality and the Role of Market Organization." *Economic Research Service* (Nov. 2004): 6–12; Prusa, Ken, and Chris Felder. "A New Definition of Pork Quality." National Swine Improvement Federation Conference (2004). *On nervous, bored, and neurotic pigs:* Grandin, Temple. "Environmental Enrichment for Confinement Pigs" (1988). http://www.grandin.com/references/LCIhand.html; "The Welfare of Intensively Kept Pigs." European Union. Report of the Scientific Veterinary Committee (Sept. 30, 1997); *On sow health:* Stalder, Ken, et al. "Genetic Factors Impacting Sow Longevity." National Swine Improvement Federation Conference (2004); McGlone, John, et al. "Review: Compilation of the Scientific Literature Comparing Housing Systems for Gestating Sows and Gilts Using Measures of Physiology, Behavior, Performance, and Health." *The Professional Animal Scientist* 20, no. 2 (April 1, 2004): 105–117. *On the spread of violence from animals to humans:* Ascione, Frank. *The International Handbook of Animal Abuse and Cruelty* (Purdue University Press, 2010); Barnes, Jaclyn, et al. "Ownership of High-risk ('Vicious') Dogs as a Marker for Deviant Behaviors: Implications for Risk Assessment." *Journal of Interpersonal Violence* 21, no. 12 (Dec. 2006): 1616–1634.

CHAPTER 7

Ann Jackson of the Oregon Hospice Association spoke with me about end of life issues. Laurence Guttmacher at the University of Rochester Medical Center told me about his stepfather, Leon Eisenberg, who, it was clear, he loved deeply. The psychiatrist and educator Carola Eisenberg also told me stories that helped give flesh to my sketch of her late husband. The doctor Jennifer Wilson suggested pheochromocytoma as a good example of a physical problem that looks like a cultural problem. *The following books were useful as background:* Dubos, Rene. *Mirage of Health* (Rutgers University Press, 1987); Fadiman, Anne. *The Spirit Catches You and You Fall Down* (Farrar, Straus and Giroux, 1998); Martensen, Robert. *A Life Worth Living* (Farrar, Straus and Giroux, 2009). *On the harm and costs of overtreatment:* Brownlee, Shannon. *Overtreated* (Bloomsbury, 2008); Fox, Maggie. "Healthcare System Wastes up to $800 Billion a Year." *Reuters* (Oct. 26, 2009); Lazarou, J., et al. "Incidence of Adverse Drug Reactions in Hospitalized Patients: A Meta-analysis of Prospective Studies." *JAMA* 279, no. 15 (April 15, 1998): 1200–1205. *On the number of deaths caused by lack of health insurance:* Committee on the Consequences of Uninsurance. "Care without Coverage: Too Little, Too Late" (National Academies Press, 2002). *On Fosomax and antiviral therapy:* Chopra, Sanjiv. "Overview of the Management of Chronic Hepatitis C Virus Infection." *UpToDate* (Nov. 9, 2011); "Fractures in Postmenopausal Women." Cochrane Database of Systematic Reviews, no. 1 (2008); Spiegel, Alix. "How a Bone Disease Grew to Fit the Prescription." NPR (Dec. 21, 2009). *On earthing:* Chevalier, Gaétan, et al. "Earthing: Health Implications of Reconnecting the Human Body to the Earth's Surface Electrons." *Journal of Environmental and Public Health* (2012): 291541; Ghaly, Maurice, and Dale Teplitz. "The Biologic Effects of Grounding the Human Body During Sleep as Measured by Cortisol Levels and Subjective Reporting of Sleep, Pain, and Stress." *Journal of Alternative and Complementary Medicine* 10, no. 5 (Oct. 2004): 767–776. *On the placebo effect:* Abumrad, Jad. "Placebo." *Radiolab*, season 3, episode 1; Goldacre, Ben. "The Placebo Effect and the Implications for Medicine." *BBC Science and Nature*. Radio 4 (Aug. 18, 2008); Harrington, Anne. *The Placebo Effect* (Harvard University Press, 1999); Hróbjartsson, Asbjørn, and Peter C. Gøtzsche. "Placebo Interventions for All Clinical Conditions." Cochrane Database of Systematic Reviews (online), no. 1 (2010); McClain, Carla. "Mom of Soldier Killed in Iraq Dies." *Arizona Daily Star* (Oct. 5, 2004); Meador, Clifton. *Symptoms of Unknown Origin* (Vanderbilt University Press, 2005); Moerman, Daniel. *Meaning Medicine and the "Placebo Effect."* (Cambridge University Press, 2002); "Resistance Is Futile." M.D.O.D. (April 2, 2011). http://docsontheweb. blogspot.com/2011/04/resistance-is-futile.html; Samuels, Martin. "The Brain–Heart Connection." *Circulation* 116, no. 1 (July 3, 2007): 77–84; Samuels. " 'Voodoo' Death Revisited." *Cleveland Clinic Journal of Medicine* 74 Suppl 1 (Feb. 2007): S8–16; Specter, Michael. "The Power of Nothing." *New Yorker* (Dec. 12, 2011). *On percentage of treatments based on evidence:* Beeson, P.B. "Changes in Medical Therapy during the Past Half Century." *Medicine* 59, no. 2 (March 1980): 79–99, quoted in: Eisenberg, Leon. "Science in Medicine." *American Journal of Medicine* 84, no. 3 Pt 1 (March 1988):

483–491; Institute of Medicine. *Crossing the Quality Chasm* (National Academies Press, 2001). **On the Flexner Report:** Brown, Chip. *Afterwards, You're a Genius* (Riverhead Books, 2000); Galland, Leo. *The Four Pillars of Healing* (Random House, 1997); Odegaard, Charles. *Dear Doctor: A Personal Letter to a Physician* (The Henry J. Kaiser Family Foundation, 1986); White, Kerr L. *The Task of Medicine: Dialogue at Wickenburg* (Henry J. Kaiser Family Foundation, 1988). **On the architecture of hospitals prioritizing technology:** Sternberg, Esther. *Healing Spaces* (Belknap Press, 2009). **On Leon Eisenberg:** Angell, Marcia. "The Illusions of Psychiatry." *New York Review of Books* (July 14, 2011); Carey, Benedict. "Dr. Leon Eisenberg, Pioneer in Autism Studies, Dies at 87." *New York Times* (Sept. 24, 2009); Eisenberg, Leon, and Laurence B. Guttmacher. "Were We All Asleep at the Switch? A Personal Reminiscence of Psychiatry from 1940 to 2010." *Acta Psychiatrica Scandinavica* 122, no. 2 (Aug. 2010): 89–102; Knowles, John. *Doing Better and Feeling Worse* (W. W. Norton, 1977). **On the decline and fall of primary care:** Flower, Joe. "Change the Model." Hospitals & Health Networks (July 7, 2008); Hasley, Ashley. "Primary-Care Doctor Shortage May Undermine Health Reform Efforts." *Washington Post* (June 20, 2009); Pauli, H.G., et al. "Medical Education, Research, and Scientific Thinking in the 21st Century." *Education for Health* 13, no. 2 (2000): 173–186; Sataline, Suzanne, and Shirley S. Wang. "Medical Schools Can't Keep Up." *Wall Street Journal* (April 12, 2010); White, Kerr, et al. "The Ecology of Medical Care." *New England Journal of Medicine* 265 (Nov. 2, 1961): 885–892; Wilder, Venis, et al. "Income Disparities Shape Medical Student Specialty Choice." *American Family Physician* 82, no. 6 (Sept. 15, 2010): 601. **On time spent with primary care physicians:** Bindman, Andrew, et al. "Diagnostic Scope of and Exposure to Primary Care Physicians in Australia, New Zealand, and the United States." *BMJ* 334, no. 7606 (June 16, 2007): 1261. **On healers caring about patients:** Berkowitz, Edward. "History of Health Services Research Project: Interview with Kerr White" (March 12, 1998). http.//www.nlm.nih.gov/hmd/nichsr/white.html; Kaptchuk, Ted, et al. "Components of Placebo Effect." *BMJ* 336, no. 7651 (May 3, 2008): 999–1003. **On protestant witch burning:** Thomas, Keith. *Religion and the Decline of Magic* (Scribner's, 1971): 494–498. **On the importance of community in health:** Illich, Ivan. *Medical Nemesis* (Pantheon, 1976): 114; Putnam, Robert. *Bowling Alone* (Touchstone Books, 2001); Umberson, Debra, and Jennifer Karas Montez. "Social Relationships and Health." *Journal of Health and Social Behavior* 51, no. 1 (Nov. 1, 2010): S54–S66.

CONCLUSION

On infant sleep and SIDS: Horsley, Tanya, et al. "Mother-infant Cosleeping, Breastfeeding and Sudden Infant Death Syndrome." *American Journal of Physical Anthropology*, Suppl 45 (2007): 133–161; Moon, Rachel Y. "SIDS and Other Sleep-Related Infant Deaths." *Pediatrics* 128, no. 5 (Nov. 1, 2011): e1341–e1367; Sampson, Margaret, et al. "Benefits and Harms Associated with the Practice of Bed Sharing." *Archives of Pediatrics & Adolescent Medicine* 161, no. 3 (March 1, 2007): 237–245. **On the dual ways of thinking, and the importance of togetherness:** McGilchrist, Iain. *The Master and His Emissary* (Yale University Press, 2010); Krakauer, Jon. *Into the Wild* (Anchor Books, 1997).

INDEX

Boldface references indicate illustrations.